neuroanatomy

The National Medical Series for Independent Study

neuroanatomy

William DeMyer, M.D.

Professor of Child Neurology
Indiana University
  School of Medicine
Indianapolis, Indiana

A WILEY MEDICAL PUBLICATION
JOHN WILEY & SONS
New York • Chichester • Brisbane • Toronto • Singapore

Harwal Publishing Company, Media, Pennsylvania

Library of Congress Cataloging-in-Publication Data

Neuroanatomy.

(The National medical series for independent study)
(A Wiley medical publication)
    Includes index.
    1. Neuroanatomy—Outlines, syllabi, etc. 2. Neuro-
anatomy—Examinations, questions, etc.   I. DeMyer,
William, 1924–   . II. Series. III. Series: A Wiley
medical publication. [DNLM: 1. Neuroanatomy—ex-
amination questions. 2. Neuroanatomy—outlines.
WL 18 N4908]
QM451.N47 1988   611′.8′0202   87-36211
ISBN 0-471-82923-4

10 9 8 7 6 5 4 3 2 1

Contents

Preface

First-year medical students usually feel harassed by neuroanatomy because of an excess of nomenclature and detail. I simplify nomenclature by defining new terms as I introduce them and by historical notes that explain their origin and application. I introduce the structure of the parts of the nervous system through the logic of embryology and phylogeny. The sections of the text follow an orderly progression from definition through embryology to the final structure of each part. Then, the text explains the connection of each part with the rest of the nervous system and finally its clinical relevance. Although in outline form, the text endeavors to teach neuroanatomy conceptually rather than as isolated details. I summarize difficult topics with rational mnemonics. At the end of the text, the student should have the knowledge to understand the clinical neurologic examination and the effects of disease on neurologic function.

After all, the nervous system is the site of our personhood. It makes me me and you you. The text, then, presents what the organ that thinks has discovered about its own structure.

William DeMyer

Acknowledgments

I am grateful first of all to my wife, Dr. Marian DeMyer, who while pursuing her own full-time academic career has always fully supported mine.

And then to my mentors in neuropathology, Drs. Wolfgang Zeman and Jans Muller, whose insatiable curiosity about anatomy reinforced my own interest.

And then to the Harwal staff: to James Harris, the publisher, whose foresight established the outline series; to editor Jane Velker, who blue-penciled many bad sentences; and to Wieslawa B. Langenfeld for her medical artistry.

To David DeMyer for assistance with several of the drawings.

And then to Terry Wenzel, who diligently word processed the original manuscript yet retained her sanity through all of the I, A, 1, a, (1), (a)'s of the outlining.

Publisher's Note

The objective of the *National Medical Series* is to present an extraordinarily large amount of information in an easily retrievable form. The outline format was selected for this purpose of reducing to the essentials the medical information needed by today's student and practitioner.

While the concept of an outline format was well received by the authors and publisher, the difficulties inherent in working with this style were not initially apparent. That the series has been published and received enthusiastically is a tribute to the authors who worked long and diligently to produce books that are stylistically consistent and comprehensive in content.

The task of producing the *National Medical Series* required more than the efforts of the authors, however, and the missing elements have been supplied by highly competent and dedicated developmental editors and support staff. Editors, compositors, proofreaders, and layout and design staff have all polished the outline to a fine form. It is with deep appreciation that I thank all who have participated, in particular, the staff at Harwal/Wiley Medical—Debra L. Dreger, Jane Edwards, Gloria Hamilton, Judy Johnson, Susan Kelly, Wieslawa B. Langenfeld, Keith LaSala, June Sangiorgio Mash, Jane Velker, and Elizabeth Waddington.

The Publisher

Introduction

Neuroanatomy is one of ten basic science review books in the *National Medical Series for Independent Study*. This series has been designed to provide students and house officers, as well as physicians, with a concise but comprehensive instrument for self-evaluation and review within the basic sciences. Although *Neuroanatomy* would be most useful for students preparing for the National Board of Medical Examiners examinations (Part I and FLEX) and FMGEMS, it should also be useful for students studying for course examinations. These books are not intended to replace the standard basic science texts but, rather, to complement them.

The books in this series present the core content of each basic science, using an outline format and featuring 300 study questions. The questions are distributed throughout the book, at the end of each chapter and in a post-test. In addition, each question is accompanied by the correct answer, a paragraph-length explanation of the correct answer, and specific reference to the outline points under which the information necessary to answer the question can be found.

We have chosen an outline format to allow maximal ease in retrieving information, assuming that the time available to the reader is limited. Considerable editorial time has been spent to ensure that the information required by all medical school curricula has been included and that the question format parallels that of the National Board examinations. We feel that the combination of the outline and the board-type study questions provides a unique teaching device.

We hope you will find this series interesting, relevant, and challenging. The authors and the staff at Harwal/Wiley Medical welcome your comments and suggestions.

Gross Subdivisions of the Nervous System

I. GROSS SUBDIVISIONS OF THE NERVOUS SYSTEM

A. Gross appearance of the nervous system. Figure 1-1 shows the nervous system as it appears when dissected free from the body.

B. Major subdivisions of the nervous system

1. The nervous system has two main parts:
   a. **Central nervous system (CNS)**
   b. **Peripheral nervous system (PNS)**

2. The PNS commences with the **nerve roots**.
   a. To free the CNS from the PNS, we snip the nerve roots just at their attachment to the CNS (Fig. 1-2).
   b. The nerve roots combine into peripheral nerves to connect the CNS with the rest of the body.

II. GROSS ANATOMY OF THE CENTRAL NERVOUS SYSTEM

A. Gross subdivisions of the CNS

1. The CNS, or **neuraxis**, consists of two main subdivisions:
   a. **Brain** (encephalon)
   b. **Spinal cord** (myelon)

2. To free the brain from the spinal cord, we cut across the CNS at the level of the foramen magnum of the skull (Fig. 1-3).

B. Anatomical definition of the brain and its subdivisions

1. The **brain** is that part of the CNS rostral to a cut through the foramen magnum. The spinal cord is caudal to the cut.

2. The **subdivisions of the brain** (see Fig. 1-3) are:
   a. **Cerebrum**
   b. **Diencephalon**
   c. **Brainstem**
   d. **Cerebellum**

3. **Historical note on the definition of cerebrum and brainstem.** The original Basle *Nomina Anatomica* (BNA; 1895) defined the diencephalon and midbrain as part of the cerebrum, a practice uncommon today. Conversely, some authors include the diencephalon or even the basal ganglia with the brainstem. This text follows the Mexico City *Nomina Anatomica* (5th edition; 1980) and assigns the basal ganglia to the cerebrum. The diencephalon stands separately, and the midbrain, pons, and medulla oblongata comprise the brainstem (the truncus encephali).

C. Gross anatomy of the cerebral surface

1. **Fissures of the cerebrum**
   a. The cerebrum consists of mirror-image halves called **cerebral hemispheres**, which are separated by an **interhemispheric fissure** (Fig. 1-4; see also Fig. 1-6).
   b. Each cerebral hemisphere has a major fissure, the **sylvian** or **lateral fissure**, seen best on the lateral side (see Fig. 1-4A).

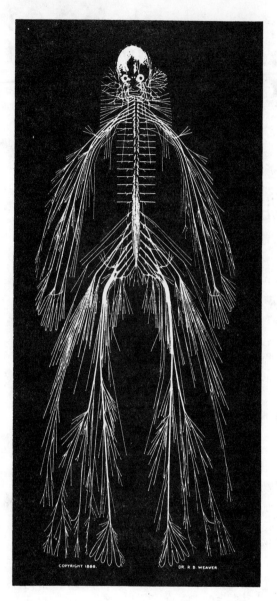

COPYRIGHT 1888.   DR. R.B. WEAVER.

Figure 1-1. Frontal view of the nervous system dissected free from the body. This figure, although extensive, does not include the profusion of finer peripheral branches to the body wall and viscera. (Courtesy of Dr. P. Amenta, Hahnemann University School of Medicine, Philadelphia, Pennsylvania.)

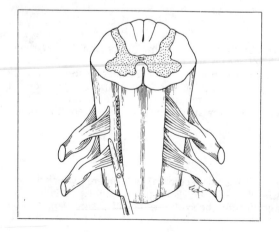

Figure 1-2. Frontal view of the spinal cord and nerve roots. The *scissors' cut*, precisely through the attachment of the nerve roots, separates the peripheral nervous system (PNS) from the central nervous system (CNS).

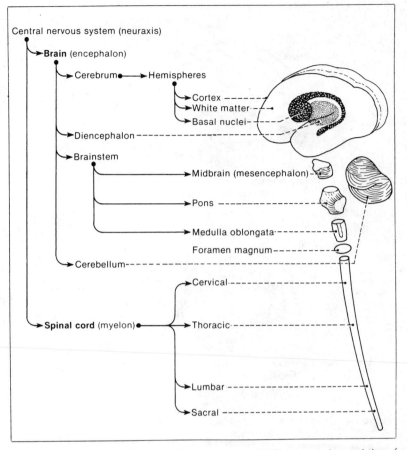

Figure 1-3. Lateral view of the central nervous system (CNS), or neuraxis, consisting of the brain, spinal cord, and their subdivisions.

   c. Bundles of nerve fibers and neural tissue unite the two hemispheres deep in the interhemispheric fissure (see Fig. 1-6).

2. Sulci and gyri of the cerebrum
   a. The general surface of each cerebral hemisphere displays smaller crevices, called **sulci**, which separate elevations of the surface, called **gyri**.
   b. Locate the **central sulcus**, the **calcarine sulcus**, and the **parieto-occipital sulcus** in Figure 1-4.
      (1) The central sulcus separates two gyri, a precentral gyrus and a postcentral gyrus.
         (a) The **precentral gyrus** is mainly a **motor area**, which directs volitional movements.
         (b) The **postcentral gyrus** is mainly the **sensory receptive area** for body sensation.
      (2) The gyri around the calcarine sulcus constitute the **visual receptive area**.
      (3) Gyri buried under the posterior part of the sylvian or lateral fissure, the **transverse temporal gyri**, constitute the **auditory receptive area**.

3. Lobes of the cerebrum
   a. Fissures, sulci, and certain arbitrarily selected lines divide each cerebral hemisphere into five lobes:
      (1) Frontal lobe
      (2) Parietal lobe
      (3) Temporal lobe
      (4) Occipital lobe
      (5) Limbic lobe
   b. On the lateral surface of a hemisphere (see Fig. 1-4A), notice the following.
      (1) The plane of the **central sulcus** divides the **frontal lobe** from the **parietal lobe**.
      (2) The **sylvian fissure** anteriorly divides the **frontal lobe** from the **temporal lobe**, and posteriorly, the sylvian fissure partially divides the **parietal lobe** from the **temporal lobe**.

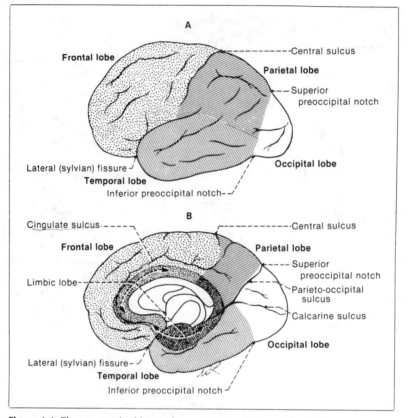

Figure 1-4. The two cerebral hemispheres. (*A*) Lateral view of the left hemisphere. (*B*) Medial view of the right hemisphere.

    (3) An arbitrary line from the superior **preoccipital notch** to the inferior preoccipital notch divides the **occipital lobe** from the **parietal lobe** above and from the **temporal lobe** below.

    (4) An arbitrary line from the midpoint of the foregoing line to the sylvian fissure completes the separation of the **parietal lobe** from the **temporal lobe** posteriorly.

  c. On the medial surface of a hemisphere (see Fig. 1-4*B*), notice the following.

    (1) An imaginary extension of the central sulcus divides the **frontal lobe** from the **parietal lobe**.

    (2) The **parieto-occipital sulcus** divides the **parietal lobe** from the **occipital lobe**. The parieto-occipital sulcus cuts the superomedial margin of the hemisphere at the superior preoccipital notch.

    (3) An arbitrary line extended from the junction of the parieto-occipital sulcus and the calcarine sulcus to the inferior preoccipital notch divides the **temporal lobe** from the **occipital lobe**.

    (4) The forward extension of the calcarine sulcus divides the **temporal lobe** from the **parietal lobe**.

  d. Limbic and olfactory lobes (Fig. 1-5)

    (1) Neuroanatomists recognize another lobe, the **limbic lobe**, shown stippled in Figure 1-5. It can be regarded as parts of the first four lobes, or it can be listed as a separate entity.

    (2) Yet another lobe, the **olfactory lobe**, is sometimes defined. It nestles concentrically inside of the limbic lobe, as shown in black in Figure 1-5.

D. Cross-sectional anatomy of the cerebrum

  1. A coronal slice through a cerebral hemisphere discloses the **four gross hemispheric components** (Fig. 1-6):

    a. Surface gray matter

    b. Deep white matter

    c. Deep gray matter (basal ganglia and thalamus)

    d. Ventricular cavities

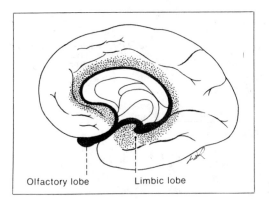

Figure 1-5. Medial aspect of the right cerebral hemisphere, showing the limbic lobe (*stippled*) and the olfactory lobe (*black*).

2. Gray matter

    a. The gray matter looks gray because it consists of masses of nerve cell bodies that contain pigment and organelles.

        (1) On the surface of the cerebrum, nerve cell bodies form a continuous sheet, which is called a **cortex**.

        (2) Deep in the hemispheres, the nerve cell bodies accumulate as nuclear masses, or **nuclei**, which surround the ventricular cavities.

    b. Explanatory note

        (1) A **nucleus** is a fairly compact group of nerve cell bodies, which are more or less similar in form and function, located **inside the CNS**.

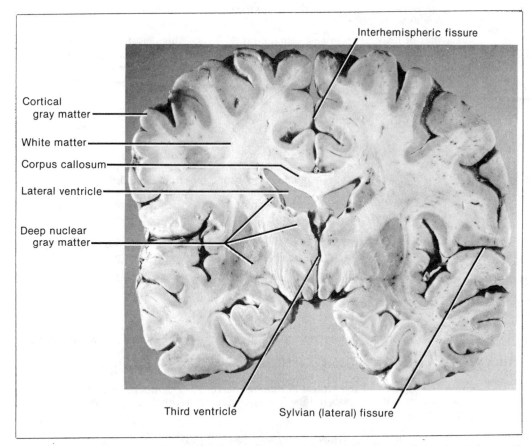

Figure 1-6. Gross photograph of the unstained coronal section of the cerebrum showing the two hemispheres with their gray and white matter and ventricles. White matter, called the corpus callosum, composed of nerve fiber bundles, connects the two hemispheres across the bottom of the interhemispheric fissure.

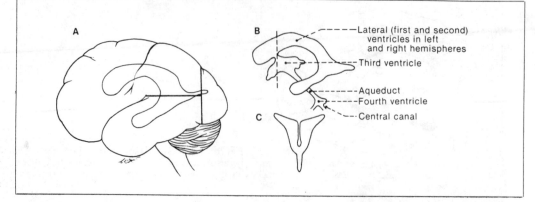

Figure 1-7. The cerebral ventricles. (A) Lateral aspect of the left cerebral hemisphere showing the contour of the lateral ventricles and their relation to the cerebral lobes. (B) Lateral outline of the four ventricles. (C) Frontal (coronal) section of the lateral and third ventricles at the level of the *dotted line* (B) showing their communicating interventricular foramen.

    (2) A **ganglion** is a similar group of nerve cell bodies located **outside the CNS**. The term **basal ganglia** is a holdover from the early days of neuroanatomy. These structures should properly be called **basal nuclei**, but the archaic term persists.

  3. White matter. Gleaming white material called white matter separates the cortex from the deep nuclear masses.

    a. It consists of nerve fibers and their coverings, called **myelin sheaths**.

    b. The **myelin**, a fatty substance, causes the white appearance, just as fat gives mammalian milk its white color.

  4. Cavities of the cerebrum and spinal cord (Fig. 1-7). Although the brain looks solid when viewed from the outside, it originates embryologically as a tubular structure, and it retains the original lumen as the ventricles. The ventricles conform to the shape of the hemispheres and brainstem (see Fig. 1-7A).

    a. The **ventricular system** consists of:

      (1) Paired **lateral ventricles** in the cerebral hemispheres

      (2) A slit-like **third ventricle** in the sagittal plane of the diencephalon (see Fig. 1-7)

      (3) A narrow tubular **aqueduct**, which runs in the sagittal plane through the midbrain (see Fig. 1-7B)

      (4) An expanded portion called the **fourth ventricle**, located in the pons and medulla just ventral to the cerebellum (see Fig. 1-7B)

    b. A small central cavity, called the **central canal**, runs from the fourth ventricle to the tip of the spinal cord.

    c. During life, the ventricles and the central canal contain a clear fluid, which is called **cerebrospinal fluid (CSF)**.

E. Cross-sectional anatomy of the brainstem, cerebellum, and spinal cord

  1. The **brainstem** is a mixture of deep nuclei and superficial white matter (Fig. 1-8; see Fig. 1-8A). Although some neurons are located more superficially, they do not form a cortex.

  2. The **cerebellum** has surface cortex and deep nuclear masses, which are separated by white matter (see Fig. 1-8B).

  3. The **spinal cord** has a central, H-shaped core of gray matter that consists only of nuclear masses. The spinal cord has no cortex. The periphery of the cord is all white matter.

III. GROSS ANATOMY OF THE PERIPHERAL NERVOUS SYSTEM

A. Gross components of the typical peripheral nerve. Although peripheral nerves do differ in composition and distribution, most follow a common plan with the same gross components (Fig. 1-9).

B. The PNS has three main types of nerves.

  1. The **cranial nerves** all attach to the cerebrum or brainstem, except for cranial nerve (CN) XI,

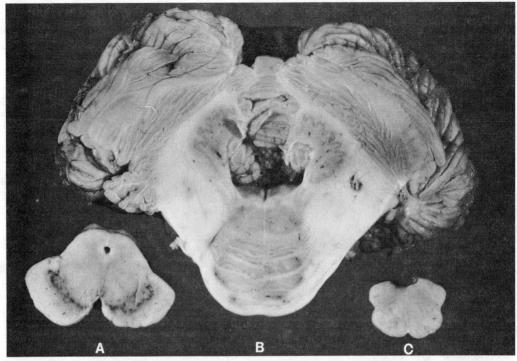

Figure 1-8. Gross photograph of unstained transverse sections of the brainstem and cerebellum. (*A*) Midbrain with aqueduct. (*B*) Pons connected to the overlying cerebellum by white matter. The cerebellum has a cortical surface surrounding its deep white matter. Deep nuclei surround the fourth ventricle. (*C*) Medulla with fourth ventricular cavity dorsally, with the roofing membrane torn away.

which arises from the rostral part of the spinal cord. (Chapter 8 discusses the complicated origin and classification of cranial nerves.)

2. The **spinal nerves** all attach to the spinal cord.
   a. All have dorsal and ventral roots, except for the first cervical nerve, which may have no dorsal root.
   b. Spinal nerves innervate skeletal muscles and sensory receptors and, in part, convey visceral nerves.

3. The **autonomic (visceral) nerves** run through the roots of cranial or spinal nerves to ganglia or to autonomic plexuses in the walls of the viscera (see Figs. 6-1 and 6-2).
   a. Then the nerves run to smooth muscles or glands.
   b. The autonomic nerves return impulses to the CNS from the sensory receptors in the viscera.

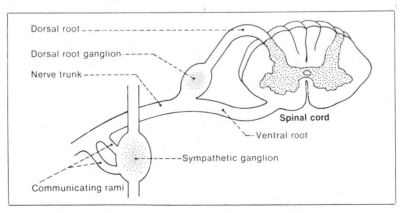

Figure 1-9. Gross components of the typical peripheral nerve.

STUDY QUESTIONS

Directions: Each question below contains five suggested answers. Choose the **one best** response to each question.

1. The largest crevice on the lateral surface of the cerebrum is the

(A) central sulcus
(B) sylvian fissure
(C) superior temporal sulcus
(D) transverse fissure
(E) primary fissure

2. White matter appears white because of

(A) myelin sheaths
(B) profusion of astrocytic processes
(C) axoplasm
(D) large amount of fluid
(E) numerous blood vessel walls

3. A complete section through the midpoint of the cerebrum either in the horizontal or coronal plane would disclose all of the following EXCEPT

(A) a thin covering of cortex
(B) lateral ventricles
(C) basal ganglia
(D) thick layer of deep white matter
(E) parieto-occipital fissure

4. All of the following landmarks form an extensive part of the boundary of the parietal lobe EXCEPT

(A) the sylvian fissure
(B) the central sulcus
(C) a line from the superior preoccipital notch to the inferior preoccipital notch
(D) the calcarine sulcus
(E) the limbic lobe

Directions: Each question below contains four suggested answers of which **one or more** is correct. Choose the answer

A if **1, 2, and 3** are correct
B if **1 and 3** are correct
C if **2 and 4** are correct
D if **4** is correct
E if **1, 2, 3, and 4** are correct

5. The definition of the brain includes which of the following?

(1) Basal ganglia
(2) Diencephalon
(3) Mesencephalon
(4) Cerebellum

6. The current definition of the brainstem includes which of the following?

(1) Cerebellum
(2) Deep cerebral white matter
(3) Basal ganglia
(4) Mesencephalon

Directions: The groups of questions below consists of lettered choices followed by several numbered items. For each numbered item select the **one** lettered choice with which it is **most** closely associated. Each lettered choice may be used once, more than once, or not at all.

Questions 7–10

For each vernacular or common term, match the correct technical term.

(A) Hypothalamus
(B) Truncus encephali
(C) Mesencephalon
(D) Encephalon
(E) Myelon

7. Brain
8. Spinal cord
9. Midbrain
10. Brainstem

Questions 11–16

Match the cerebral lobes listed below with the landmarks that completely or partly divide them.

(A) Central sulcus
(B) Lateral (sylvian) fissure
(C) Line from the superior preoccipital notch to the inferior preoccipital notch
(D) Cingulate sulcus
(E) None of the above

11. Frontal lobe separated from temporal lobe
12. Parietal lobe separated from temporal lobe
13. Limbic lobe separated from olfactory lobe
14. Parietal lobe separated from occipital lobe
15. Parietal lobe separated from limbic lobe
16. Frontal lobe separated from parietal lobe

ANSWERS AND EXPLANATIONS

1. The answer is B. (*II C 1 b*) The lateral surface of the cerebrum is covered by numerous sulci of varying size and depth. Only one major fissure can be seen on the lateral surface, the sylvian fissure, which separates the frontal lobe from the temporal lobe anteriorly and the parietal lobe from the temporal lobe posteriorly.

2. The answer is A. (*II D 3*) The white matter of the brain appears white because of the myelin sheaths around axons. The myelin sheaths consist of oligodendroglial cell membranes, which wrap around the axons. The sheaths contain fat molecules, which give the white color, just as the fat gives the white color to mammalian milk.

3. The answer is E. [*II D 1, 2 a (1), b (2), 4 a (1)*] A section through the midpoint of the cerebrum in either the horizontal or coronal plane discloses a thin surface covering of cortex, an adjacent thick layer of deep white matter, basal ganglia, and lateral ventricles. The parieto-occipital fissure is too far posterior to be shown in a coronal section of the cerebrum through its middle third.

4. The answer is D. (*II C 3 b, c; Figures 1-4, 1-5*) The parietal lobe bounds the frontal lobe at the central sulcus and the temporal lobe at the sylvian fissure, and it is separated from the occipital lobe by an arbitrary line from the superior to the inferior preoccipital notches. Depending on definitions, the limbic lobe can be considered as a lobe that borders on the parietal lobe or as part of the parietal lobe. The calcarine sulcus splits the occipital lobe medially, and although it contacts the isthmus between the parietal and temporal lobes, it does not itself demarcate an extensive boundary of the parietal lobe.

5. The answer is E (all). (*II B 1, 2*) The definition of the brain includes all structures rostral to the level of the foramen magnum. Thus, it would include the entire brainstem, cerebellum, diencephalon, basal ganglia, white matter, and cerebral cortex.

6. The answer is D (4). (*II B 3, E 1*) The definition of the brainstem has undergone changes over the years. Currently, the brainstem is defined to include the mesencephalon, pons, and medulla. It has never included any parts of the cerebrum rostral to the basal ganglia, such as the deep cerebral white matter, and it has never included the cerebellum.

7–10. The answers are: 7-D, 8-E, 9-C, 10-B. (*II A 1, B 3*) The parts of the nervous system often have two names, a common, or vernacular, name and a technical name. The technical name is often more precisely used and precisely defined than the vernacular term. In addition, the technical term can be used as a combining form in order to describe changes in the portions of the nervous system under consideration. For example, the term myelon is the technical term for the spinal cord. To describe inflammation of the spinal cord, one would speak of myelitis rather than spinal corditis. Similarly, the term would be encephalitis rather than brainitis. The brainstem has had a variety of definitions over the years, whereas the term truncus encephali is now precisely defined in the latest *Nomina Anatomica*. Redundancy in terminology and imprecision in the use of terms have always been problems in anatomy, and the purpose of the precise definition of technical terms is to avoid confusion. Even now, however, there is really no universally accepted guiding principle for developing the most descriptive and accurate terms and ones that can be most readily remembered.

11–16. The answers are: 11-B, 12-B, 13-E, 14-C, 15-D, 16-A. (*I C 3*) The lobes of the cerebrum were originally named because they underlie the skull bones previously named. They are an arbitrary and artificial subdivision of the cerebrum, but their accurate delineation allows description of normal variations in the regions of the brain as well as the exact sites of lesions.

The central sulcus separates the largest lobe of the cerebrum, the frontal lobe, from the parietal lobe. This sulcus cuts the crest of the hemisphere just rostral to the ascending ramus of the cingulate gyrus and extends ventrally and somewhat anteriorly along the lateral side of the cerebral wall. It divides the motor cortex of the precentral gyrus from the sensory cortex of the postcentral gyrus.

The sylvian, or lateral, fissure is not a sulcus but is formed by the evagination of the temporal lobe from the primitive telencephalon. After the stem of the sylvian fissure runs from the vallecula to the lateral surface of the brain, it forms a relatively horizontal ramus, which separates the frontal lobe in front from the temporal pole and the parietal lobe behind from the posterior part of the temporal lobe. Thus, the temporal lobe sits beneath the sylvian fissure, under the posterior inferior part of the frontal lobe and under the inferior margin of the parietal lobe.

The occipital lobe is divided from the parietal lobe by an arbitrary line from the superior to the inferior preoccipital notch. This notch occurs at the site where a bridging vein runs to the superior sagittal sinus from the preoccipital notch and from the inferior preoccipital notch to the transverse sinus.

On the medial hemispheric wall, the cingulate sulcus roughly divides the limbic lobe from the parietal and frontal lobes, which occupy the medial hemispheric wall dorsal to the limbic lobe.

2
Structure and Function of Neurons and Their Supporting Tissues

I. CHARACTERISTICS OF NEURONS

A. Structure of neurons (Fig. 2-1)

   1. A **neuron** is a cell consisting of:
     a. A **nucleus** (karyon)
     b. A **cell body** (perikaryon)
     c. One or more **processes**, which typically consist of an **axon** and **dendrites**.
        (1) Axons typically are long and have relatively few branches.
           (a) The branches of an axon are **collaterals**.
           (b) The terminals of the axon or its collaterals are **end feet**.
        (2) Dendrites are typically much shorter than axons and usually branch extensively, forming dendritic trees.

   2. Neurons are the parenchymal cells of the nervous system. The supporting cells are **glia**.

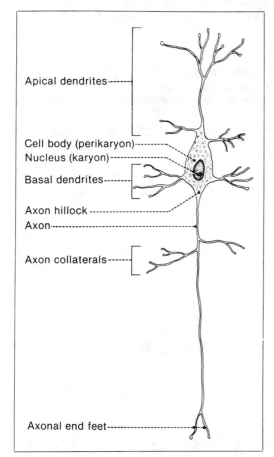

Apical dendrites - - - - - -

Cell body (perikaryon) - - - - - - -
Nucleus (karyon) - - - - - -
Basal dendrites - - - - - - -

Axon hillock - - - - - - - - -
Axon - - - - - - - - - -

Axon collaterals - - - - - -

Axonal end feet - - - - - - - - - - - - - - - - -

Figure 2-1. Typical components of a multipolar neuron.

B. Morphologic types of neurons

1. Neurons are classed as **unipolar**, **bipolar**, or **multipolar**, depending on the configuration of their processes (Fig. 2-2). Although almost all neurons fall into one of these three types, the various types of neurons differ in shape (Fig. 2-3).

2. Neurons are also classified by axon length.
   a. **Golgi type I neurons** have long axons (see Fig. 2-3). The longest in the central nervous system (CNS) of man extend from the cerebral cortex to the tip of the spinal cord, a distance of 50 cm to 70 cm.
   b. **Golgi type II neurons** have short axons (see Fig. 2-3). The shortest axons terminate only a few micra from the perikaryon.
   c. **Amacrine neurons**, an unusual cell type, lack axons.

C. Nerve impulses. Neurons function by the production, propagation, and transfer of nerve impulses, much in the manner of units in electrical circuits.

1. Various stimuli activate neurons from their resting state and cause them to produce nerve impulses. In neurology, a **stimulus** is any change that causes a neuron to produce a nerve impulse. The change may be a physical event, a chemical event, or an electrical event.
   a. **Resting potential.** At rest, a neuron maintains a difference in potential (i.e., voltage) of about -50 mV to -80 mV between the inside and outside of its surface membrane. Thus, the cell surface is **polarized** in respect to the cell interior.
   b. **Action potential.** If a stimulus excites a site on the surface membrane, the resting potential at that point drops to zero or even overshoots slightly. Then, like a sequence of falling dominoes, the depolarization wave, now called an **action potential**, propagates along the surface membrane of the neuron.
   c. The term **nerve impulse** describes all of the **biologic and electrical events** involved in the passage of a neuronal message. The term **action potential** describes only the **electrical component** of the nerve impulse.

2. Typically, the nerve impulse begins with excitation in the dendritic tree or perikaryon of a neuron and then travels distally along the axon to its terminals. Thus, neurons are anatomically arranged into a **receiving end** and a **sending end**.
   a. **Dendrites** are specialized to **receive** nerve impulses.
   b. **Axons** are specialized to **convey** nerve impulses away from the perikaryon.

3. A single neuron (e.g., a neuron isolated in a tissue culture) is functionally useless. To function, a nerve impulse must affect the next cell in line in a circuit.
   a. The next cell in line at the axonal end feet may be another neuron, or it may be an effector cell.

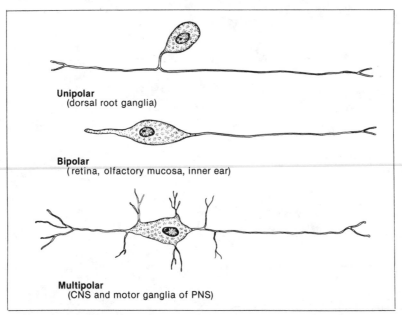

Unipolar
(dorsal root ganglia)

Bipolar
(retina, olfactory mucosa, inner ear)

Multipolar
(CNS and motor ganglia of PNS)

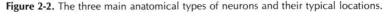

Figure 2-2. The three main anatomical types of neurons and their typical locations.

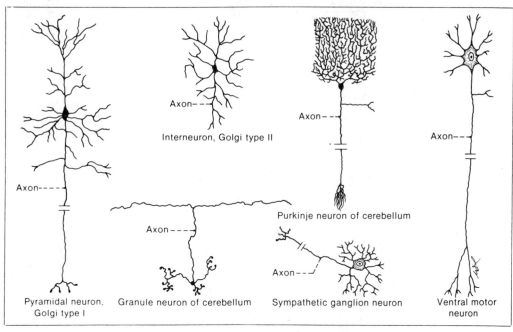

Axon - - -

Interneuron, Golgi type II

Axon - - -

Purkinje neuron of cerebellum

Axon - - - -

Axon - - - -

Axon - - -

Axon - - -

Pyramidal neuron, Golgi type I   Granule neuron of cerebellum   Sympathetic ganglion neuron   Ventral motor neuron

Figure 2-3. Variety of shapes of multipolar neurons.

   b. Effector cells are:
      (1) Skeletal muscle cells
      (2) Smooth muscle cells
      (3) Cardiac muscle cells
      (4) Gland cells

D. Synapses and neurotransmitters

  1. Definition: A **synapse** is the **site of functional contact** between the axonal membrane of one neuron and the membrane of the neuron or effector cell next in line. Synapses thus are the **anatomical basis of intercellular communication** by neurons.
    a. Location and morphologic classification of synapses
      (1) The axon of one neuron can synapse on the dendritic tree of another neuron, on its perikaryon, or, less commonly, on its axon hillock or even its axon. Thus, synapses are called **axodendritic, axosomatic** (soma means body or perikaryon), and **axoaxonic** (Fig. 2-4).
      (2) Apparently, some neurons are connected by dendrodendritic synapses, a fact that tends to blur the classic distinction between axons and dendrites [e.g., the amacrine neurons of the retina (see Fig. 10-4) and olfactory bulb lack axons as such].
    b. Typical synapses (Fig. 2-5) consist of:
      (1) A **presynaptic membrane** provided by the axonal terminal
      (2) A **synaptic cleft**
      (3) A **postsynaptic membrane** provided by the next cell in line

  2. The arrival of the nerve impulse at the synaptic terminal of the axon releases a stored chemical substance into the synaptic cleft (see Fig. 2-5).
    a. The chemical substance unites with chemical receptors on the postsynaptic membrane.
    b. Because the chemical transmits the effect of the stimulus to the next cell in line, it is called a **neurotransmitter**.

  3. Neurotransmitters are of two types, **excitatory** and **inhibitory**.
    a. Excitatory neurotransmitters tend to **depolarize** the cell membrane and **excite** that cell. Excitatory neurotransmitters cause a neuron to discharge a nerve impulse or cause an effector to act. Most synapses in the peripheral nervous system (PNS) are excitatory; that is, they cause a muscle cell to contract or a gland cell to secrete.
    b. Inhibitory neurotransmitters tend to **hyperpolarize** the next cell in line. They **inhibit the production of a new impulse** by making membrane depolarization more difficult. These transmitters cause inhibitory reflexes, such as slowing of the heart or inhibition of neurons in the CNS that are causing a muscular contraction.

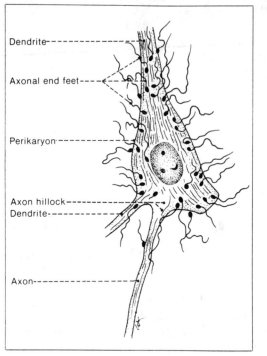

Figure 2-4. Axonal end feet on a neuron forming axo-dendritic, axosomatic, and axoaxonic synapses.

4. Each CNS neuron, in general, receives thousands of synapses, some excitatory and some inhibitory. Whether a given neuron will generate an impulse or not depends on the summation of the excitatory and inhibitory transmitters acting upon its surface at any particular time.

E. Polarization of impulse flow

1. Because dendrites receive impulses and axons send them, nerve impulses normally flow in one direction; that is, to the axonal tip. At the tip, the impulse crosses the synapse in one direction, as if the system were a one-way valve. This one-way arrangement is called **neuronal polarization** (as contrasted to membrane polarization).

2. Under pathologic or experimental conditions, a neuronal membrane may be stimulated abnormally.
    a. For example, in an experiment, a stimulating electrode might be applied halfway along an axon. In that case, a wave of depolarization will sweep in two directions: **distally** toward the axonal tip (**orthodromic conduction**) and **proximally** toward the perikaryon (**antidromic conduction**).
    b. The impulse will cross the synapse at its own axonal tip but will not cause retrograde stimulation of the synapses on the perikaryon or dendrites made by axons from other neurons. The postsynaptic neuronal membrane at these sites, specialized to receive messages, will not release a transmitter to act in the wrong direction.

F. The terms **polar** and **polarization** have now been used in three senses:

1. To classify neurons anatomically as **unipolar**, **bipolar**, or **multipolar**

2. To describe **membrane polarization**, the electrical charge across the membrane of the resting neuron (the terms **hyperpolarization** and **depolarization** apply only to membrane polarization)

3. To describe **neuronal polarization** in the sense of the usual one-way transmission of nerve impulses

G. Afferent and efferent impulses

1. The terms **afferent** and **efferent** describe the relative direction of impulse flow in neurons and their circuits.
    a. Impulses that flow **from** a designated point on a neuronal membrane or neural circuit are called **efferent**.

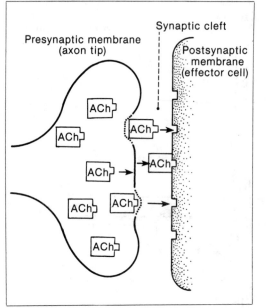

Figure 2-5. Diagram of a synapse showing the release of a neurotransmitter, in this case, acetylcholine (ACh).

     b. Impulses that flow **toward** a designated point on a neuronal membrane or neuronal circuit are called **afferent**.

    2. These terms describe nothing about the properties or results of the impulse, only the direction of flow relative to some arbitrarily designated site.

II. FUNCTIONAL CHARACTERISTICS AND FUNCTIONAL CIRCUITS OF NEURONS

    A. Functional types of neurons

       1. All neurons can be grouped into one of **three types** on the basis of their functional roles.
         a. Primary sensory neurons receive stimuli and transmit **afferent** impulses to the CNS.
         b. Interneurons (syn: internuncial neurons) form circuits in the CNS.
         c. Motoneurons deliver **efferent** impulses out through the PNS to the effectors to carry out the actions directed by the CNS.

       2. This functional classification reflects the basic plan of the nervous system, with the afferent neurons sending information to the CNS. There, countless interneurons integrate the afferent information and ultimately direct the motoneurons to activate effectors (Fig. 2-6).

    B. Characteristics of all primary sensory neurons (afferent neurons)

       1. General considerations
         a. The skin, eyes, ears, tongue, nose, viscera, and skeletomuscular structures contain nerve endings called **receptors**, designed to detect various stimuli. The distal receptor tip may end freely or may become encapsulated by cells to form a sensory **end organ** (see Fig. 7-14). Some specialized CNS cells may respond to internal chemical stimuli; however, they are not classed as primary sensory neurons.
         b. All primary sensory neurons are **bipolar or unipolar** in form. Bipolar primary sensory neurons are found only in the retina and in olfactory, vestibular, and auditory ganglia, which mediate special senses.
         c. With the major exception of the retina (and a few minor exceptions), primary sensory neurons have their perikarya located outside the CNS.

       2. Characteristics of unipolar primary sensory neurons
         a. The unipolar neurons mediate all general sensation from the parietes and viscera.
         b. The perikarya of unipolar primary sensory neurons are located in a **dorsal root ganglion** of a spinal nerve or a corresponding ganglion of a cranial nerve.
         c. The unipolar process bifurcates into **peripheral** and **central branches**.
           (1) The **peripheral process** runs out through a nerve trunk to the skin, skeletomuscular apparatus, or viscus.
           (2) The **central process** enters the CNS via a dorsal root. It ends on a motoneuron or an in-

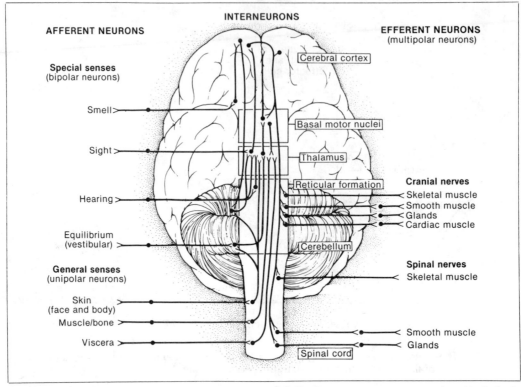

Figure 2-6. Basic plan of the nervous system seen as a series of afferent neurons, an interneuronal pool in the brain and spinal cord, and a series of efferent neurons.

terneuron. Characteristically, it **branches** many times to terminate on many different CNS neurons.

(3) No primary sensory axon returns to the PNS after entering the CNS.

d. Both the peripheral and central processes of unipolar neurons are called **axons** because they are long and slender and have few branches.

e. The **peripheral process** of a unipolar neuron is **dendritic** in function because it conveys the nerve impulse **toward** the perikaryon. The **central process** is **axonal** both **in structure and function** because it conveys the nerve impulse **away** from the perikaryon.

C. Characteristics of interneurons

1. With a few exceptions, interneurons are **multipolar**.

2. Their dendrites and axons **remain within the CNS**. No interneurons send axons into the PNS.

3. The **perikarya and dendrites** of interneurons, along with **motoneurons**, form the **gray matter** of the brain and spinal cord. The number of interneurons greatly exceeds the number of primary sensory neurons and motoneurons combined.

4. The **axons** of interneurons with their **myelin sheaths** form most of the **white matter** of the CNS.

D. Characteristics of motoneurons (efferent neurons)

1. Motoneurons are **multipolar**.

2. Their **perikarya** are located in the **gray matter** of the brainstem or spinal cord.

3. The **efferent axons** exit from the CNS through a ventral root of a spinal nerve or corresponding part of a cranial nerve.

4. Motoneuron impulses reach their effectors directly or indirectly.

a. The axons from motoneurons for **skeletal muscle** run uninterruptedly to the muscle cells, forming a **direct, one-neuron pathway**.

b. The axons from motoneurons for **smooth and cardiac muscle and glands** synapse first on motor ganglia in the PNS, which in turn send axons to the effector cells, forming an **indirect, two-neuron pathway**.

E. Human behavior as expressed through motoneurons to the effectors

1. Behavioral psychologists may choose to disregard the mental activity produced by the interneuronal pool of the brain. By ignoring thought processes and emotions, which are private and unobservable, they may study behavior per se. Behavior per se means any **observable change** produced by neural activation of an effector.

2. Nerve impulses can produce behavior in only two ways:
   a. By causing a gland to secrete something
   b. By causing muscle fibers to shorten
   (1) Shortening of muscle fibers may change the diameter of an orifice or internal organ or activate a skeletomuscular lever.
   (2) By stopping the flow of nerve impulses, the nervous system can stop the shortening of muscle fibers but it cannot actively lengthen them. That happens because muscles act in antagonistic pairs.

3. Thus, all of our behavior consists of shortening muscle fibers and secreting substances.

F. Reflex arcs

1. **Definition.** A reflex is an observable, reproducible, nearly automatic, neurally mediated response to a stimulus.

2. In **monosynaptic reflexes**, incoming axons of unipolar sensory neurons synapse directly on a motoneuron. Excitation of the motoneuron causes a twitch of a skeletal muscle fiber or activates a gland (Fig. 2-7).

3. In **polysynaptic reflexes**, one or more interneurons, excitatory or inhibitory, intervenes between the afferent impulses and the motoneuron (Fig. 2-8). Polysynaptic reflexes may involve a single muscle or the whole body (e.g., when postural reflexes adjust the body to changes in position).

G. Axonal transport. Small structures in the perikaryon called **organelles** produce most of the energy and conduct most of the metabolism of the neuron. Since the axons lack most of the organelles necessary for cell metabolism, transport mechanisms move critical **metabolic substances** and **neurotransmitters** down the axon.

1. The axonal volume may exceed the perikaryal volume by a ratio of as much as 2000:1 in Golgi type I neurons.

2. Slow and rapid axonal transport mechanisms provide for the flow of materials down the axon from the perikaryon as well as back up to the perikaryon. Dendritic flow also occurs.

3. If metabolic and toxic disorders interfere with the axonal transport mechanisms, metabolites cannot reach the entire axon. The distal tips of the longest axons then suffer, causing a **"dying back"** neuropathy.

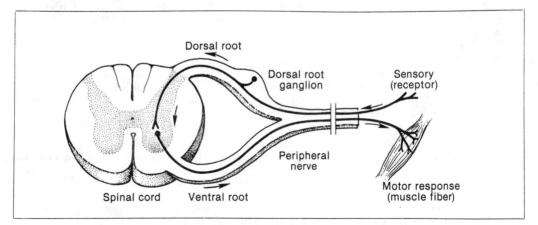

Figure 2-7. Monosynaptic reflex arc, consisting of a primary sensory neuron activating a motoneuron by a direct synapse.

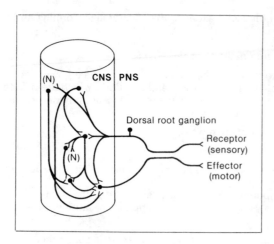

Figure 2-8. Polysynaptic reflex arc consisting of a primary sensory neuron, any number of interneurons (N), and a motoneuron.

III. PATHOLOGIC REACTIONS OF NEURONS

A. Doctrine of selective vulnerability of neurons

1. **Metabolic diversity of neurons**
   a. Nerve cells have a greater diversity of structure, function, and metabolic characteristics than all of the other cells of the body together.
   b. Each type of neuron is genetically programmed to have its particular structure and critical metabolic pathways.
      (1) Some neurons produce large quantities of pigment, others virtually none.
      (2) Some neurons respond to chemical stimuli, others to physical stimuli.
      (3) Some neurons produce excitatory transmitters, others produce inhibitory transmitters.

2. **Selective vulnerability of neurons**
   a. Because of metabolic differences, various types of neurons exhibit **differential susceptibility to pathogens**; for example, some neurons are especially susceptible to hypoxia, others to hyperbilirubinemia.
      (1) Certain viruses attack only specific groups of neurons (e.g., the poliomyelitis virus prefers motoneurons over all other CNS neurons).
      (2) Genetic defects may produce types of neurons that lack an enzyme critical for their function. These disorders are called inborn errors of metabolism.
   b. The selective vulnerability of neurons leads to **systematized degeneration** of related neuronal populations.
      (1) If the pathogen selectively affects retinal neurons, the patient becomes blind. If it affects auditory neurons, the patient becomes deaf. If it selects motoneurons, the patient becomes paralyzed.
      (2) In theory, and it is almost ratified by practice, a toxic, viral, or genetic disease could exist for each anatomically and metabolically different group of neurons. (This text mentions some of these diseases as parts of the nervous system are described.)

B. Neuronal death

1. **Direct neuronal death**
   a. Interruption of the metabolic machinery in the perikaryon may cause the neuron to die.
   b. The entire neuron—dendrites, perikaryon, and axon with all its collaterals—dies, but neighboring neurons, including the next neuron in line, generally survive unless the disease also affects them directly.

2. **Transsynaptic neuronal death**
   a. Ordinarily, each neuron dies as a unit, and the next cell in line survives.
   b. In the CNS, the next neuron in line may undergo **transsynaptic degeneration** (atrophy or cell death) if it has no or few other sources of afferent fibers. For example, the retina supplies most of the axons that synapse on the neurons of a nucleus called the lateral geniculate body. Transection of the optic nerve, which conveys retinal axons to the geniculate body, results in degeneration of the optic nerve fibers. Denuded of all synapses, the geniculate body neurons undergo transsynaptic degeneration.
   c. Since most CNS neurons have multiple sources of synapses, they do not die after destruction of one source of synapses.

    d. When an axon to a muscle cell dies, the muscle cell has no other source of stimulation and it will then undergo atrophy. If denervated for months, the muscle cell itself will die, an example of transsynaptic degeneration in the PNS.

    e. Denervated glands may undergo transsynaptic atrophy and death.

C. Wallerian degeneration

  1. Definition. Wallerian degeneration is the dissolution of the distal part of an axon and its myelin sheath that follows separation of the axon from the perikaryon. In fact, any bit of living neuron that becomes separated from the metabolic machinery in the perikaryon will die (Fig. 2-9).

    a. After axonal injury, the axon may also degenerate for varying distances back toward the perikaryon.

    b. Wallerian degeneration of the distal segment of the axon always occurs, but the centripetal degeneration varies. Usually, it extends backward to the first collateral above the transection.

    c. If the axon has no collateral or the axon is severed close to the perikaryon, the whole neuron may die.

  2. Neuroanatomists use wallerian degeneration to determine the course of axonal pathways. After destroying neuronal perikarya or transecting nerve fibers, the observer can selectively stain degenerating myelin or axoplasm to trace the course of nerve fibers through serial sections to their termination (see Chapter 4, section IV D).

D. Chromatolysis. After axonal injury, the neuronal perikaryon shows **nuclear eccentricity** and **cytoplasmic swelling**, with pallor of Nissl bodies (Fig. 2-10).

  1. The Nissl bodies stain less intensely than is the case in the normal neuron, but their endoplasmic reticulum is merely diluted by cytoplasmic swelling and is not destroyed.

  2. The cytoplasmic swelling also displaces the nucleus to the side of the neuron opposite the axon hillock (**nuclear eccentricity**).

E. Regeneration of neurons

  1. Mature neurons, which are the most specialized cells of the body, do not regenerate themselves, but they do have a limited capacity to regenerate axons after axonal death. Although the severed distal part of an axon always undergoes wallerian degeneration, the proximal

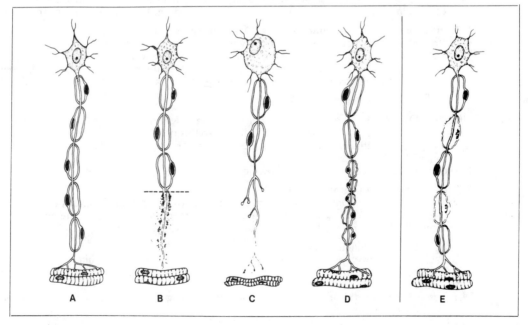

Figure 2-9. Wallerian degeneration. (*A*) Normal neuron with myelinated axon. (*B*) Degeneration of the axon and myelin sheath distal to its point of transection. (*C*) Regeneration of the axon after removal of axonal and myelin debris. (*D*) Irregular remyelination of regenerated axon. (*E*) Segmental demyelination (described later in the text).

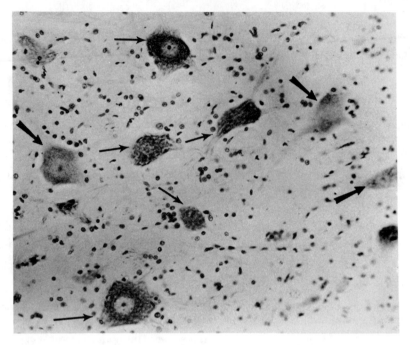

Figure 2-10. Microphotograph of Nissl-stained motoneurons. The *thin arrows* indicate normal motoneuron perikarya showing Nissl bodies. The *thick arrows* indicate motoneuron perikarya undergoing chromatolysis, with dissolution of Nissl bodies.

stump, which still retains contact with the perikaryon, may grow out again to reestablish synaptic connection with an effector.

    a. In the PNS, both motor and sensory neurons may regenerate axons and reestablish synaptic connections.

    b. Although in theory any neuron might be able to regenerate its axon, **neurons in the CNS of humans** do not regenerate axons, or at least they **do not regenerate axons effectively**.

2. Transplantation of embryonic neurons. One of the most exciting areas of research involves the transplantation of bits of embryonic nervous tissue to the CNS of a mature animal. For example, after destruction of a part of the brain, the transplantation of embryonic tissue of the same type may allow functional regeneration to occur. Whether such an approach is biologically possible in humans, or morally justifiable in terms of obtaining human fetal tissue, is still unsettled.

IV. NEURON DOCTRINE. The neuron doctrine of Santiago Ramón y Cajal summarizes neuron structure and function, and it recapitulates this chapter to this point. The neuron doctrine is a special case of the general theory that the cell is the basic unit of living organisms.

    A. The neuron doctrine consists of the following **six tenets**.

        1. Each neuron is an anatomical unit.

            a. A neuron is a cell consisting of a **nucleus**, a **perikaryon**, and **axonal/dendritic processes**.

            b. The perikaryon and its processes are enclosed by a membrane that keeps the neuron anatomically distinct from all other cells and from the extracellular fluid.

        2. Each neuron is a genetic unit.

            a. Each neuron develops from an independent embryonic cell, a **neuroblast**.

            b. Each neuron contains a **genetic code**, which specifies its **structure**, **metabolism**, and **connections**.

            c. Some variability of connections may result from learning, but the brain connections are genetically programmed.

        3. Each neuron is a functional unit.

            a. A neuron is the smallest unit capable of receiving a **stimulus** and generating and transmitting a **nerve impulse**.

        b. Each neuron forms a unit in a **communication circuit**. A neuron in isolation, such as one growing in a tissue culture, is functionally useless.

        c. Intercellular communication between neurons or effectors occurs after a stimulus generates a nerve impulse. The nerve impulse affects the next cell in line by a terminal structure called a **synapse**.

           (1) Neurons synapse on other neurons or effectors.

           (2) A chemical **neurotransmitter** released at the synapse transmits the effect of the nerve impulse to the next cell in line.

           (3) The neurotransmitter may inhibit (hyperpolarize) or excite (depolarize) the next cell in line. Whether any given neuron generates a nerve impulse depends on the algebraic summation of inhibitory and excitatory effects.

        d. A neuron generates a nerve impulse according to an **all or none law**. It either produces an impulse or it does not. The impulse, considered as a depolarization wave, is always the same.

    4. Each neuron is a polarized unit.

        a. The neuron, when stimulated under normal conditions, conducts nerve impulses in **one direction**, from dendrite, to perikaryon, to axon, and to synaptic endings at the axonal tips.

        b. If a stimulus excites a neuronal membrane at some site other than its normal afferent source, the membrane may conduct the nerve impulse in both directions from the site of stimulation, but it will transmit impulses to other neurons only at the synapse.

    5. Each neuron is a pathologic unit.

        a. Each neuron reacts to injury as a unit. If severely enough injured, the whole neuron—dendrites, perikaryon, and axon—will die as a cellular unit.

        b. Although each neuron reacts individually when injured, populations of **similar neurons** are **selectively vulnerable** to various toxins, metabolic derangements, viral infections, or genetic defects. This leads to **systematized degeneration** of structurally and metabolically similar neurons in response to certain specific pathogens or genetic defects.

        c. Any bit of cytoplasm, dendritic or axoplasmic, that is separated from its perikaryon will die, although the remainder of the cell itself may survive. The process of degeneration of the axon and its myelin sheath distal to a site of transection is called **wallerian degeneration**.

    6. Each neuron is a regenerative unit.

        a. Although neurons cannot divide to replenish their numbers, some may grow new axons if the axon is severed.

        b. In a practical sense in human disease, the only axons that regenerate are those that run in the PNS. **Tracts of the CNS do not regenerate** effectively in man.

B. The **neuron doctrine** can be summarized in one sentence: The neuron is the **anatomical, genetic, functional, polarized, pathologic,** and **regenerative unit** of the nervous system.

V. SUPPORTING TISSUES OF THE NERVOUS SYSTEM

  A. Functions of supporting tissues

    1. Because of their extreme specialization for their unique kind of intercellular communication, neurons cannot also support and maintain the structural integrity of the nervous system.

    2. Supporting tissues are, therefore, needed to:

        a. Provide a scaffolding to keep the neurons in place and hold them in contact

        b. Produce protective coverings, which absorb and distribute blows

        c. Produce intercellular fluids and cerebrospinal fluid (CSF) that coat, support, and protect neurons

        d. Form a blood–neuronal (blood–brain) barrier

        e. Proliferate to form scars to heal the nervous tissue after injury

        f. Produce myelin sheaths

  B. Classification of supporting tissues

    1. The body contains **two main types of supporting tissue, fibrous connective tissue** and **glia**.

        a. The **PNS** contains only **fibrous connective tissue**.

        b. Within the **CNS** proper, all of the connective tissue is **glia**. However, fibrous connective tissue forms coverings around the CNS called **meninges** and accompanies the larger blood vessels that penetrate the CNS.

2. Fibrous connective tissue consists of:
   a. Fibrocytes
   b. Collagen and elastic fibrils
   c. Intercellular fluid
   d. Miscellaneous types of cells, including Schwann cells, in peripheral nerves

3. Glial connective tissue consists only of cells and intercellular fluid. It contains no extracellular fibrils and relatively little extracellular fluid.
   a. Types of glial cells (Table 2-1)
      (1) Glia consist of **astrocytes, oligodendrocytes, microglia**, and **ependyma**. The glial cells differ in location, size, shape, and function (Fig. 2-11).
      (2) Ependymal cells form simple columnar epithelium, which lines the ventricular cavities and central canal of the spinal cord. Ependymal cells have the simplest contours of any of the glia.
      (3) Astrocytes, oligodendroglia, and **microglia** have complicated, branched contours (see Fig. 2-11).
   b. Perineuronal satellite cells
      (1) Three types of glial cells, **astrocytes, oligodendroglia**, and **microglia** send processes that contact the membrane of neuronal perikarya in the CNS (Fig. 2-12).
      (2) Although these contacts are not known to function as actual synapses, they may influence neurons by transfer of metabolites.

C. Blood–brain (blood–neuronal) barrier and extracellular space in the CNS

1. Ehrlich, in the last century, discovered that dye injected into the vessels would stain almost all organs and tissues except the CNS. Apart from a few tiny regions, the CNS remained uncolored (i.e., the dye did not penetrate the CNS from the blood).

2. It is now known that some substances—oxygen, carbon dioxide, glucose, certain amino acids—enter the CNS readily from the blood, whereas barrier mechanisms exclude other substances, particularly large molecules like protein.

3. This **blood–brain barrier** may provide for active transport of some molecules and passive diffusion, or active rejection, of other molecules.

4. The anatomical structures that collectively constitute the blood–brain barrier include the following:

Table 2-1. Types of Glial Cells, Their Locations and Normal Functions

Cell Type	Location	Normal Function
Astroglia (astrocytes) Protoplasmic Fibrous	Gray matter (perineuronal satellites) White matter	Provide supportive scaffolding for the CNS, end feet against vessels and meninges; may function as extracellular space of the CNS and as part of the blood–neuronal barrier
Oligodendroglia	Perineuronal satellites	One of the cell types that surround the neuron, perhaps acting to influence its metabolism or polarization
	White matter (interfascicular oligodendroglia)	Oligodendroglia membranes surround the axons to form myelin sheaths in the CNS; Schwann cells form myelin sheaths in the PNS
Microglia	Perineuronal satellites Diffuse in white matter but concentrated around blood vessels	One of the cell types that surround the neuron, perhaps acting to influence its metabolism or polarization; classic doctrine holds that microglia form macrophages, but they are now thought to come from blood monocytes
Ependyma	Line cavities of the CNS	Serve as an epithelial barrier between CNS tissue and the CSF within the CNS cavities; may act in part to control volume, secretion, and composition of the CSF

CNS = central nervous system; PNS = peripheral nervous system; CSF = cerebrospinal fluid.

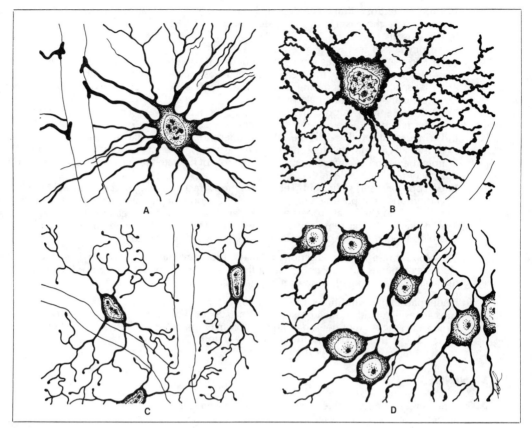

Figure 2-11. Branched glial cells. (*A*) Fibrous astrocyte. (*B*) Protoplasmic astrocyte. (*C*) Microgliocyte. (*D*) Oligodendrocyte.

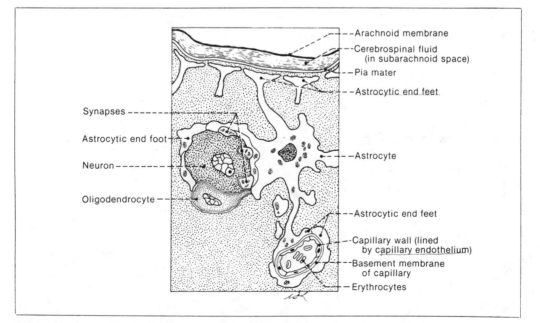

Figure 2-12. Relationship of astrocytic processes to the pial surface, blood vessels, and neurons. (After De Robertis E, Gershenfeld HM: Submicroscopic morphology and function of glial cells. In *International Review of Neurobiology*, vol 3. Edited by Pfeiffer CC, Smythies, JR. New York, Academic Press, 1961, p 20.)

a. Capillary endothelium. The endothelial cells of CNS capillaries have very tight junctions that oppose the passage of some substances.
b. Vessel walls
c. Astrocytic end feet (see Fig. 2-12)
   (1) End feet of astrocytes form a continuous covering on the external capillary wall. Only tiny spaces separate the membranes of the astrocytes. Just how much of this extracellular space is present during life and whether the astrocytic cytoplasm functions as extracellular space remain at issue today.
   (2) Because the astrocytic end feet form a continuous covering on the blood vessels, they form part of the blood–brain barrier.
d. Perineuronal satellite cells (i.e., the oligodendroglia, microglia, and astrocytes). The contacts of all glia with the neuronal surface may act to transmit or exclude specific substances from the neuronal surface membrane. The role of the satellite cells in modulating neuronal activity remains unclear.
e. Glycoprotein and sialic acid. These form the **surface covering of the neuronal membrane** and are the final possible components of the blood–brain barrier. They would make the physical and chemical properties of the neuronal membrane itself the final censor of what is to affect it. In this sense, the barrier would best be called a **blood–neuronal barrier**, not a blood–brain barrier, but the latter is the conventional language.

5. The **blood–brain barrier functions to make the neuronal surface a privileged site**. It excludes extraneous substances, ensuring that only the appropriately released neurotransmitters will affect the polarization of neuronal membranes.

6. Under **pathologic conditions**, the blood–brain barrier breaks down. Then normally excluded substances like fluid or metabolites from the CSF or blood can leak into the CNS.
   a. The ensuing state of neuronal intoxication may inhibit or excite neuronal discharges.
   b. The accumulation of fluid in the cells, a state called edema, may cause rupture of cell membranes and interrupt their function.

VI. MENINGES

A. The **meninges** consist of three concentric but distinct fibrous connective tissue membranes, which ensheathe the CNS (Fig. 2-13).

1. The **three membranes** are the following.
   a. The **pia mater**, which literally means soft mother, is the innermost membrane.

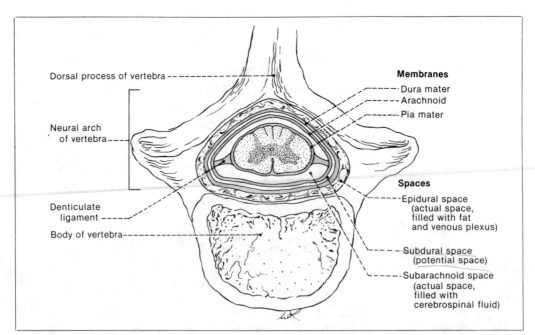

Figure 2-13. Cross section through a vertebra showing the vertebral canal with its contained epidural space, meninges, and spinal cord.

    b. The **arachnoid membrane**, which literally means spidery membrane, is the intermediate membrane.

    c. The **dura mater**, which literally means hard mother, is the outermost.

  2. Both the pia mater and the arachnoid membrane are relatively thin and delicate. Hence, together they are called the **leptomeninges** (lepto means thin and delicate).

B. Pia mater

  1. The pia mater is the innermost meningeal sheath. Its inner surface closely adheres to the external surface of the CNS, covering each bump and entering each crevice as if sprayed on.

  2. Since the **astrocytic end feet** adhere to the inner surface of the pia (see Fig. 2-12), no space, actual or potential, exists between the pia and the neural tissue. Because the astrocytic end feet form a continuous lining on the pia, they form a part of a CNS–CSF barrier (the blood–brain barrier).

C. Arachnoid membrane and subarachnoid space

  1. The arachnoid membrane is inside the dura mater and surrounds the pia mater.

  2. The **subarachnoid space**, an **actual space**, separates the inner surface of the arachnoid membrane from the outer surface of the pia mater (Fig. 2-14).

    a. Numerous fibrous trabeculae bridge the subarachnoid space.

    b. The subarachnoid space contains blood vessels and CSF.

  3. **Blood vessels** penetrate the CNS from its surface (see Fig. 2-14), hence they must penetrate the pia mater.

    a. As the blood vessels penetrate the pia mater, they receive a **fibrous connective tissue investment** from the pia.

    b. This connective tissue, forming the external part of the blood vessel wall, is the only fibrous connective tissue central to the pia mater. All remaining connective tissue of the CNS is glial.

D. Dura mater

  1. The **dura mater**, the outermost of the three meningeal membranes, is thick and very tough, in contrast to the leptomeninges.

  2. The **subdural space**, the space between the dura and the arachnoid membrane, contains no free fluid. It is a **potential space**, like the pleural space. Hence, it can become distended with tissue fluids, blood, or pus.

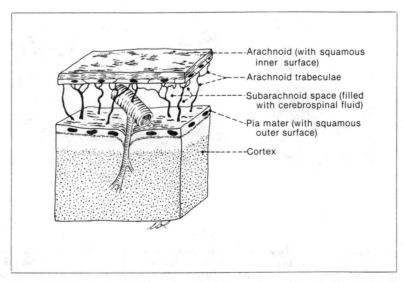

Arachnoid (with squamous inner surface)

Arachnoid trabeculae

Subarachnoid space (filled with cerebrospinal fluid)

Pia mater (with squamous outer surface)

Cortex

Figure 2-14. Section through the subarachnoid space, formed between the arachnoid membrane and the pia mater.

3. Epidural space
   a. Within the skull, the external surface of the dura mater normally adheres to the bone, forming in fact the periosteum. Under pathologic conditions, blood, pus, or tissue fluid may separate the dura from the skull bones (Fig. 2-15), creating an actual space from the potential space.

   b. At the vertebral level, an actual **epidural space** extends caudally along the vertebral column, separating the external dural surface from the vertebral periosteum (see Fig. 2-13). Fat and an epidural plexus of veins occupy this actual epidural space. Pus, blood, or neoplasms in this **vertebral epidural space** may compress the spinal cord.

E. Fossae of the skull. The base of the skull displays three hollows, or fossae—the **anterior, middle**, and **posterior fossae** (see Fig. 8-13).

   1. Anterior fossa. The orbital plates of the **frontal bone** form the floor of the anterior fossa. The undersurface of the **frontal lobe** rests in the anterior fossa.

   2. Middle fossa. The **temporal bone** forms the floor of the middle fossa. The undersurfaces of the temporal and occipital lobes rest in the middle fossa.

   3. Posterior fossa. The **temporal** and **occipital bones** form the posterior fossa. The bony floor of the posterior fossa underlies the **pons** and **medulla oblongata**.

F. Dural compartments of the skull. Within the skull, **dural folds** called the **cerebral falx** and the **cerebellar tentorium** partition the space into compartments (Fig. 2-16).

   1. The **cerebral falx** is a fold of dura mater in the midsagittal plane, inserted into the interhemispheric fissure. It partitions the skull into right and left halves.

   2. The **cerebellar tentorium**, inserted between the cerebellum and the inferomedial surfaces of the temporal and occipital lobes, forms a tent-like configuration.
   a. Anteriorly, the halves of the tentorium separate to form the **tentorial notch**.
   b. The **space above the tentorium**, the **supratentorial space**, contains the cerebrum.
   c. The **space below the tentorium** is the **infratentorial space**, or **posterior fossa**, and it contains the brainstem and cerebellum. The tentorial notch admits the passage of the midbrain from the infratentorial to the supratentorial space (see Fig. 2-16).
   d. Figure 2-16 shows that the rostral tip of the cerebellum also extends slightly into the supratentorial space.

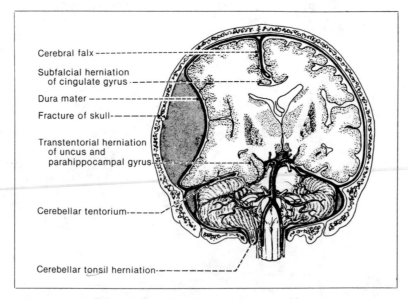

Cerebral falx

Subfalcial herniation of cingulate gyrus

Dura mater

Fracture of skull

Transtentorial herniation of uncus and parahippocampal gyrus

Cerebellar tentorium

Cerebellar tonsil herniation

Figure 2-15. Coronal section of the head showing an epidural hematoma causing internal herniation of the cerebrum across the midline and of the cerebellar tonsil down through the foramen magnum. (Adapted from Netter F: *Ciba Symposia*, vol 18, 1966, plate XI.)

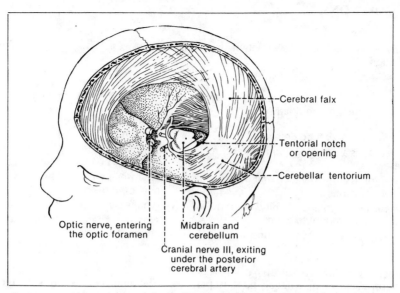

Figure 2-16. Oblique view of the skull with the hemicranium and hemispheres removed to show the cerebral falx and cerebellar tentorium, formed by the dura mater.

STUDY QUESTIONS

Directions: Each question below contains five suggested answers. Choose the **one best** response to each question.

1. Current evidence has most modified which tenet of the classic neuron doctrine?

(A) The neuron is a genetic unit
(B) The neuron is a pathologic unit in reacting to disease
(C) The neuron is a regenerative unit in regard to regrowth of axons
(D) The neuron is a polarized unit with impulses flowing from dendrite to axon
(E) The neuron is an anatomical unit

2. In order to withdraw cerebrospinal fluid (CSF) [i.e., perform a spinal tap], a needle tip must pass successively through the

(A) pia mater, dura mater, epidural space, and arachnoid membrane
(B) arachnoid membrane, epidural space, dura mater, and subdural space
(C) subdural space, dura mater, epidural space, and arachnoid membrane
(D) arachnoid membrane, subdural space, dura mater, and epidural space
(E) epidural space, dura mater, subdural space, and arachnoid membrane

3. The one true statement about synapses is

(A) synapses are more common on axons than dendrites
(B) synapses act usually by transmitting electrical messages across the gap
(C) synapses permit the two-way transmission of nerve impulses
(D) synapses may be excitatory or inhibitory
(E) synapses characteristically consist of a pre- and postsynaptic membrane, one of which is derived from a glial cell

4. The ultimate function of the blood–brain barrier is to

(A) exclude small molecules
(B) actively transport proteins
(C) keep out white blood cells
(D) control the ingress of cholesterol into myelin
(E) protect the polarization of the neuronal membrane

Directions: Each question below contains four suggested answers of which **one or more** is correct. Choose the answer

A   if **1, 2, and 3** are correct
B   if **1 and 3** are correct
C   if **2 and 4** are correct
D   if **4** is correct
E   if **1, 2, 3, and 4** are correct

5. In contrast to dendrites, axons typically

(1) are longer
(2) are thinner
(3) produce one or more synaptic end feet
(4) receive more synaptic contacts

6. A stimulus that excites nerve impulses may consist of a

(1) chemical event
(2) change in temperature
(3) an electrical event
(4) physical blow

7. Effector cells as defined behaviorally include

(1) neurons
(2) skeletal muscle cells
(3) squamous epithelium
(4) gland cells

8. The cerebral falx is a fold of dura mater that can be described as

(1) separating the right and left temporal lobes
(2) consisting of glial cells
(3) soft and yielding
(4) occupying the interhemispheric fissure

ANSWERS AND EXPLANATIONS

1. The answer is D. *(IV A 1, 2, 4, 5, 6)* The original neuron doctrine as advocated by Ramón y Cajal is generally regarded as correct, although some of the tenets have been modified by newer information. The original idea that the neuron is a strictly polarized unit with impulses flowing from dendrites to axons has had to be modified with the demonstration of a number of dendrodendritic contacts in the nervous system, which appear to be synapses. In addition, some nerve cells have only dendritic processes without axons. Nevertheless, for the majority of neurons, the original statements of the neuron doctrine are generally true.

2. The answer is E. *(VI A 1, C 1, D 2, 3)* The physician can insert a needle into the subarachnoid space to withdraw cerebrospinal fluid (CSF) for diagnostic analysis. The needle tip passes successively through the epidural space, the dura mater, the subdural space, and the arachnoid membrane. The CSF is between the arachnoid membrane and the pia mater, the innermost of the three meningeal sheaths.

3. The answer is D. *(I D)* Synapses typically consist of a presynaptic membrane from an axonal terminal, a postsynaptic membrane from a dendrite or perikaryon, and an intervening synaptic cleft. Synapses typically act by releasing a chemical substance into the synaptic cleft between the two membranes. The released neurotransmitter may excite or inhibit the next cell in line when it attaches to the postsynaptic membrane.

4. The answer is E. *(V C 5)* The ultimate function of the blood–brain barrier is to protect the surface membrane of the neuron. It excludes a variety of substances that might enter the CNS from the blood and that might alter the electrical potential of the neuronal membrane, causing the neuron to function inappropriately. The neuron should function only in response to the appropriate release of neurotransmitters from its synaptic contacts.

5. The answer is A (1, 2, 3). *[I A 1, D 1 a (1)]* Axons typically are longer and thinner than dendrites and produce one or more synaptic end feet. Although there are axoaxonic synapses, far fewer synapses occur on the axon itself than upon the dendrites or perikaryon of the neuron.

6. The answer is E (all). *(I C 1)* A variety of stimuli may induce a neuron to produce a nerve impulse. Stimuli may be chemical substances, temperature changes, electricity, or a simple physical blow (as occurs by tapping a nerve). Many other events such as light and the pull of gravity on hair cells in the labyrinth may also initiate nerve impulses.

7. The answer is C (2, 4). *(I C 3 b; II E 1, 2)* Effector cells are the final cells that ultimately respond to produce the behavior that originates in the CNS. The effectors are either gland cells or muscle cells. The three types of muscle cells are smooth, cardiac, and skeletal. The only behavior that the nervous system can produce is to shorten muscle fibers and to secrete something.

8. The answer is D (4). *(VI F 1)* The dura mater forms two flat membranes within the cranial cavity, the cerebral falx and the cerebellar tentorium. The falx is inserted in the interhemispheric fissure between the frontal, parietal, and occipital lobes. The cerebellar tentorium is inserted between the cerebellum and the inferior aspect of the temporo-occipital region. The falx consists solely of fibrous connective tissue, not glia.

3
Embryology of the Nervous System

I. BASIC MECHANISMS OF MORPHOGENESIS

A. Stages of morphogenesis. For convenience, morphogenesis can be divided into three stages: **cytogenesis**, **histogenesis**, and **organogenesis** (Table 3-1).

B. Configuration of developing cells. The geometric configurations that developing cells assume are few in number, although the forms are almost infinitely variable in their detailed expression. The cells can form into:

1. Solid or hollow balls

2. Sheets or layers on or beneath surfaces

3. Nodular masses or protrusions

4. Rod-like masses, which may remain solid or canalize

5. Tubes, which may then evaginate or fold over upon themselves

C. Embryonic development. The human embryonic disk and the embryo that develops from it show the sequence of cytogenesis, histogenesis, and organogenesis and the formation of the basic cell configurations.

1. Origin of the embryonic disk (cytogenesis to histogenesis) [Fig. 3-1]
   a. The fertilized ovum multiplies to form a berry-like mass, a **morula**.
   b. The morula forms a fluid-filled ball, a **blastocyst**.
   c. Cells at one pole of the blastocyst multiply to form a **polar mass**, or **inner cell mass**.

Table 3-1. Three Stages of Morphogenesis

Cytogenesis
Formation of gametes by mitosis and meiosis, followed by fertilization

Cell multiplication at proper time and site

Cell differentiation into various parenchymal and supporting cells

Programmed death of certain cell populations

Histogenesis
Orientation of cells to each other and their supporting tissues

Establishment of intercellular contacts (synapses)

Migration of cell populations

Arrangement of migrating, multiplying, and differentiating parenchymal and connective tissue cells, and blood vessels, into tissues

Organogenesis
Blending of tissues into organs

Shaping of the external contour of organs

Shaping of the internal contour of organs

Growth to complete the somatotype of the individual

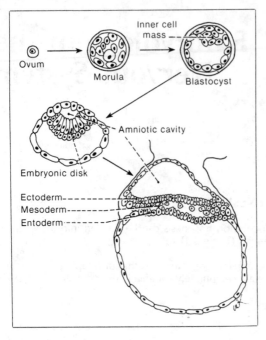

Figure 3-1. Development of ovum into morula, blastocyst, and embryonic disk, with lamination of the latter into ectoderm, mesoderm, and entoderm.

d. The polar mass secretes additional fluid, which separates it from the surface cells, forming a partition called the **embryonic disk**. This disk becomes the embryo proper.

2. **Origin of the three basic embryonic layers in the embryonic disk** (histogenesis)
   a. By proliferation, differentiation, and orientation of its cells, the embryonic disk forms into three layers, the **ectoderm**, **mesoderm**, and **entoderm**. The ectoderm and entoderm are sheets of cells on the dorsal and ventral surface of the mesoderm (see Fig. 3-1).
   b. The **ectodermal layer** becomes the epidermis and the nervous system.
   c. The **mesodermal layer** produces bone, muscle, fibrous connective tissue, the circulatory system, and much of the genitourinary tract.
   d. The **entodermal layer** becomes the gastrointestinal tract and its appendages and the lungs.

II. DEVELOPMENT OF THE EXTERNAL CONTOUR OF THE NEURAXIS (ORGANOGENESIS)

A. Major organogenetic events of the neuraxis [central nervous system (CNS)]

1. The **fundamental event** in organogenesis of the neuraxis is the rolling up of the monolayer of ectodermal cells to form the **neural tube**. Thus, the neuraxis commences as a tube; subsequent events shape the tube into the final form of the brain and spinal cord.

2. The organogenetic events consist of:
   a. Closure of the neural tube (neurulation)
   b. Transverse segmentation of the neural tube
   c. Evagination of the neural tube walls
   d. Flexion of the neural tube
   e. Protrusion of masses: cerebellum, olivary eminences, quadrigeminal bodies, and so forth
   f. Fissuring and **sulcation** of the cerebrum and cerebellum
   g. Growth to adult size of the parts already formed

B. Neurulation or closure: formation of the neural tube. Although neurulation and some of the other organogenetic events proceed simultaneously, this text, for conceptual simplicity, describes these events as if they occurred separately.

1. The first indication of neural organogenesis is the appearance of the **primitive streak** and **primitive node** along the dorsal aspect of the embryonic disk in the sagittal plane (Fig. 3-2; see Fig. 3-2A).

2. Next, a median **neural groove** flanked by **neural folds** appears in the sagittal plane of the embryonic disk (Fig. 3-3).

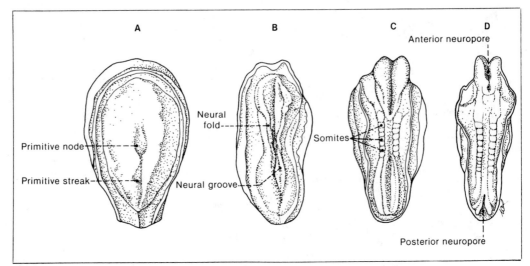

Figure 3-2. Dorsal view of the embryonic disk showing elevation and fusion of the neural folds to form the neural tube. (Adapted from Streeter GL: Factors involved in the formation of the filum terminalis. *Am J Anat* 25:1–11, 1919.)

3. **Closure** or **fusion** of the dorsal margins of the neural folds then follows (see Figs. 3-2 and 3-3).
   a. The fusion of the neural folds allows the neural tube to separate from the remainder of the surface ectoderm.
   b. The neural folds first come into contact in the lower cervical and upper thoracic region. From that site, the closure of the neural folds proceeds rostrally and caudally (see Fig. 3-3).
   c. Figure 3-2C and 3-2D shows the incompletely closed ends of the neural tube. These ends, the last to close, are called the **anterior** and **posterior neuropores**.

4. **Fusion of the neuropores**, the end of neurulation, completes the transformation from a single cell to a ball of cells, to a sheet of cells, to a tube of cells. The neuraxis now is a simple fluid-filled tube sealed at the ends.

C. **Transverse subdivision of the neural tube** proceeds as the neuropores close. Figure 3-4 shows that:

1. The brain first exhibits three transverse subdivisions or units.

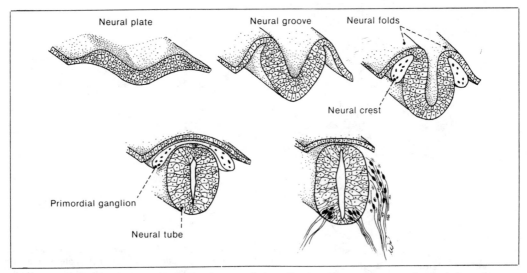

Figure 3-3. Formation of the neural tube by closure or fusion of its dorsal lips and sequestration from the surface ectoderm.

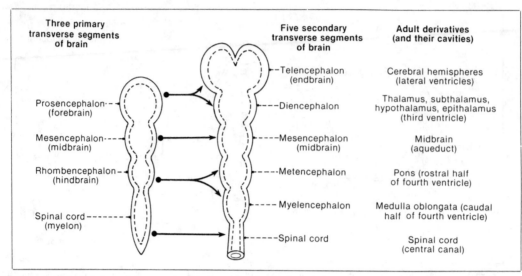

Three primary transverse segments of brain	Five secondary transverse segments of brain	Adult derivatives (and their cavities)
	Telencephalon (endbrain)	Cerebral hemispheres (lateral ventricles)
Prosencephalon (forebrain)	Diencephalon	Thalamus, subthalamus, hypothalamus, epithalamus (third ventricle)
Mesencephalon (midbrain)	Mesencephalon (midbrain)	Midbrain (aqueduct)
Rhombencephalon (hindbrain)	Metencephalon	Pons (rostral half of fourth ventricle)
	Myelencephalon	Medulla oblongata (caudal half of fourth ventricle)
Spinal cord (myelon)	Spinal cord	Spinal cord (central canal)

Figure 3-4. Dorsal view of the neural tube after closure, showing transverse segmentation into three and then five gross divisions.

2. The first and third units then split into two each, making five final brain units.

3. The midbrain and spinal cord do not undergo further transverse subdivision.

4. The original fluid-filled lumen of the neural tube remains throughout its length.

D. Evagination of the neural tube walls

1. Along with closure and transverse subdivision, the neural tube starts to show evaginations.
   a. Evagination involves the outpouching of the entire wall of the neural tube.
   b. The lumen extends out into the evaginations, as shown in the development of the telencephalon in Figures 3-4 and 3-5.

2. Evagination produces the **pineal body**, **hypophysis**, the **optic** and **olfactory bulbs**, and the **cerebral hemispheres** themselves (see Fig. 3-5).
   a. Figure 3-5, a lateral view of the neuraxis, depicts only the forebrain (diencephalon and telencephalon) because only the forebrain produces evaginations.

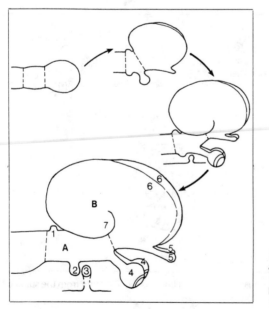

Figure 3-5. Lateral view of the forebrain (diencephalon and telencephalon) with the evaginations numbered. (*1*) Pineal body. (*2*) Neurohypophysis. (*3*) Adenohypophysis. (*4*) Optic bulb. (*5*) Olfactory stalks and bulb. (*6*) Cerebral hemispheres. (*7*) Temporal lobe.

b. Also, the figure depicts evagination as occurring after closure and segmentation, whereas in fact evagination begins before the completion of these events.

3. The **pineal body evaginates dorsally** in the median plane near the junction of the diencephalon with the midbrain (see Fig. 3-5, *1*).

4. **Hypophysis (pituitary gland)**
   a. The **neurohypophysis (posterior pituitary) evaginates ventrally** in the median plane near the junction of the diencephalon with the midbrain (see Fig. 3-5, *2*).
   b. The neurohypophysis meets another evagination, **Rathke's pouch,** which comes from the roof of the mouth. Rathke's pouch becomes the **adenohypophysis (anterior pituitary)** [see Fig. 3-5, *3*].
   c. The stalk of the neurohypophysis remains in continuity with the neuraxis. The adenohypophyseal stalk atrophies. Thus, the adenohypophysis loses its connection with its origin.

5. **Optic stalks**
   a. The optic stalks **evaginate from the diencephalon ventrally** in the median plane and bifurcate (see Fig. 3-5, *4*). The pineal body and neurohypophysis also evaginate in the median plane, but they do not bifurcate.
   b. The optic stalks produce the retinas at their distal ends and become the **optic nerves**.
      (1) Like the neurohypophysis, the optic stalks retain their neural connections and blood supply with the neuraxis. Thus, both the optic stalks and the neurohypophysis originate from the neuraxis and remain part of the CNS.
      (2) The **optic nerves**, being evaginations of the brain wall, have glial supporting cells. The myelin of the optic nerves comes from oligodendroglia. Hence, the demyelinating diseases that affect the CNS, such as multiple sclerosis, may affect the optic nerves. Conversely, the pure peripheral nerve diseases spare the optic nerve.
      (3) The **term optic nerve is thus a misnomer** embryologically, histologically, and pathologically.
   c. Originally, the lumen of the neural tube extended into the pineal, neurohypophyseal, and optic evaginations, but it is obliterated during maturation.

6. **Cerebral hemispheres**
   a. Two evaginations, the **cerebral hemispheres, extend laterally from the telencephalon** (see Fig. 3-5, *6*).
   b. The fissure between the hemispheres is the **interhemispheric fissure**.
   c. The two olfactory bulbs (see Fig. 3-5, *5*) and the temporal lobes (see Fig. 3-5, *7*) can be regarded as secondary evaginations from the original hemispheric evaginations. However, if we interpret our cerebrum phylogenetically, we can regard the cerebral hemispheres as evaginating from the olfactory bulbs, not the other way around (see Fig. 13-10).
   d. The cerebral hemispheres and temporal lobes retain the original lumen of the neural tube as the **lateral ventricles**. The original lumen that extended into the olfactory bulbs is obliterated.

E. Flexions

1. As the neural tube elongates, the brain undergoes a series of flexions that fit it more compactly into the intracranial space (Fig. 3-6).

2. These flexions and the evaginations and protuberances explain why the final form of the brain differs from a simple linear tube.

F. Protuberances

1. Proliferation of cells into masses at particular sites in the wall of the neural tube produces thickenings or actual protuberances.

2. The difference between protuberances in the wall and evaginations is that the ventricular lumen does not extend out into the protuberances. They are solid masses.

3. The **largest protuberance**, the **cerebellum**, grows from the dorsal aspect of the metencephalon (pons).

4. Additional protuberances include the:
   a. Inferior olivary eminence of the medulla
   b. Nuclei of the basis pontis
   c. Four elevations of the quadrigeminal plate of the midbrain
   d. Mamillary bodies of the diencephalon

G. Formation of fissures and sulci (see Chapter 13, section I D)

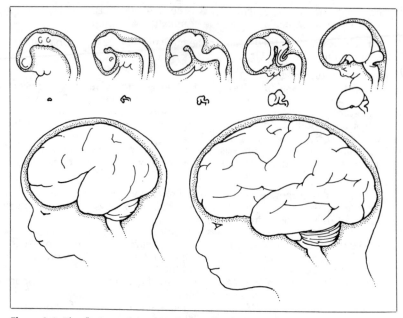

Figure 3-6. The flexions of the neural tube that fit the brain into the skull. (Adapted from Cowan WM: The development of the brain. *Sci Am* 241:113–133, 1979.)

III. CYTOGENESIS AND HISTOGENESIS IN THE WALL OF THE NEURAL TUBE

A. Cytogenesis of neurons and glia (Fig. 3-7)

1. As the neural tube closes, multiplying cells in the periventricular zone produce **neuroblasts** and **glioblasts**.

   a. Theoretically, glioblasts and neuroblasts have a common precursor cell, which is pluripotential until a certain number of cell divisions have occurred.

   b. The blast cell then becomes "determined": It "breeds true" and produces only one type of mature glial cell or neuron.

2. Although most neurons and glia arise from the periventricular zone, some CNS cells derive from the neural crest (see section IV D).

3. After the fetal period, the periventricular cells lose their capacity to produce new neuroblasts and glioblasts, but some glial cells, notably astrocytes, retain their proliferative capacity. The ependymal cells, which ultimately line the ventricles, are mature cell forms with little proliferative capacity.

B. Cytogenesis and neoplasia. The theory of neural cytogenesis shown in Figure 3-7 is used in the classification of CNS neoplasms.

1. CNS neoplasms are composed of cell types that resemble the cell lineages seen during normal embryogenesis.

2. One theory of CNS neoplasia assumes that certain cells, perhaps nests of primitive embryonic cells, later undergo mitosis unrestrained by the normal controlling influences that govern cell division during the embryonic period.

3. An alternative theory holds that neural cells, after differentiation into mature forms, can "dedifferentiate" to resemble their embryonic precursors.

C. Cytogenesis of neurons (Fig. 3-8)

1. In differentiating, the neuroblast initially produces protoplasmic expansions at opposite poles. Most neuroblasts are thought to pass through this **bipolar state**.

2. One of the bipolar processes continues to grow out, producing an **axon**, which seeks out its genetically determined synaptic contacts.

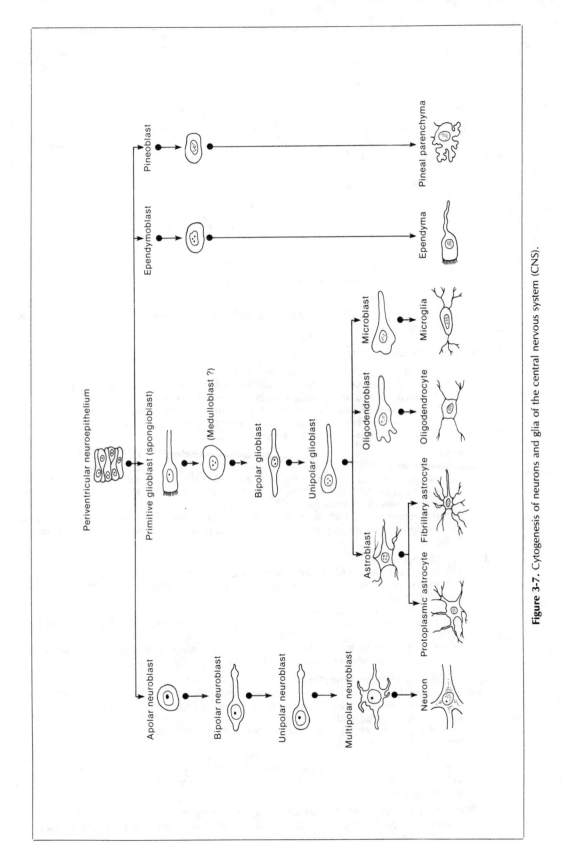

Figure 3-7. Cytogenesis of neurons and glia of the central nervous system (CNS).

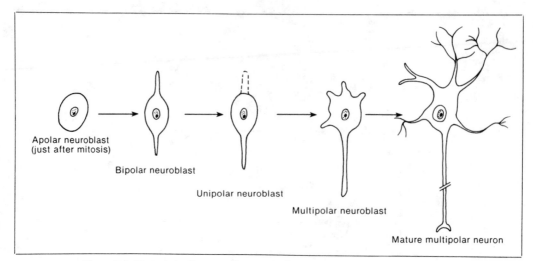

Figure 3-8. Typical developmental stages in the cytogenesis of a multipolar neuron.

3. The other bipolar process undergoes atrophy. A **dendritic tree** replaces it, then forming a **multipolar neuron**.

D. Histogenesis of CNS gray matter

1. Disposition of neuronal perikarya in gray matter

    a. In the CNS, the perikarya of neuroblasts arrange themselves into one of three forms of gray matter: **nuclei**, **reticular formation**, or **cortex** (Fig. 3-9; see Fig. 3-9A–C).

    b. In the peripheral nervous system (PNS), the neuronal perikarya of differentiating neuroblasts arrange themselves into ganglia, paravertebral or near the organs they innervate, and plexuses in the walls of viscera (see Fig. 3-9D).

2. Migration of neuroblasts. In the CNS, the neuroblasts undergo mitosis in the periventricular matrix zone, after which many migrate outward.

    a. The neuroblasts that remain in the region surrounding the periventricular zone of the spinal cord, brainstem, cerebellum, or cerebrum form **nuclei**. In the brainstem, they form, in addition, **reticular formation**.

    b. In the cerebrum and cerebellum, many neuroblasts separate from the periventricular nucleated zone. They migrate further outward to the surface, where they form **cortex** (Fig. 3-10).

3. Disposition of nuclei

    a. The nucleate arrangement extends from the caudal tip of the spinal cord up through the brainstem, diencephalon, and basal nuclei to the basal region of the cerebrum known as the rhinencephalon.

    b. All gray matter of the cerebral surface otherwise is cortex.

    c. In the diencephalon, nuclei, covered by ependyma, form most of the wall of the third ventricle.

    d. In the telencephalon, the caudate nuclei of the basal ganglia, covered by ependyma, form most of the lateral wall of the anterior horn of the lateral ventricle.

4. Disposition of reticular formation

    a. The reticular formation is the next step up from nuclei in complexity of neuronal disposition. It consists of loosely arranged neuronal groupings surrounding the denser nuclei proper, intermingled with numerous axonal connections and dendrites (see Fig. 3-9B).

    b. The reticular formation proper commences in the rostral part of the cervical cord and extends up through the midbrain and, possibly, diencephalon.

    c. The reticular formation provides integrative polysynaptic reflex circuits for activities more complex than are possible through simple nuclear connections. It mediates activities such as breathing, swallowing, and hiccuping as well as pulse rate, blood pressure, and even consciousness itself.

5. Disposition of cortex and its relationship to underlying nuclei

    a. Cortex consists of layers of neuronal perikarya alternating with layers of dendrites and axons (see Figs. 3-9C and 13-32).

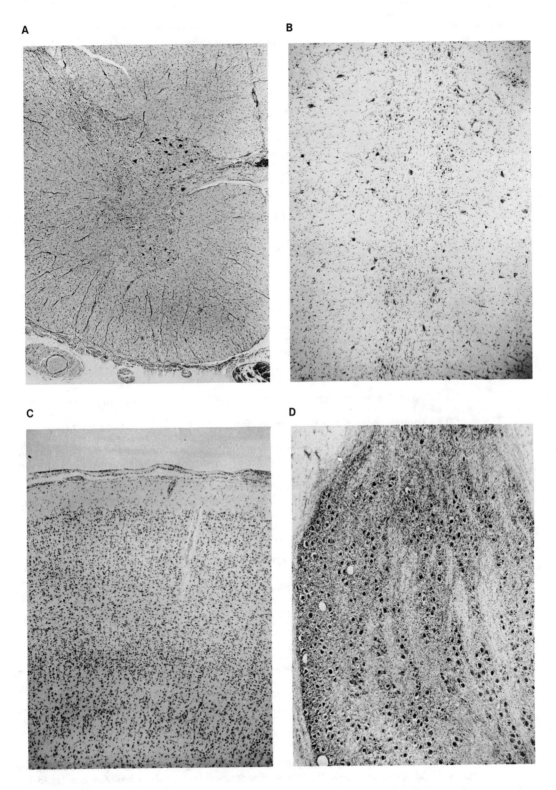

Figure 3-9. Microphotograph of four fundamental arrangements of neuronal perikarya (Nissl stain). (A) Nuclei in ventral horn of spinal cord (25 ×). (B) Reticular formation (40 ×); section of the rostral medullary raphe and paramedian reticular formation. (C) Cerebral cortex (40 ×). (D) Dorsal root ganglion (25 ×). A–C occur only in the central nervous system (CNS); D occurs only in the peripheral nervous system (PNS).

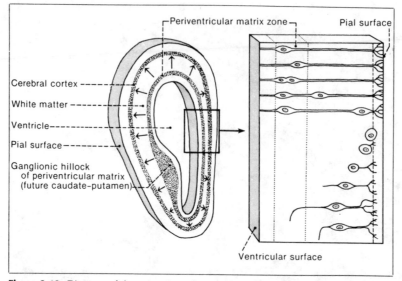

Figure 3-10. Diagram of the migration of neuroblasts from the periventricular matrix zone to the subpial zone to form cerebral cortex. After the nuclei migrate to the pial surface, the elongated cytoplasmic connection separates to form two individual cells from the preceding binucleate phase. The neuroblasts that remain along the ventricular lumen form the future caudate–putamen of the basal ganglia.

(1) In the cerebrum and cerebellum, neuroblasts form the cortex by migrating to the surface.

(2) By contrast, neuroblasts that remain close to the ventricular lumina form nuclei.

   (a) Those in the cerebellum form the **deep nuclei of the cerebellum**.

   (b) Those in the forebrain form the nuclei of the **diencephalon** and the **basal ganglia**.

(3) The cerebellar and cerebral cortices then form extensive axonal connections with their respective deep nuclei.

  b. The cerebellum and cerebrum contain the only true cortex. A stratified arrangement of neurons occurs in a few other sites, namely the retina, olfactory bulbs, and quadrigeminal plate of the midbrain, but these are not true cortices.

  c. Cortex furnishes the ultimate in plasticity and variety of interneuronal circuits, allowing for more complex neural activity than either nuclei or reticular formation.

IV. CYTOGENESIS AND HISTOGENESIS OF THE SPINAL CORD

  A. Three concentric layers of the spinal cord. After closure of the neural tube, the spinal portion of the tube develops, from the inside out, three concentric layers: the **ependymal layer**, the **mantle layer**, and the **marginal layer** (Fig. 3-11; see Fig. 3-11A).

    1. The **ependymal layer** remains as monocellular epithelium surrounding the central canal.

    2. The **mantle zone** becomes nucleated gray matter as neuroblasts differentiate within it.

    3. The **marginal zone** becomes the white matter as axons invade it from the dorsal root ganglia, the spinal cord nuclei, and the brainstem and cerebral cortex.

  B. Glial framework of the spinal cord. Glial cells, both ependymal and otherwise, extend their processes from the deepest layer of the cord to the surface (Fig. 3-12).

  C. Configuration of spinal gray matter (see Fig. 3-11B–D)

    1. The neuroblasts invade and thicken the mantle zone to form paired **alar plates** dorsally and paired **basal plates** ventrally. The plane of separation is the **sulcus limitans** (see Fig. 3-11B and C).

    2. The paired alar and basal plates thicken progressively to form the four limbs of the **H-shaped gray matter**, but the roof and floor plates remain thin.

      a. The **crossbar** of the H-shaped gray matter surrounds the central canal.

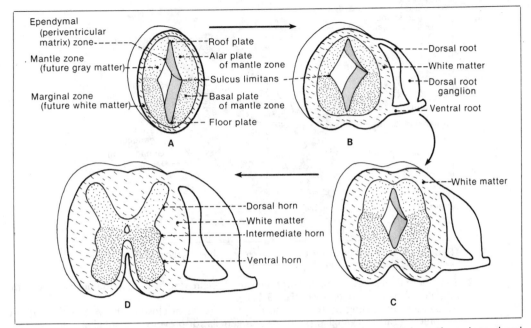

Figure 3-11. Cross section of developing spinal cord. (A) Early stage showing the marginal, mantle, and ependymal (periventricular matrix) zones. (B) and (C) Intermediate stages showing the fate of the sulcus limitans and the roof, floor, alar, and basal plates. (D) Final contour of the spinal cord.

       b. The **four major limbs** of the H **become dorsal and ventral horns** of gray matter. Just ventral to the plane of the central canal, an **intermediate** (intermediolateral) **horn** appears as neuroblasts thicken the region.

  D. Neural crest. The neural crest consists of two longitudinal bands of cells with nodular thickenings that develop along the dorsolateral aspect of the neural tube, where surface ectoderm and neural ectoderm join (see Fig. 3-3).

     1. The neural crest consists of two parts:
       a. Rostral (cranial) neural crest, adjacent to the brain
       b. Caudal (spinal) neural crest, adjacent to the spinal cord

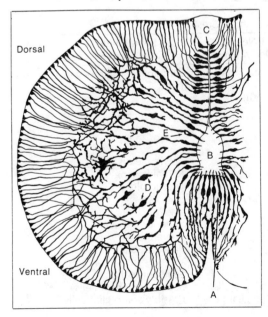

Figure 3-12. Cross section of the embryonic spinal cord showing the ependymal and astrocytic framework. (A) Ependyma of the floor plate. (B) Central canal. (C) Ependyma of the dorsal part of the central canal and roof plate. (D) Astroblasts. (E) Ependyma of the midpart of the central canal. (Adapted with permission from Chambers W, Liu C: Anatomy of the Spinal Cord. In *The Spinal Cord*, 2nd ed. Edited by Austin G. Springfield, IL, Thomas Publishing, 1972, p 12.)

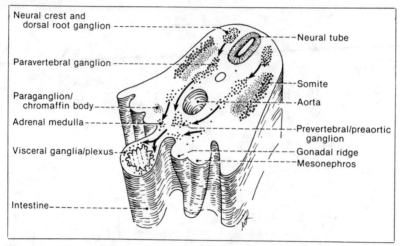

Figure 3-13. Cross section of the trunk of an embryo showing the migratory pathway of sympathetic neuroblasts from the neural crest.

2. Some neural crest cells remain near their site of origin, dorsolateral to the neural tube. Others migrate varying distances away (Fig. 3-13).

   a. The cells remaining dorsolateral to the neural tube or close to the vertebral column become dorsal root ganglia, paravertebral ganglia, or prevertebral ganglia.

   b. The cells migrating away from the paravertebral region become the more peripheral ganglia or plexuses in the walls of the viscera.

   c. Table 3-2 lists the neural derivatives of the spinal and cranial neural crest. Figure 3-14 depicts the cytogenesis of the neural and non-neural derivatives of the neural crest.

E. Sources of neurons

   1. As a general rule, all neurons whose perikarya lie outside of the CNS derive from the neural crest, and all neurons whose perikarya lie within the CNS derive from the neural tube (ectoderm).

   2. Thus, neural crest cells produce the neurons of the dorsal root afferent system and the neurons of the autonomic ganglia and plexuses.

   3. Although these rules are true in general, recent studies suggest greater intermingling of peripheral and central precursor cells than previously appreciated.

Table 3-2. Neural Derivatives of the Neural Crest

Derivative Structure	Cranial Neural Crest Derivatives	Spinal Neural Crest Derivatives
Sensory ganglia	Trigeminal (V)	All spinal dorsal root ganglia
	Geniculate (VII) Superior (IX) Vagus (X)	
Autonomic ganglia		
Parasympathetic ganglia	Ciliary Pterygopalatine Otic Submandibular	Pelvic plexus Remak's ganglion Enteric plexus
Sympathetic ganglia	None	Superior cervical Prevertebral Paravertebral
Supporting cells	Schwann cells Some meningeal cells Possibly some glial cells	Schwann cells Some meningeal cells Possibly some glial cells

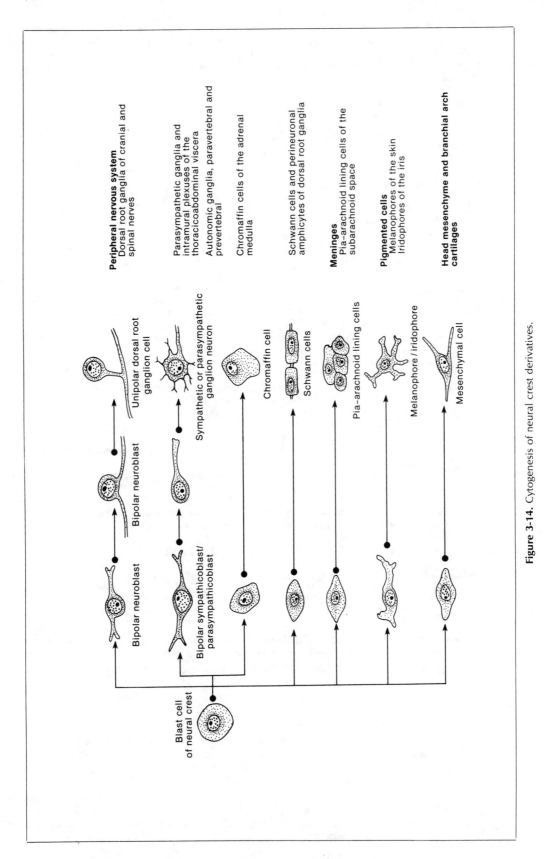

Figure 3-14. Cytogenesis of neural crest derivatives.

V. DEVELOPMENT OF THE SPINAL NERVES. The spinal cord has 31 pairs of spinal nerves. These are attached at regular intervals corresponding to the paired somites (see section VII) and to the paired nodules of the neural crest. Each spinal nerve is similar in developmental sequence, structure, and fundamental plan. **Each derives from dorsal and ventral roots**, which unite to form a **nerve trunk**.

A. Formation of the dorsal roots

1. Each paired nodule of neural crest produces neuroblasts for a dorsal root ganglion. Each neuroblast in the dorsal root ganglion produces a process that bifurcates into **peripheral and central branches** (Fig. 3-15).
    a. The **central branch** pierces the dorsolateral aspect of the spinal cord, forming the dorsal root (see Fig. 3-15).
       (1) Upon entering the spinal cord, the dorsal root axon characteristically branches.
       (2) The branches then may run up or down the cord, but at the level of entry, the axon synapses variously on dorsal horn sensory neurons, spinal interneurons, and ventral horn motoneurons.
    b. The **peripheral branch** extends to a receptor in the skin or viscera.

B. Formation of the ventral roots

1. Neuroblasts in the ventral horn gray matter differentiate and produce axons that exit from the ventrolateral aspect of the spinal cord (see Fig. 3-15).
2. Two types of axons enter the ventral roots—axons destined for **skeletal muscles** and axons destined for **autonomic ganglia** (Fig. 3-16).
    a. The **axons going to skeletal muscles** issue from motoneurons in the **ventral** horns. They travel directly to the muscle without further synapses.
    b. The autonomic axons issue from neurons in the **intermediate** horn.
       (1) These autonomic axons do not run directly to their glands or smooth muscles. Instead, the autonomic axons synapse upon a peripheral neuron in a ganglion or a plexus. The peripheral neuron then innervates the effector.
       (2) Thus, the autonomic pathway of the PNS involves two neurons; the skeletal muscle pathway involves only one (see Fig. 3-16).
       (3) Figure 3-16 shows that the **preganglionic** autonomic neuron runs to the ganglion by a small ramus from the peripheral nerve trunk. The **postganglionic** axons rejoin the trunk by another ramus.
       (4) After traveling varying distances in the nerve trunk, the postganglionic axon departs from the spinal nerve to reach its end station.

C. Table 3-3 summarizes the histologic elements of the PNS and their embryologic origin from one of three sources—neural ectoderm, neural crest, and mesoderm.

VI. FUNCTIONAL CLASSIFICATION OF PERIPHERAL NERVE FIBERS

A. Division into sensory and motor axons

1. Since **dorsal roots** conduct sensory impulses **to** the CNS and **ventral roots** conduct motor impulses **away from** the CNS, a functional classification begins with these two categories of nerve fiber.
2. The fact that the **dorsal roots are afferent**, or sensory, while the **ventral roots are efferent**, or motor, is called the **Law of Bell and Magendie**.
3. The spinal cord gray matter reflects the division of function between dorsal and ventral roots.
    a. The alar plates, or **dorsal horns**, are primarily **sensory** in function.
    b. The basal plates, or **ventral horns**, are primarily **motor** in function.

B. Division into somatic and visceral axons

1. In their course distal to the nerve trunk, the **sensory axons innervate either a somatic or visceral structure**. Although no special region of the dorsal root ganglion is known to be devoted to either somatic or visceral neurons, the fibers do separate upon entering the spinal cord and in reaching their somatic or visceral end stations.
2. In their course distal to the nerve trunk, the **motor axons** also innervate either a somatic or visceral effector, but their perikarya of origin occupy different nuclear sites in the efferent plate of the spinal cord. Hence, the two groups of efferent axons commence separately, unite in the nerve trunk, then separate again peripherally.

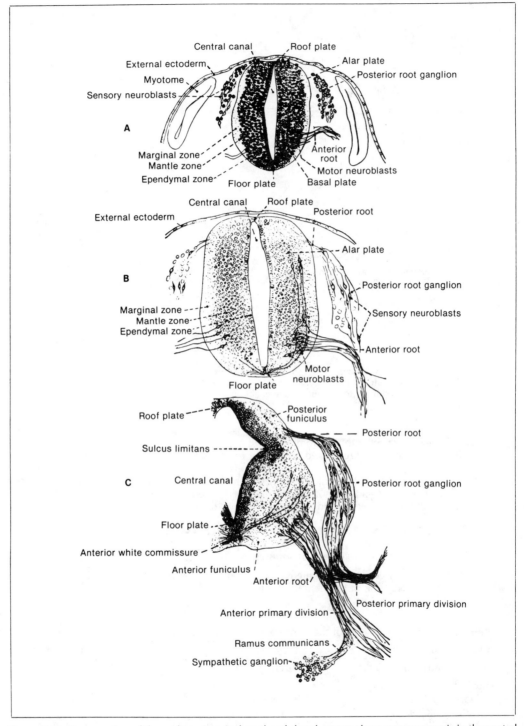

Figure 3-15. Cross section of the embryonic spinal cord and dorsal root to show neuronogenesis in the ventral horns and dorsal root ganglia. (Adapted with permission from Larsell O: *Anatomy of the Nervous System,* 2nd ed. New York, Appleton-Century-Crofts, 1951, p 56.)

C. Theory of nerve components

1. The theory of nerve components combines the motor/sensory and somatic/visceral dichotomies to recognize **four functional types of axons** in spinal nerves (Fig. 3-17).

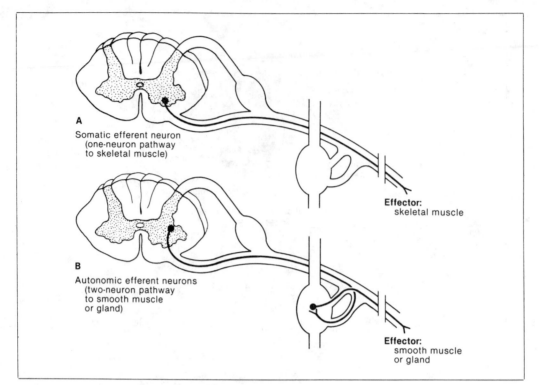

Figure 3-16. Spinal cord with an attached spinal nerve to contrast (*A*) the one-neuron pathway to skeletal muscles and (*B*) the two-neuron pathway to the autonomic effectors.

   2. Those nerve fibers running from autonomic ganglia or in visceral plexuses are all classified as **general visceral efferents and all belong to the autonomic nervous system.**

   D. Although functionally different, the individual motor and sensory axons in the peripheral nerves look exactly alike and cannot be distinguished when viewed microscopically. However, in general, autonomic axons and nerves are smaller than somatic ones and less well myelinated.

VII. THE DEVELOPMENT AND INNERVATION OF SOMITES

   A. Composition and arrangement of somites

   1. Somites, or **mesodermal segments**, develop as a series of regular, paired lumps or corrugations on each side of the neural tube (see Figs. 3-2 and 3-18).

Table 3-3. Histologic Elements of the Peripheral Nervous System and Their Embryologic Origin

Histologic Components	Function	Embryologic Origin
Axons of ventral roots	Purely motor	Neural ectoderm
Ganglia		
Dorsal root ganglia	Purely sensory	
Autonomic ganglia	Purely motor	
Plexuses (located in sheets in the walls of viscera)	Smooth muscle contraction and glandular secretion	Neural crest
Schwann cells	Produce myelin sheaths	
Fibrous connective tissue	Supports and strengthens the peripheral nervous system	Mesoderm
Blood vessels and lymphatic channels	Circulation of fluids	

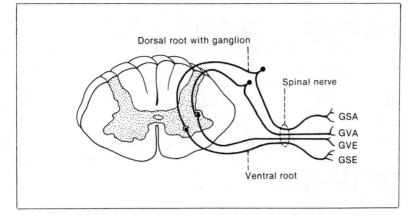

Figure 3-17. Four functional components of the typical spinal nerve. *GSA* = general somatic afferent; *GVA* = general visceral afferent; *GVE* = general visceral efferent; *GSE* = general somatic efferent.

   2. Somites produce the parietes, or somatic structures of the body, because their mesoderm differentiates into dermatomes, myotomes, and sclerotomes (Fig. 3-18).
      a. The **dermatome** produces the dermis, the deep layer of skin beneath the epidermis. The epidermis derives from surface ectoderm.
      b. The **myotome** differentiates into skeletal muscle.
      c. The **sclerotome** differentiates into the skeleton and related connective tissues.

B. Extent of the somite plan and the segmental part of the nervous system

   1. The somites extend from the caudal end of the spinal cord to the midbrain level.

   2. At the spinal level, the somites form a continuous series.

   3. At the brainstem level, the somites are discontinuous because some retrogress and disappear during the complicated developmental events that form the face.
      a. The rostral-most somite is opposite the midbrain, and the rostral-most somite cranial nerve is the CN III.
      b. Reflecting this fact, the **brainstem and spinal cord constitute the segmental part** of the nervous system, and the **diencephalon and cerebrum are the suprasegmental part**.
         (1) The brainstem has alar and basal plates, just as the spinal cord has (see Fig. 3-11). Thus, the brainstem can be interpreted simply as expanded spinal cord.
         (2) The development of the diencephalon and cerebrum differs from the basic developmental plan of the segmental nervous system. If the basal or efferent plate stops at the midbrain, as some authorities hold, then the cerebrum proper develops from expanded alar (afferent) plates, as an elaborate interneuronal pool.

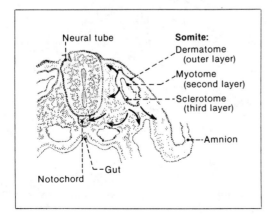

Figure 3-18. Cross section of the embryonic neural tube (spinal cord) and adjacent body wall showing the three derivatives of a somite: the dermatome, myotome, and sclerotome. The *arrows* show pathways of migration of the cells from the myotomes and sclerotomes to form muscles, bones, and connective tissue.

C. Innervation of the somites

1. Each somite receives one somite nerve from the spinal cord or brainstem. It also receives a single artery from the aorta. Hence, each somite has one primary nerve and one primary artery. Since somites are paired, the spinal nerves and spinal arteries are paired.

2. Each **somite nerve** innervates all of the tissues derived from its original somite and only those tissues.
   a. It innervates the dermis derived from the particular somite's dermatome, the muscles derived from the somite's myotome, and the bone derived from its sclerotome.
   b. This rule holds even when the somite derivatives migrate and undergo extensive transformations in the arm and leg regions.
   c. Figure 3-19 shows the transformation of the dermatomes. Only the thoracic region retains the original somite simplicity since it is unaltered by face, arm, or leg growth.

3. Opposite each somite, a single paravertebral autonomic ganglion forms, but some ganglia coalesce in the cervical region. The single-somite–single-ganglion arrangement is confined roughly to the thoracic region.

D. Formation of somatic nerve plexuses

1. Figure 3-20A shows that a spinal nerve trunk upon entering a plexus contains axons from only one spinal nerve serving only one spinal segment. The axons of the individual nerve trunks intermingle in the plexus, but each axon retains its own identity and does not anastomose with axons of another segment.

2. Figure 3-20B shows that the peripheral nerves issuing from a somatic plexus may contain axons from more than one nerve trunk or spinal segment.

3. Three plexuses
   a. Nerve trunks form three plexuses along the spinal cord: the **cervical**, **brachial**, and **lumbosacral** (see Fig. 7-1).
   b. The brachial and lumbosacral plexuses are the largest because the somite derivatives, the dermatomes, myotomes, and sclerotomes, undergo the greatest redistribution in the limb buds, which form the arms and legs. No plexuses occur in the thoracic region, where the somites retain their original serial simplicity.

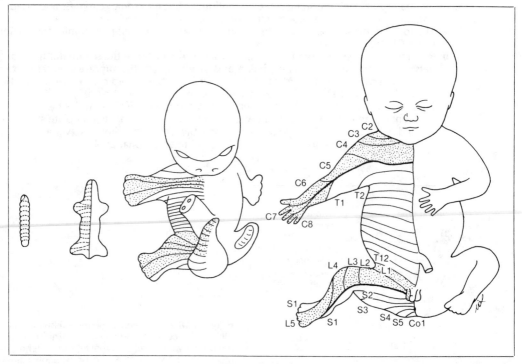

Figure 3-19. Transformation of dermatomes during the outgrowth of the limb buds. *C* = cervical; *T* = thoracic; *L* = lumbar; *S* = sacral.

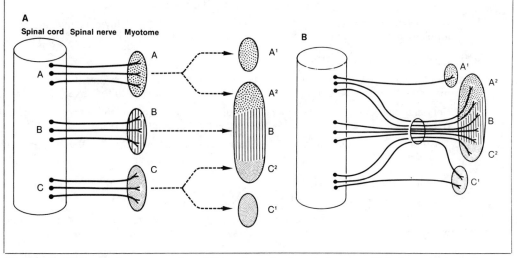

Figure 3-20. Diagrammatic representation of plexus formation by spinal nerves. (A) Each myotome receives one spinal nerve, but the myotome may split to contribute to a composite muscle. See A^1 and A^2 and C^1 and C^2. (B) The axons that innervate a composite muscle still reach their original myotome but first run through a plexus (circled) to form a common nerve or nerves.

VIII. MYELINATION IN THE PNS AND CNS

A. Jelly-roll hypothesis of myelin formation

1. The axons of the CNS and PNS initially grow out as naked cytoplasmic extensions. Many then receive a myelin sheath, while others remain unmyelinated.

2. In the **PNS**, Schwann cells, derived from neural crest, form the myelin sheaths. In the **CNS**, oligodendroglial cells, derived from the neural ectoderm, form the myelin sheaths.

3. In the **PNS**, the Schwann cells myelinate the axons by a lip of cytoplasm that encircles the axon in a "jelly roll" manner topologically (Fig. 3-21). The myelin sheath thus consists of layers of Schwann cell membrane.
    a. The axons that remain unmyelinated are imbedded in Schwann cell cytoplasm, but the lips of the Schwann cell do not encircle the fiber (see Fig. 3-21).
    b. Any given Schwann cell may accommodate both myelinated and unmyelinated fibers.

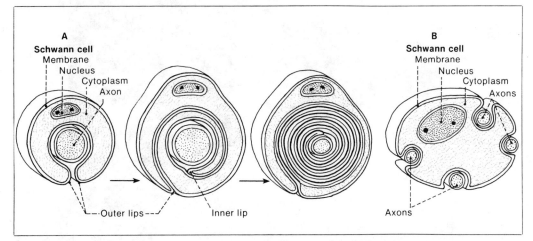

Figures 3-21. Cross section of a myelinating axon in the peripheral nervous system (PNS). (A) Three stages in the encircling of the axon by a lip of Schwann cell to form a "jelly roll" myelin sheath. (B) The nonmyelinated axons indent the surface membrane of the Schwann cell but do not receive a jelly roll wrapping.

c. In the PNS, the structure of the peripheral nerve is completed by the formation of blood vessels and fibrous connective tissue sheaths from the mesoderm.

4. In the **CNS**, the membranes of the oligodendroglial cells form the myelin lamination, but the topology of the investment is more complicated than it is in the PNS.

B. Junction of the CNS and PNS

1. The Schwann cells and fibrous connective tissue of the PNS stop abruptly within a few millimeters of the site where a dorsal or ventral nerve root attaches to the CNS.

2. Central to this junction, glial connective tissue comprised of oligodendrocytes and astrocytes replaces the Schwann cells and fibrous connective tissue of the PNS.

3. The junction of the two different types of connective tissues is called the **Obersteiner-Redlich zone** (Fig. 3-22).

C. Timetable of myelination in the CNS

1. Various tracts or regions myelinate in an orderly, regular sequence (Fig. 3-23).

2. Myelination slightly precedes assumption of function in the nerve fibers. Hence, the degree of myelination in the developing nervous system is one measure of its maturation.

D. Demyelination

1. Some diseases attack the myelin sheath but tend to spare the axons. Since most of the axons remain, the disease is called a **demyelinating disease**. In multiple sclerosis, the most common demyelinating disease of young adults, patches of demyelination are scattered at various sites in the CNS white matter. The patient has a variety of signs and symptoms, depending on the site of the white matter lesions. Commonly, the demyelinating patches affect the optic nerves, brainstem, cerebellar pathways, and spinal cord.

2. Similar demyelination may affect individual Schwann cells in the PNS, resulting in segmental demyelination (see Fig. 2-9E), with corresponding loss of sensory or motor function of the peripheral nerves.

3. Remyelination may occur in the PNS (see Fig. 2-9) and possibly to some extent in the CNS. The Schwann cells or oligodendroglia then recapitulate the embryologic process of myelination.

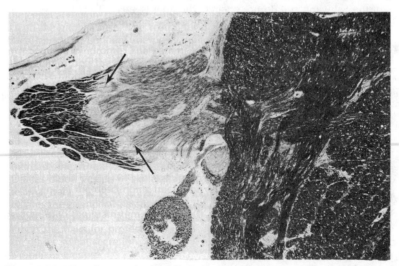

Figure 3-22. Microphotograph of myelin-stained section of nerve root attaching to the medulla. The central myelin meets the peripheral myelin at the Obersteiner-Redlich zone (*arrows*).

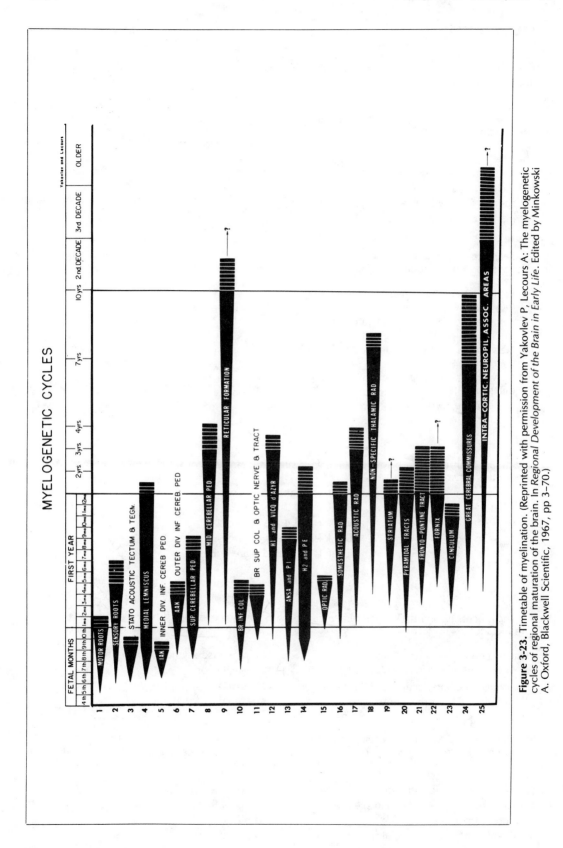

Figure 3-23. Timetable of myelination. (Reprinted with permission from Yakovlev P, Lecours A: The myelogenetic cycles of regional maturation of the brain. In *Regional Development of the Brain in Early Life*. Edited by Minkowski A. Oxford, Blackwell Scientific, 1967, pp 3–70.)

STUDY QUESTIONS

Directions: Each question below contains five suggested answers. Choose the **one best** response to each question.

1. The junction between the CNS and the PNS occurs at or near the

(A) nerve trunk
(B) dorsal root ganglion
(C) intervertebral foramina
(D) surface of the white matter
(E) margin of the gray matter

2. Select the statement that best describes the relationship of nerve roots to somites.

(A) Somites retain their original nerve root when they migrate
(B) Somites receive their innervation from the level to which they migrate
(C) Nerve roots migrate rostrally or caudally with their somites
(D) Nerve roots exchange somites when the somites migrate
(E) None of the above

3. Demyelination is defined as

(A) patchy loss of axons and myelin sheaths in equal degree
(B) loss of myelin with relative preservation of axons
(C) removal of all or most axons and myelin sheaths from a region
(D) patchy loss of random axons
(E) none of the above

Directions: Each question below contains four suggested answers of which **one or more** is correct. Choose the answer

A if **1, 2, and 3** are correct
B if **1 and 3** are correct
C if **2 and 4** are correct
D if **4** is correct
E if **1, 2, 3, and 4** are correct

4. The process of neurulation or neural tube closure includes

(1) elevation of the neural folds
(2) segmentation
(3) fusion of the dorsal margins of the neural folds
(4) elevation of the primitive streak

5. Destruction of the neural crest in an embryo would result in absence of which of the following structures?

(1) Afferent nerve fibers in the spinal nerves
(2) Parasympathetic ganglia and plexuses
(3) Adrenal medulla
(4) Blood vessels in peripheral nerves

6. Major events of CNS organogenesis, as contrasted to cytogenesis and histogenesis, consist of

(1) transverse segmentation
(2) evagination
(3) flexion
(4) axonal and dendritic sprouting

7. Structures having glial supporting tissue include the

(1) optic nerve
(2) infundibulum of the neurohypophysis
(3) olfactory tract
(4) pineal body

8. True statements about the basal plates include which of the following?

(1) They extend throughout the length of the neuraxis

(2) They are ventral to the plane of the sulcus limitans

(3) They produce the cerebellum

(4) They produce the ventral roots

Directions: The group of questions below consists of lettered choices followed by several numbered items. For each numbered item select the **one** lettered choice with which it is **most** closely associated. Each lettered choice may be used once, more than once, or not at all.

Questions 9–13

Match the adult derivative as specifically as possible with the embryologic units.

(A) Telencephalon
(B) Rhombencephalon
(C) Diencephalon
(D) Mesencephalon
(E) Myelencephalon

9. Thalamus

10. Pons

11. Medulla

12. Midbrain

13. Cerebrum

ANSWERS AND EXPLANATIONS

1. The answer is D. (*VIII B 1; Chapter 1 I B 2; II D 1, 3*) The junction between the CNS and the PNS occurs near the site of attachment of the nerve roots to the surface of the white matter of the stem and spinal cord. Histologically, the junction is defined by the presence of oligodendroglial cells proximally and Schwann cells distally. These cells form the myelin sheaths for the CNS and PNS, respectively.

2. The answer is A. (*VII C 2*) One of the most important principles of the development of the PNS is the fact that somites retain axons from their original spinal cord levels when they migrate to different locations. The axons, which in the primitive state would run directly laterally from the spinal cord to the somite, rearrange their course as they go through the cervical, brachial, and lumbosacral plexuses to reach those somites that change their position as a result of migration.

3. The answer is B. (*VIII D*) Demyelination refers to the selective loss of myelin sheaths and the relative preservation of axons. This distinction is important because several diseases characteristically affect the myelin sheath of either the CNS or PNS, leaving the axons intact. Remyelination occurs more readily in the PNS than in the CNS. It may restore the axons to normal function.

4. The answer is B (1, 3). (*II B 1–3; Figures 3-2, 3-3*) Neurulation, or neural tube closure, comes about after the neural folds elevate on either side of the neural groove. The dorsal margins of the neural folds then fuse, and a tube composed of surface ectoderm splits away from the surface. The open ends of the tube, the anterior and posterior neuropores, then fuse.

5. The answer is A (1, 2, 3). (*I C 2 b; II B 3 a*) The neural crest develops on each side of the neural tube as it closes and splits away from the surface ectoderm. Cells of the neural crest produce the dorsal root ganglia, which provide afferent nerve fibers for the spinal nerves, and the peripheral ganglia of the autonomic and parasympathetic systems. Since the adrenal medulla corresponds to a sympathetic ganglion, destruction of the neural crest would result in its absence.

6. The answer is A (1, 2, 3). (*II A 2, C–E; III A, C; Figure 3-7*) Embryogenesis can be divided into cytogenesis, histogenesis, and organogenesis. Cytogenesis refers to the formation of cells, which, in the case of neurons, involves the sprouting of axons and dendrites. Organogenesis consists of several events, including transverse segmentation, evagination, flexion, and, most fundamental of all, neural tube closure. Some gross defects in organogenesis, like failure of neural tube closure, can occur even though cytogenesis proceeds normally, showing a certain independence of the cytogenetic and organogenetic events.

7. The answer is E (all). (*II A, D; Chapter 2 V B 1 b*) All structures that develop as evaginations from the wall of the neural tube have glial supporting tissue since they are basically CNS tissue. These structures include the optic nerve, infundibulum, olfactory tract, and pineal body.

8. The answer is C (2, 4). (*IV C 1, 2; Figure 3-11*) The basal plates and the alar plates form the major plates of the segmental part of the nervous system. The sulcus limitans divides the two plates, with the basal plate being ventral. A roof plate connects the alar plates dorsally, and a floor plate connects the basal plates ventrally. Ventral roots come from the basal plates; the cerebellum comes from the alar plates. If the neural tube fails to close, the alar plates will have a widely separated or absent roof plate, whereas the floor plate will still hold the basal plates together along their ventromedial margins.

9–13. The answers are 9-C, 10-B, 11-E, 12-D, 13-A. (*Figure 3-4*) Transverse segmentation of the neural tube produces embryologic subdivisions, which then give rise to adult segments. The forebrain or prosencephalon divides into the telencephalon and diencephalon, which produce the cerebrum and thalamus, respectively. In addition, the diencephalon produces the epithalamus, subthalamus, and hypothalamus. One transverse segment of the CNS, the mesencephalon, does not undergo further segmentation but remains as the definitive midbrain of the adult CNS. The hindbrain, or rhombencephalon, becomes the metencephalon and myelencephalon. The metencephalon becomes the pons, and the myelencephalon becomes the medulla oblongata. From the level of the medulla to the tip of the spinal cord no further transverse segmentation occurs, although the spinal nerve roots attach at orderly intervals corresponding to the somites. Transverse segmentation is already beginning by the time the neural tube is closing.

The pons in turn gives rise to a protuberance called the cerebellum. It is a solid structure that grows from the dorsum of the pons and is created neither by transverse segmentation nor by evagination.

The original cavity, which extends from the rostral end of the forebrain to the tip of the spinal cord, continues through the various embryologic segments and their adult derivatives. The original cavity includes the lateral ventricles in the cerebrum, the third ventricle in the diencephalon, the aqueduct in the midbrain, the fourth ventricle in the pons and medulla, and the central canal of the spinal cord.

4
Neuroanatomical Methodology

I. INTRODUCTION TO THE GOALS AND METHODS OF NEUROANATOMY

A. The **immediate goal** of neuroanatomy is to identify the spatial arrangement of individual neurons and how they relate to each other, to their supporting glial cells and blood vessels, to the structures that they innervate, and to the membranes and bones that enclose them.

B. The **ultimate goal** is to interpret how the special structure of the nervous system relates to its functions.

C. To achieve these goals, the neuroanatomist seeks to:

   1. Discover the ontogenetic and phylogenetic sequences of the nervous system

   2. Identify the location and configuration of neurons and classify them into their various arrangements as nuclei, reticular formation, and types of cortex

   3. Identify the course of axons, their synaptic distributions, or afferent and efferent terminals

   4. Recognize the types, configuration, and disposition of glia

   5. Describe the internal structure of neurons and glia

   6. Identify the neurotransmitters and chemically specify the axonal pathways

   7. Describe the distribution of the veins and arteries of the nervous system

   8. Correlate anatomical lesions with deficits in neural function

   9. Develop a rational nomenclature that promotes rather than obstructs learning

D. Each goal requires its special techniques.

   1. Gross anatomy supplies only a limited amount of information.

   2. The major advances have depended on microscopy and staining techniques that demonstrate the normal tissue elements and alterations in the normal elements induced by surgical lesions, natural diseases, or chemical reactions.

II. TYPES OF MICROSCOPY

A. The two main types of microscopy are **light microscopy** and **electron microscopy**.

   1. Light microscopy has an effective magnification of 1200 ×.

   2. Electron microscopy has an effective magnification up to 200,000 ×, but it is ordinarily used at 3000 × to 100,000 ×.

B. Types of light microscopy

   1. In **ordinary light microscopy**, ordinary light is passed through tissue that has been mounted on a slide and stained to enhance some particular cell type or histologic feature.

   2. Phase contrast microscopy utilizes the difference in the refractive index of tissues. It may be used to examine unstained tissue mounted on slides or to observe living tissue directly.

   3. Flourescence microscopy. Either a naturally occurring compound, usually a catecholamine, can be made fluorescent or flourescent dye may be injected, which enters the perikaryon and is distributed to the neuronal processes. In either event, the neurons stand out brightly against a dark background.

C. Electron microscopy

1. Electron microscopy with its great magnification allows only a tiny field of view. The thinness of the sections (600 Å) and the very limited field size make it impossible to follow very far along the branches of nerve cells and glia. Hence, it is difficult to study dendritic patterns and axonal distributions or to survey the general organization of tissues.

2. The great advantage of electron microscopy is its **ability to show cell membranes**, either the surface membranes and intercellular relations such as synapses or the deep intracellular membranes of the cytoplasmic organelles.

III. PROCESSING TISSUE FOR MICROSCOPY. The preparation of tissue for microscopy requires a sequence of **fixation** of the tissue, **embedding** it, **thin-sectioning**, **mounting** on a slide, and **staining** it or treating it with **metallic impregnation** before **viewing** with the appropriate microscope.

A. Fixation

1. Fixatives preserve the cells in as near their living state as possible.

2. They generally work by denaturing protein, thus blocking the action of the autolytic enzymes that are released by lysosomes when cells die.

3. **Alcohol, formaldehyde**, and **freezing** are used for light microscopy; **glutaraldehyde** is used for electron microscopy.

B. Embedding, sectioning, and mounting

1. After fixation, tissue is **embedded** in a substance to give it **support** while it is cut into thin sections and mounted on slides.
   a. For light microscopy, tissue is usually embedded in paraffin or celloidin.
   b. For electron microscopy, tissue is usually embedded in a plastic.

2. If frozen, the tissue is usually cut directly on the microtome without embedding.

3. If embedded, the tissue is **sectioned** on a microtome.
   a. For light microscopy, sections are usually cut at 3 to 30 μ in thickness.
   b. For electron microscopy, sections are usually 600 Å thick.

4. The tissue is usually **stained** after mounting on a slide, but some methods involve staining before embedding and mounting.

C. Staining

1. **Overview.** Staining enhances the various elements of the tissue, providing contrast for better visualization.
   a. Many staining methods employ true dyes, while other methods do not, although all are generically referred to as staining.
   b. The affinity of dyes (or other agents) for the tissue component varies with the methods of fixation, embedding, and mordanting applied. Depending on the staining technique, only one cell type or one tissue element such as axons or myelin sheaths will stain selectively, standing out against an unstained background.

2. **Types of dyes**
   a. **Nissl cellular stains**
   (1) Basic aniline dyes such as **hematoxylin** have a selective affinity for the nuclei of cells and for Nissl substance (DNA and RNA).
   (2) Generically called **Nissl stains** (see Figs. 2-10 and 5-2A), these dyes show the distribution of neuronal perikarya into nuclear groups, cortical laminae, and so on (see Fig. 3-9).
   b. **General-purpose stains**
   (1) General-purpose stains display most of the tissue elements, nuclei, perikarya, processes, and fibers.
   (2) The two most common are:
      (a) The **Ehrlich hematoxylin and eosin (H&E) stain**, which uses hematoxylin to stain nuclei and Nissl bodies and esoin to stain the remaining tissue components
      (b) The **Masson trichrome stain**

    c. **Iron–hematoxylin for myelin sheaths.** Mordanting the neural tissue with iron salts reduces the affinity of hematoxylin for nuclear material and enhances its affinity for myelin sheaths, which then stand out against an unstained background (see Fig. 5-2*D*).

    d. **Phosphotungstic acid–hematoxylin** (PTAH) stains astrocytes especially well.

3. In addition to dyes, the methods of special interest for neuroanatomy include:
    a. Metallic impregnation
    b. Enzyme histochemistry
    c. Immunohistochemistry
    d. Radioactive tracers and autoradiography
    e. Combinations of these

4. **Metallic impregnation.** Several heavy metals, notably silver, gold, and osmium, enhance tissue components by their property of precipitating on membranes, either the surface membranes of cells or fibers or the membranous organelles inside the cell.
    a. **Osmium** is the most useful metal for **electron microscopy**.
    b. **Silver** is most useful for **light microscopy**.
        (1) Its advantages are its ease of chemical reduction and its affinity for precipitating on membranes or other surfaces. These are also the reasons that silver is used in photographic and x-ray film and to make mirrors by precipitation on a glass surface.
        (2) Varying the fixatives, the reducing agent, or the conditions of exposure of the tissue to the silver salt will cause the silver ion to precipitate on specific tissue elements. Thus, by use of different silver impregnation methods, the cells of the glial series can be shown selectively, as can neurons or fibrous connective tissue (Table 4-1).

5. **Histochemical reactions**
    a. **Enzyme histochemistry** involves exposure of the tissue to an enzymatic substrate. The end product then can be stained to demonstrate the location of the enzyme. This method can display perikarya and certain neurotransmitters.
    b. The location of cells that metabolize specific radioactive substrates can be disclosed by autoradiography of tissue slices.

IV. METHODS FOR TRACING NERVE TRACTS

A. Gross dissection. Many of the larger tracts can be followed by gross dissection along the fiber pathway.

B. Phylogenetic comparison. Certain tracts stand out very clearly in some animals and may show an increase or decrease in size depending on the phylogenetic rank of the animal.

C. Embryologic methods

1. **Silver impregnation for axons (neurofibrillary impregnation).** The outgrowth and ultimate connections of axons may be directly observed in embryos of successive ages subjected to

Table 4-1. Metallic Impregnation Methods for Demonstrating Neural Elements by Light Microscopy

Element to be Demonstrated	Originator and Method
Normal axons	Bodian protargarol method Ramón y Cajal neurofibrillary impregnation Hortega neurofibrillary impregnation Glees neurofibrillary impregnation Bielschowsky neurofibrillary impregnation
Degenerating axons	Nauta-Gygax silver impregnation method
Astrocytes	Ramón y Cajal gold chloride sublimate Hortega silver impregnation method (I)
Microglia/oligodendroglia	Hortega silver impregnation method (II)
Entire individual neurons	Golgi silver impregnation method
Reticulin	Laidlaw silver impregnation for reticulin

silver impregnation for axons. The method works best for tracts that appear early, before other pathways grow out and cause confusion.

2. **Myelination.** Tracts that myelinate early can be followed with myelin stains before adjacent tracts myelinate (see Fig. 3-23).

3. The **Golgi method.** A special silver impregnation recipe causes entire cells—perikarya, dendrites, and axonal processes—to stand out against an unstained background (see Fig. 13-32*B*). Although best applied to an immature central nervous system (CNS), it also works with the mature CNS.

D. **Wallerian (anterograde) degeneration.** Some methods for tracing nerve tracts disclose wallerian degeneration in nerve fibers that have been transected experimentally or by natural disease.

1. **Axonal degeneration methods**
   a. The silver impregnation method of Nauta-Gygax selectively shows degenerating axoplasm, without staining normal axons, giving a positive trail of the degenerating tract.
   b. Silver impregnation of degenerating synaptic end feet shows the sites of synaptic termination of a severed tract.

2. **Myelin degeneration methods**
   a. **The Marchi method.** Osmic acid reacts with degenerating myelinated fibers so that they show up against an unstained background, giving a **positive trail** of the degenerating tract.
   b. **Iron–hematoxylin method.** After a myelinated tract has degenerated, iron–hematoxylin staining shows the surrounding fibers intact while the tract in question stands out as an unstained void, giving a **negative trail** of the tract.

E. **Nuclear reaction methods**

1. **Nissl chromatolysis method.** After transection of a tract, the perikarya of origin of the axons can be identified by chromatolysis.

2. **Gudden method.** After transection of a tract of axons, the nuclear group of origin may undergo complete (retrograde) degeneration. Nissl staining then shows a void of neurons at the nuclear site of origin of the tract. The method works best in immature animals.

F. **Injection-tracer methods.** A variety of substances can be injected near or directly into the neuronal perikarya. Axoplasmic transport mechanisms then distribute the substance through the neuronal perikarya, dendrites, and axons, where it can be seen by microscopy, either directly or after the tissue is subjected to a chemical reaction.

1. **Horseradish peroxidase**, when injected around the perikarya or axonal terminals, is picked up by the neuron and distributed to all of its processes. An enzymatic reaction then shows the distribution, allowing one to see the axons and dendrites of individual perikarya.

2. **Procion yellow dye** is picked up by neurons, allowing demonstration by fluorescence microscopy.

3. **Radioactive metabolites**, when introduced into neuronal perikarya, can be demonstrated in the neuronal processes by autoradiography of tissue slices.

G. **Electrophysiologic methods**

1. Electrical impulses induced by stimulating neurons can be detected along the course of their axons. As applied clinically, responses evoked by stimulating visual, auditory, or somatosensory afferents can be recorded by surface electrodes placed along the course of the pathway. The observer can then determine objectively whether the sensory pathway is intact or interrupted.

2. Alternatively, stimulation of a tract enables retrograde (antidromic) potentials to be recorded at the site of the perikarya of origin.

5

Nerve Roots, Plexuses, and Peripheral Nerves

I. MICROSCOPIC ANATOMY OF PERIPHERAL NERVES

A. Cross sections of peripheral nerve

1. Cross sections of a peripheral nerve disclose round fascicles of nerve fibers separated by connective tissue sheaths that transmit blood vessels (Fig. 5-1).

2. The fascicles (Fig. 5-2) contain:
   a. Schwann cells and fibrocytes (see Fig. 5-2A)
   b. Axons (see Fig. 5-2B)
   c. Myelin sheaths (see Fig. 5-2D)
   d. Collagen fibrils of the endoneurium (see Fig. 5-2C)
   e. Blood vessels (see Fig. 5-2D)

3. **Axons in peripheral nerve**
   a. Axons vary in diameter from less than 1 μ to 15 μ.
   b. **Relation of axons to Schwann cells**
      (1) Many axons in peripheral nerves merely indent the surface membrane of Schwann cells, forming **unmyelinated axons** (Fig. 5-3; see Fig. 3-21).
      (2) Other axons receive circular wrappings by the surface membrane of Schwann cells, forming **myelinated axons** (see Figs. 5-3 and 3-21).
      (3) One Schwann cell may accommodate myelinated and unmyelinated fibers.

4. **Connective tissue sheaths in peripheral nerve**
   a. Connective tissue forms three sheaths in peripheral nerve, from inside out called the endoneurium, perineurium, and epineurium.

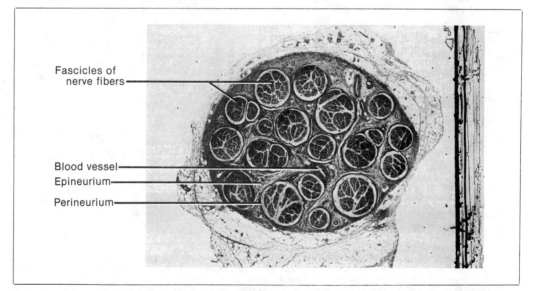

Fascicles of
nerve fibers

Blood vessel
Epineurium
Perineurium

Figure 5-1. Low-power microphotograph (25 ×) of silver-impregnated cross section of peripheral nerve, showing round *fascicles* of nerve fibers separated by connective tissue, consisting of the ring-like *perineurium* and the looser *epineurium*, containing *blood vessels*.

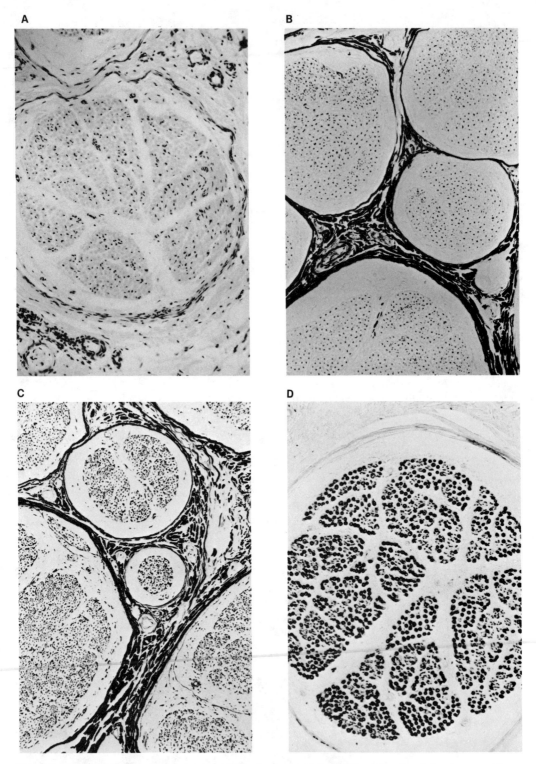

Figure 5-2. Medium-power microphotographs (160 ×) of cross sections of fascicles of peripheral nerve with surrounding perineurial sheaths. (*A*) Nissl stain, showing nuclei of Schwann cells and fibrocytes. Perineurial fibrocytes encircle the entire fascicle. Note blood vessels in the epineurium. (*B*) Selective silver impregnation showing axons. The surrounding myelin sheaths and endoneurium are unstained, but the perineurium and epineurium are well shown. (*C*) Less selective silver impregnation showing axons and endoneurium. (*D*) Selective iron–hematoxylin stain for myelin sheaths, which appear as a small doughnut around each axon. The axons, endoneurium, and perineurium are unstained.

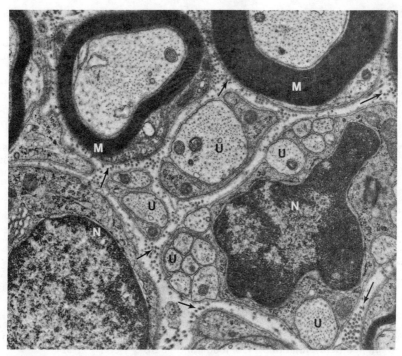

Figure 5-3. Electron microphotograph (22,500 ×) of a normal peripheral nerve in cross section. Compare with Figure 3-21. *Arrows* = endoneurial collagen fibrils cut in cross section. They are located in the extracellular space, between surface membranes of the Schwann cells. *M* = the myelin sheath enclosing a fairly large axon; notice the myelin lamination; *N* = the nucleus of a Schwann cell; *U* = Unmyelinated axons of various sizes indenting the cytoplasm of Schwann cells. Some unmyelinated axons are in groups.

- **(1)** The **endoneurium** consists of scattered fibrocytes and numerous collagen fibers, which run longitudinal to the nerve fibers (see Figs. 5-2C and 5-3).
    - **(a)** The collagen fibers of the endoneurium occupy the space between the surface membranes of the individual Schwann cells, which embed the axons.
    - **(b)** Those endoneurial collagenous fibers close to the Schwann cell contact a carbohydrate matrix that covers the cell surface, thus forming a **basal lamina**.
- **(2)** The outer surface of the Schwann cell, the basal lamina, and the immediately adjacent endoneurial fibrils form the **neurilemmal sheath** of classic light microscopy.
    - **(a)** The term **nerve fiber** designates the axon and, when present, its myelin and neurilemmal sheaths.
    - **(b)** The term **axon** refers only to the actual axoplasmic extension of the neuron and excludes the sheaths.
- **(3)** The **perineurium** divides the nerve into fascicles, which run an undulating or interweaving course.
    - **(a)** The perineurial sleeve around each fascicle consists of:
        - **(i)** Concentric lamellae of fibrocytes, flattened and oriented circumferentially (see Fig. 5-2A–C)
        - **(ii)** Collagen fibers oriented circumferentially and obliquely
    - **(b)** Electron microscopy shows that the perineural cells have a basal lamina on their inside and outside surfaces and that the cell membranes form **tight junctions** where they come into contact with each other.
- **(4)** The **epineurium** is the outermost sheath of peripheral nerves (see Fig. 5-1).
    - **(a)** The epineurium consists of fibrocytes and collagen fibers, and it conveys blood vessels and lymphatic vessels.
    - **(b)** The epineurium binds together the fascicles demarcated by the perineurium and conveys blood vessels destined for the interior of the nerve.
- **b. Functions of the connective tissue sheaths in peripheral nerve**
    - **(1)** The connective tissue sheaths with their interwoven fibers provide **strength with flexibility**.
        - **(a)** Engineers understand that a cable woven of many wires is stronger than a solid metal rod of equal diameter.

(b) The interweaving of the collagen strands and the undulating fascicles allow for stretch when the extremities move.

(2) Although peripheral nerve has great tensile strength, it lacks resistance to compression. Hence, the nerves may suffer **compression neuropathies** where they pass by bones or the edges of ligaments.

(3) The perineurium serves as a **blood–nerve barrier** in the sense of the blood–brain barrier previously described (see Chapter 2, section V C).

(a) The tight junctions of the membranes of the perineurial cells provide a selective barrier to chemical substances. They may also block the access of viruses into the fascicles and hence into the axons.

(b) The perineurium and the amphicytes (satellite cells) around neurons of the ganglia provide a continuous protective barrier along the entire surface of neuronal membranes in the peripheral nervous system (PNS), in analogy with the blood–brain barrier of the central nervous system (CNS).

B. Nodes of Ranvier and the internodal segment of Schwann cells

1. Definition. A **node of Ranvier** is the site where one Schwann cell membrane stops and the next begins (Fig. 5-4).

2. Internodal segment

a. Definition. The internodal segment is the distance between two nodes of Ranvier (see Fig. 5-4).

b. The distance between the nodes is the length of an individual Schwann cell. One Schwann cell nucleus is present for each internodal segment.

c. In some neuropathies, such as in lead poisoning, individual Schwann cells along peripheral nerves will die, while other Schwann cells will remain. The lesion is called **segmental demyelination** of Gombault and Stransky (see Fig. 2-9E).

II. CLASSIFICATION OF NERVE FIBERS

A. Anatomical versus functional classification

1. Anatomically, nerve fibers can be classified by:
   a. Diameter
   b. Length
   c. Presence or absence of a myelin sheath
   d. Cells of origin
   e. Distribution peripherally and centrally

2. Functionally, nerve fibers can be classified by:
   a. Conduction velocity
   b. Conduction direction, afferent or efferent (sensory or motor)
   c. Type of sensory modality served
   d. Type of structure innervated, visceral or somatic
   e. Type of neurotransmitter

B. Fiber diameter and conduction velocity

1. Human peripheral nerves contain fibers ranging in size from around 1μ to 20μ in diameter (myelin sheath included) and conducting at rates from about 1 to 120 m/sec.

2. In general, the larger the axon, the thicker the myelin sheath, and the longer the internodal distance, the faster the conduction velocity. All fibers conducting faster than 3 m/sec are myelinated.

3. To classify nerve fibers, physiologists use a confusing mixture of alphabetic (Latin and Greek) and Roman numeric designations.

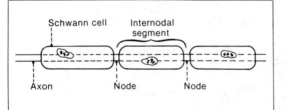

Figure 5-4. Longitudinal diagram of a myelinated axon showing the nodes of Ranvier and the internodal segment presided over by one Schwann cell and its nucleus.

      a. The simple system of Gasser and Erlanger classifies nerve fibers into groups of A, B, and C.
         (1) Group A contains all small, medium, and large myelinated afferent and efferent somatic fibers (1 μ to 20 μ in diameter).
         (2) Group B consists only of small preganglionic myelinated axons of the autonomic nervous system (ANS) [1 μ to 3 μ in diameter].
         (3) Group C consists only of small, unmyelinated fibers; visceral afferents, pain and temperature afferents, and postganglionic autonomic efferents (2 μ to 2.2 μ in diameter).
      b. The Roman numeral system as introduced by Lloyd included all afferents but now is frequently restricted to muscle afferents (Table 5-1).
      c. Larger cutaneous afferent fibers are then designated as A fibers with Greek alphabetic subscripts.

III. GROSS BRANCHES AND FIBER COMPONENTS OF THE PROTOTYPICAL SPINAL NERVE

    A. Gross branches. An intercostal nerve illustrates the gross branches of a prototypical spinal nerve (Fig. 5-5).

Table 5-1. Classification of Nerve Fibers by Diameter and Conduction Velocity

Type		Diameter (μ)*	Conduction Velocity (m/sec)	Terminal Field
Somatic and visceral efferents				
A	Alpha motoneurons	12–20	70–120	To extrafusal skeletal muscle fibers from alpha motoneurons
	Gamma motoneurons	2–8	10–50	To intrafusal muscle fibers from gamma motoneurons
B		< 3	3–15	To autonomic ganglia (preganglionic axons)
C		0.2–1.2	0.7–2.3	To smooth muscle and glands (postganglionic axons)
Cutaneous afferents				
A		12–20	70–120	From joint receptors
A		6–12	30–70	From pacinian corpuscle and touch receptors
A		2–6	4–30	From touch, temperature, and pain endings
C		< 2	0.5–2	From pain, temperature, and some mechanoreceptor endings
Visceral afferents				
A		2–12	4–70	From visceral receptors
C		< 2	0.2–2	From visceral receptors
Muscle afferents				
I$_\alpha$		12–20	70–120	From muscle spindles (annulospiral endings)
I$_\beta$		12–20	70–120	From Golgi tendon organs
II		6–12	30–70	From muscle spindles (flower-spray endings)
III		2–6	4–30	From pressure–pain endings
IV		< 2	0.5–2	From pain endings

*Myelin sheath included if present.

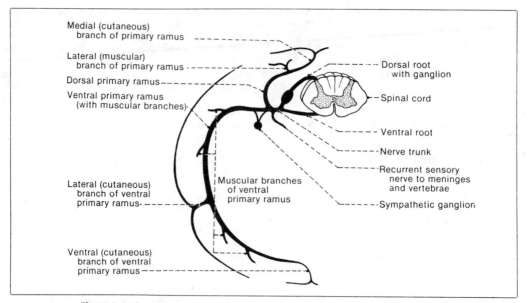

Figure 5-5. Gross components of a prototypical peripheral nerve (thoracic level).

B. Fiber components. The prototypical spinal nerve has all of the four standard nerve fiber components: general somatic afferent (GSA) axons; general visceral afferent (GVA) axons; general visceral efferent (GVE) axons; and general somatic efferent (GSE) axons (Fig. 5-6).

IV. BLENDING OF THE THREE MENINGES AND THE THREE CONNECTIVE TISSUE SHEATHS OF PERIPHERAL NERVES

A. The dorsal and ventral roots unite to exit from the vertebral canal at the intervertebral foramina. At this site, the three connective tissue sheaths of the CNS and PNS blend.

  1. The **dura mater** continues distally as the **epineurium**.

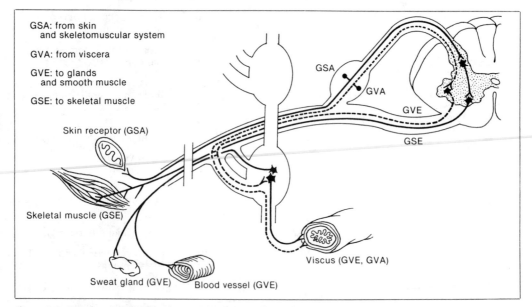

Figure 5-6. Four functional types of axons in prototypical peripheral nerve. *GSE* = general somatic efferent; *GVE* = general visceral efferent; *GVA* = general visceral afferent; *GSA* = general somatic afferent.

2. The **pia–arachnoid** or **leptomeninges** continues distally as the **perineurium** and **endoneurium**.

B. The nerve roots themselves, as they cross the subarachnoid space, lack an epineurium and a perineurial fascicular arrangement (Fig. 5-7).

   1. Lacking the tensile strength provided by the two outer sheaths, nerve roots will avulse from the cord or stretch if a peripheral nerve is pulled too hard.

   2. Traction on a baby's arm or shoulder during a difficult delivery may cause permanent paralysis.

V. GROSS ANATOMY OF THE VERTEBRAE AND VERTEBRAL COLUMN

A. The **vertebral column** consists of 24 vertebrae and the sacrum and coccyx, which are fused vertebrae. Figure 5-8 shows a prototypical vertebra.

B. Atlas and axis. At its rostral end, the vertebral column has two modified vertebrae, the atlas and the axis, which differ considerably from the prototypical vertebra.

C. Intervertebral disks

   1. Location and function. An **intervertebral disk** separates each vertebral body from its neighbor. The disks act as shock absorbers for the vertebral column.

   2. Structure. A disk consists of an **annulus fibrosus** surrounding a **nucleus pulposus** (Fig. 5-9; see Fig. 5-9A).
   a. The **annulus** is dense fibrous connective tissue.
   b. The **nucleus** is soft, pulpy material.

   3. Rupture of disks
   a. Longitudinal ligaments, which run between the vertebral bodies, hold the disk in place.
   b. The ligaments and the annulus fibrosus may rupture, allowing the nucleus pulposus to herniate into the vertebral canal.
   c. The herniated disk may impinge on a nerve root, as shown in Figure 5-9B, or it may impinge on the spinal cord. In either case, it may cause loss of sensation or paralysis, depending on the root or part of the spinal cord involved.

D. Innervation of the vertebra

   1. The vertebrae, joints, and ligaments receive sensory nerves from two sources:
   a. Direct **branches from the posterior rami** of the spinal nerves (review Fig. 5-5)

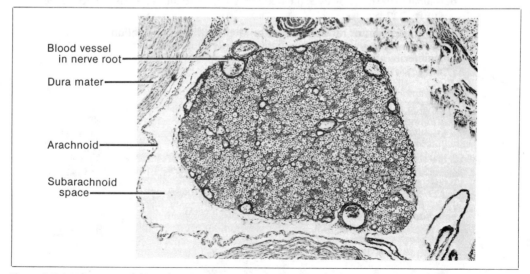

Figure 5-7. Medium-power microphotograph (160 ×) of cross section of nerve root in the subarachnoid space, silver impregnated for axons and collagen fibrils. Axons are small dots within clear spaces, which are the unstained myelin sheaths. Notice the scattered groups of small, unmyelinated axons. Compare with Figures 5-1 and 5-2B and C, and note the absence of fascicular structure and the absence of distinct epi- and perineurial sheaths.

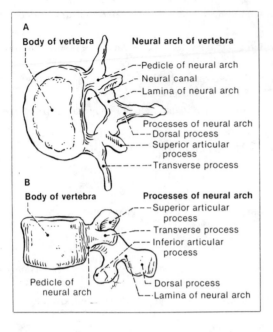

A

Body of vertebra   Neural arch of vertebra

--Pedicle of neural arch
- Neural canal
--Lamina of neural arch

Processes of neural arch
---Dorsal process
--- Superior articular
       process
---------Transverse process

B

Body of vertebra   Processes of neural arch
---Superior articular
       process
--- Transverse process
--- Inferior articular
       process

Pedicle of
neural arch   - Dorsal process
                   ---Lamina of neural arch

Figure 5-8. Typical vertebrae. (*A*) Dorsal view. (*B*) Lateral view.

> **b.** The recurrent sinu-vertebral nerve of Luschka (Fig. 5-10)

> **2.** These nerves mediate pain (backache) and proprioception from the vertebral column.

E. Relationship of nerve roots, spinal nerves, and the spinal cord to vertebral levels

1. Numbering of spinal nerves

a. The average adult has 31 to 32 pairs of spinal nerves, each one corresponding to an embryonic somite.

b. The spinal nerves are numbered in relation to the vertebrae. There are 8 pairs of cervical nerves, 12 thoracic, 5 lumbar, 5 sacral, and 1 or 2 coccygeal (Fig. 5-11).

c. There are only **7 cervical vertebrae** but **8 cervical nerves** because cervical nerve 1 (C1) comes out rostral to the first cervical vertebra and cervical nerve 8 (C8) comes out caudal to the seventh cervical vertebra.

d. Caudal to the cervical level, the numbers assigned to the vertebrae and to the spinal nerves correspond (see Fig. 5-11).

2. Effect of ascensus of the spinal cord on the length and angulation of nerve roots

a. Because the vertebral column elongates faster during gestation than the spinal cord, the caudal tip of the cord, which originally lay opposite the coccyx, comes to lie opposite the first lumbar vertebra (L1).

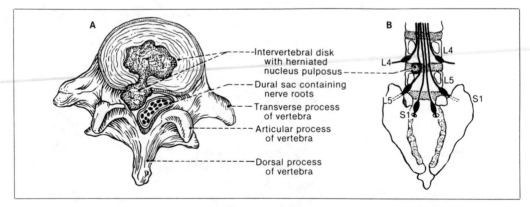

A

----Intervertebral disk
    with herniated
    nucleus pulposus ---------
----Dural sac containing
    nerve roots
-- Transverse process
   of vertebra
--- Articular process
    of vertebra

----Dorsal process
    of vertebra

B

L4
L4
L5
L5
S1
S1

Figure 5-9. Herniation of an intervertebral disk. (*A*) Horizontal section of lumbar vertebra and cauda equina. (*B*) Dorsal view of the cauda equina with the neural arches removed from the pedicles, showing lateral herniation of an intervertebral disk impinging on root L5. (Only roots L4–L5 and S1 of the cauda are shown.)

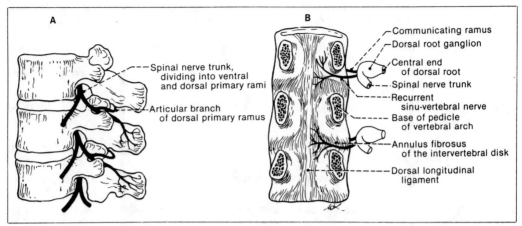

Figure 5-10. Innervation of the vertebral column. (A) Lateral view of vertebrae showing the spinal nerves branching into dorsal and ventral rami as the nerve trunks clear the intervertebral foramina just distal to the dorsal root ganglia. (B) Dorsal view of the vertebrae with their neural arches removed down to the base of their pedicles, exposing the dorsal root ganglia on the right. The ganglia were pulled laterally to emphasize the origins of the sinu-vertebral nerve of Luschka prior to the exit of the spinal nerve trunk from the intervertebral foramina. [After Pedersen HE, Blunck CFJ, Gardner E, et al: The anatomy of lumbosacral posterior rami and branches of spinal nerves (sinu-vertebral nerves). *J Bone Joint Surg* 38:377, 1956.]

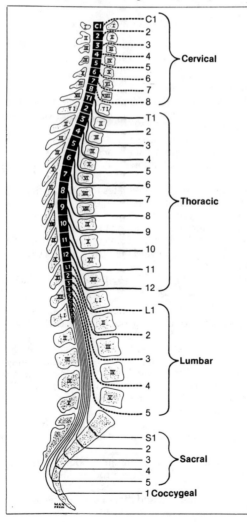

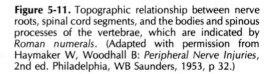

Figure 5-11. Topographic relationship between nerve roots, spinal cord segments, and the bodies and spinous processes of the vertebrae, which are indicated by *Roman numerals.* (Adapted with permission from Haymaker W, Woodhall B: *Peripheral Nerve Injuries,* 2nd ed. Philadelphia, WB Saunders, 1953, p 32.)

b. Because of this relative elevation (ascensus), the more caudal a nerve root the further it must run to reach its intervertebral foramen and the greater its downward angulation (see Fig. 5-11).

c. Since the tip of the cord lies at L1, a physician can insert a needle into the subarachnoid space at L4–L5 or L5–S1 to obtain cerebrospinal fluid (CSF) for diagnostic analysis without fear of puncturing the cord. The nerve roots will move aside and generally are undamaged by the needle.

VI. THE SEGMENTAL (SOMITE) PATTERN OF SOMATIC SENSORY AND MOTOR INNERVATION

A. Innervation of somite derivatives. Chapter 3, section VII, explains the principles of somite innervation. Briefly:

1. One spinal nerve innervates the dermatome, myotome, and sclerotome derived from one somite.

2. Wherever the somite derivative migrates during embryogenesis, it retains its original somite nerve.

3. The most extensive rearrangement of the somites is in the head, arms, and legs. The thorax retains the simple serial somite plan, undisturbed by somite rearrangements.

4. The somatic nerve plexuses redistribute the axons from the spinal nerve trunks into convenient pathways to the migrated somite derivatives of the head, arms, and legs.

B. Final distribution of somite derivatives

1. Figure 5-12 shows the final arrangements in the leg of the dermatomes, sclerotomes, and myotomes with their segmental innervation.

2. Figure 5-13 assembles all of the dermatomes to contrast them with peripheral nerve distributions shown in Figure 5-14.

3. Which dermatomal distributions to remember
a. No useful purpose is served by memorizing Figures 5-13 and 5-14. However, knowledge of some dermatomal distributions is important because of the frequency of nerve root compression syndromes in everyday clinical practice.
  (1) Spinal dermatomes begin with **C2**, which abuts on the sensory area of CN V (see Fig. 5-13). Spinal nerve C1 departs from the prototype by often lacking a dorsal root.
  (2) C3 and C4 innervate the "cape area," where a graduation cape would rest on the neck and shoulders.
  (3) C5 and C6 run down the top surface of the arm, **C7** innervates the middle finger, and T1 and T2 run up the underside of the arm. Hence, merely remember the distribution of C7; C4–T2 are arranged in an orderly plan around it.
  (4) T4 innervates the level of the nipple; **T10** innervates the level of the umbilicus.
  (5) L2, L3, and L4 creep down the front of the leg; **L5** innervates the big toe, and **S1** innervates the little toe. S2, S3, S4, and S5 converge toward the tip of the coccyx. Hence, remember L5 and S1 and the S2–S5 convergence.
b. The problem has now been reduced to remembering **C2, C7, T4, and T10; L5 and S1; and the coccygeal bull's-eye.**

4. Overlapping of dermatomal innervation. The sharp lines on the dermatomal charts (see Fig. 5-13) give a false impression of the sharpness of dermatomal boundaries as disclosed by clinical examination.
a. The sensory nerve terminals overlap considerably at the dermatomal margins (Fig. 5-15).
  (1) Anatomical overlapping explains an otherwise puzzling clinical fact: A patient may experience pain or numbness in a dermatomal distribution but the physician, upon sensory examination with a wisp of cotton or a pin, may not detect any sensory loss. Thus, the description of the area of sensory loss by a reliable patient may prove a better guide to the involved dermatome than the examination.
  (2) Touch fibers overlap more at the dermatomal margins than pain fibers do. Hence, testing the distribution of loss of pain may delineate a dermatomal loss in a single root better than testing touch.
b. Peripheral nerve boundaries are generally sharper than dermatomal boundaries. Hence, peripheral nerve lesions produce a sharper sensory border than root lesions.

C. The **segmental innervation of myotomes** is given in Table 5-2 and that of spinal reflexes is given in Table 5-3.

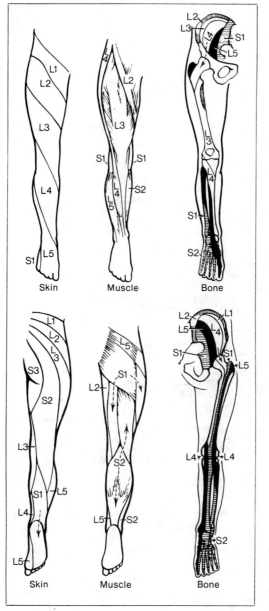

Figure 5-12. Distribution in the leg of the dermatomes (skin), myotomes (muscles), and sclerotomes (bones) by spinal segments L1 to S3. (Reprinted with permission from Bateman JE: *Trauma to Nerves in Limbs*. Philadelphia, WB Saunders, 1962, p 79.)

VII. PLEXUSES AND PERIPHERAL NERVE DISTRIBUTIONS

A. Fate of nerve trunks

1. After the dorsal and ventral roots unite to form a spinal nerve trunk, the trunk reaches its terminal distributions by one of two routes.
   a. The nerve trunk may merely extend directly to its end stations without interchanging fascicles with a neighboring nerve, as is seen in the typical intercostal nerve of Figure 5-5.
   b. The nerve trunk may interchange fascicles with neighboring trunks. The interchange of fascicles from adjacent nerves produces a **plexus** (review Figure 3-20).

2. The peripheral nerves that issue from the plexus generally convey axons from more than one somite. (Compare the dermatomal distributions in Figure 5-13 with peripheral nerve distributions in Figure 5-14.)

3. **Summary of the segmental relations among roots, plexuses, and their peripheral nerves**
   a. **Roots** convey either **sensory or motor axons of only one somite** (one segment).

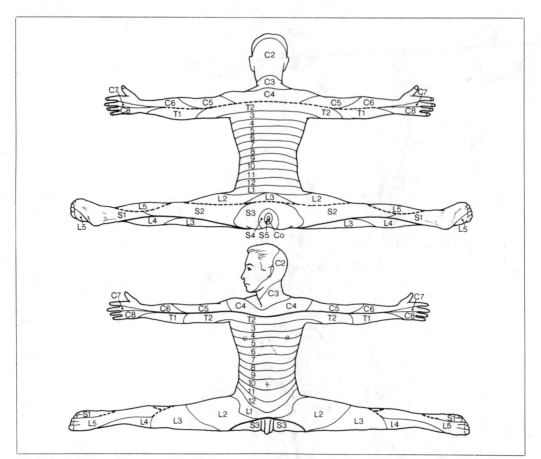

Figure 5-13. Pattern of dermatomal distributions and their innervation by the spinal roots. (Reprinted with permission from Haymaker W, Woodhall B: *Peripheral Nerve Injuries.* 2nd ed. Philadelphia, WB Saunders, 1953, p 19.)

    b. Intercostal nerves (T2–T12) convey both **sensory and motor axons of only one somite**.

    c. The **peripheral nerves** that issue **from a plexus** convey **sensory and motor axons from more than one somite**.

    d. The intercostal nerves (T2–T12) and nerve roots have no special name, only a number corresponding to their spinal cord level.

    e. The peripheral nerves that issue from a plexus always receive a name.

    f. The **histologic structure** of intercostal and plexus nerves is the same, although many plexus nerves are much larger than intercostal nerves.

B. Three plexuses. The spinal nerves form three plexuses—the **cervical, brachial,** and **lumbosacral**.

    1. Cervical plexus

        a. Anatomical pattern (Fig. 5-16)

        b. Segmental origin: C1–C4

        c. Distribution

            (1) Motor (Table 5-4)

                (a) The cervical plexus innervates muscles that turn, flex, and extend the head and open the jaw.

                (b) It shares innervation of the trapezius muscles with CN XI.

                (c) The **cervical plexus originates the phrenic nerve**, the most important spinal nerve in the body because it innervates the diaphragm, the most important muscle for breathing.

                    (i) The phrenic nerve arises from roots C3–C5 but mainly from C4 (see Fig. 5-16).

                    (ii) The nerve runs behind the anterior thoracic wall to reach the diaphragm.

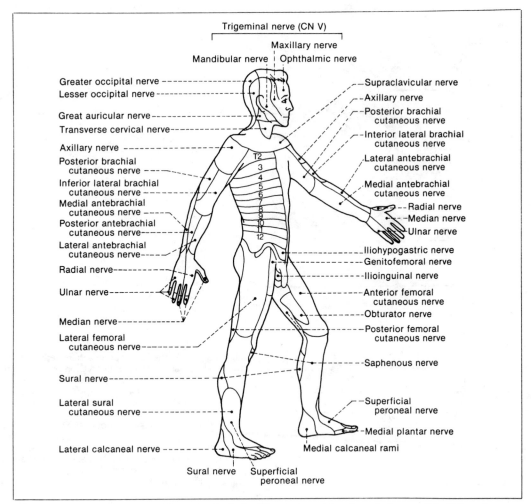

Figure 5-14. Pattern of cutaneous innervation by the peripheral nerves. Note that spinal nerves T2 to T12 receive numbers only, whereas the other nerves, which run through plexuses, receive names. (Adapted from Poeck K: *Einführung in die klinische Neurologie*, New York, Springer-Verlag, 1966, p 23.)

   (2) Sensory
      (a) The cervical plexus innervates the skin on the back of the head (C2) and the cape area of the neck and shoulders (C3 and C4).
      (b) It conveys afferents from neck muscles and adjacent vertebrae.

2. **Brachial plexus**
   a. Anatomical pattern (Fig. 5-17)
   b. Segmental origin: C5–T1
   c. Distribution
      (1) Motor. The brachial plexus innervates muscles of the shoulder girdle, upper chest wall, arms, and hands.
      (2) Sensory. It innervates skin, bone, and muscle of the shoulders, arms, and hands.
   d. Plan of the brachial plexus (Fig. 5-18; see Table 5-4)
      (1) The brachial plexus issues a number of small, short nerves, most of which branch off at acute angles to the longitudinal axis of the plexus. (Figure 5-18 shows these branches cordoned off by a dotted line.) These nerves run to muscles of the shoulder girdle and chest wall.
      (2) Apart from these nerves, the plexus involves **five nerve roots**, **three nerve trunks**, **three cords**, and **five major terminal nerves**, which extend distally in the long axis of the plexus. The five major terminal nerves (see Table 5-4 and Fig. 5-18) consist of:
         (a) One for the **shoulder**, the **axillary or circumflex nerve**

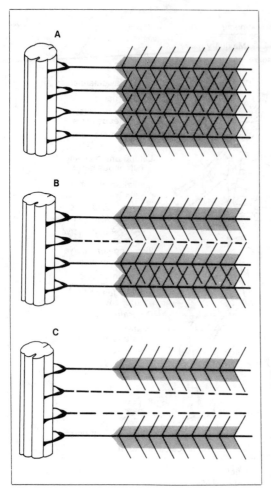

Figure 5-15. (*A*) The *herringbone pattern* represents the width of the band for touch innervation by each spinal nerve, which overlaps its neighbors. The *shaded areas* represent the narrower band of pain innervation for each spinal nerve, which does not overlap. (*B*) After destruction of one spinal nerve, testing for touch may not disclose a loss because of overlapping bands of innervation whereas a band of pain loss can be found because the pain bands do not overlap. (*C*) With two adjacent spinal nerves destroyed, the patient has a band of anesthesia for touch and pain but the band of loss of pain is wider than the band of loss of touch.

Table 5-2. Segmental Innervation of Myotomes

Segment	Structures Innervated
C1–C4	Neck muscles
C3–C5	Diaphragm
C5–C6	Biceps
C7–C8	Triceps; long muscles of the forearm
C8–T1	Some long muscles for finger and wrist movements; the small intrinsic muscles of the hand
T2–T12	Axial musculature; intervertebral muscles; muscles of respiration; abdominal muscles
L1–L2	Flexors of the thigh
L2–L3	Quadriceps of the thigh
L4–S1	Extensors of the foot and great toe
L5–S1	Gluteal muscles
S1–S2	Plantar flexors of the foot (calf muscles); intrinsic foot muscles
S3–S5	Muscles of the pelvic floor, bladder, sphincters, and external genitalia

Table 5-3. Segmental Innervation of Spinal Reflexes

Deep Muscle Reflexes	Superficial Reflexes	Methods of Elicitation	Normal Results	Segment Traversed
Biceps		Tap biceps tendon	Flexion of the forearm at the elbow	C5–C6
Triceps		Tap triceps tendon	Extension of the forearm at the elbow	C6–C7
Brachioradial		Tap styloid process of the radius, with forearm held in semipronation	Flexion of the forearm at the elbow	C7–C8
Finger flexion		Flick palmar surface of the tip of the finger	Flexion of the fingers	C7–T1
Abdominal muscle		Tap lowermost portion of the thorax or abdominal wall; or tap symphysis pubis	Contraction of the abdominal wall or, when the symphysis is tapped, adduction of the leg	T8–T12
	Abdominal skin and muscle	Stroke skin of the upper abdominal quadrants	Contraction of the abdominal muscles and retraction of the umbilicus to the stimulated side	T8–T12
	Cremaster	Stroke skin of the upper and inner thigh	Upward movement of the testicle	L1–L2
Adductor		Tap medial condyle of the tibia	Adduction of the leg	L2–L4
Quadriceps		Tap tendon of the quadriceps femoris	Extension of the lower leg	L2–L4
Triceps surae		Tap tendon Achillis	Plantar flexion of the foot	L5–S2
	Plantar	Stroke sole of the foot	Plantar flexion of the toes	S1–S2
	Anal	Prick skin of the perianal region	Constriction of the anal sphincter—"anal wink"	S4–Co1
	Bulbocavernous	Prick skin of the glans penis	Contraction of the bulbocavernosus muscle and constrictor urethrae	S3–S4

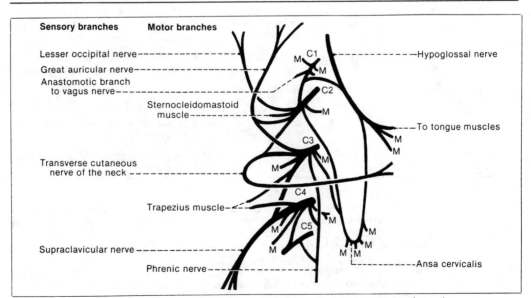

Figure 5-16. Frontal view of the right cervical plexus. *M* = motor to striated muscle.

Table 5-4. Summary of the Motor Distributions of the Major Nerves of the Cervical, Brachial, and Lumbosacral Plexuses

Major Terminal Nerves	Segment of Origin	Distribution and Function
Cervical plexus	C1–C4	Supplies neck muscles that turn the head and open the jaw; shares trapezius muscle with CN XI
Phrenic nerve	C3–C5	Innervates diaphragm
Brachial plexus	C5–T1	
Axillary (circumflex) nerve	C5–C6	Elevates the arm (deltoid action); aids in sweeping arm forward and backward
Musculocutaneous nerve	C5–C7	Flexes arm at the shoulder and forearm at the elbow (except for brachioradialis muscle)
Radial nerve	C5–C8	Extensor nerve of the elbow, wrist, and fingers; supplies the brachioradialis muscle, a forearm flexor; extends the digits, except for the distal phalanges, which are extended by the intrinsic hand muscles
Median nerve	C6–C8, T1	Flexor nerve of the wrist (aided by the ulnar nerve) and of the distal phalanges of the fingers, innervates five hand muscles: the three thenar muscles (the flexor brevis, abductor, and opponens) and the two lumbricals (to the second and third digits)
Ulnar nerve	C7–C8, T1	Main mover of the fingers; innervates the flexor carpi ulnaris of the forearm and all interossei, the lumbricals to the fourth and fifth digits, the adductor pollicis, and part of the flexor pollicis brevis. (Lumbricals, supplied by the median and ulnar nerves, flex the proximal phalanges and extend the distal phalanges; the interossei waggle the fingers laterally and flex the proximal phalanges and extend the distal. The actions of the thumb test all three long nerves of the brachial plexus: extension, radial; opposition to the little finger, median; and adduction, ulnar.)
Lumbosacral plexus	T12–S5	
Obturator nerve	L2–L4	Adductor nerve of the thigh
Femoral nerve	L2–L4	Extensor nerve of the knee
Sciatic nerve	L4–L5, S1–S3	Flexor nerve of the knee; flexor and extensor nerve of the foot and toes; in the popliteal space, it divides into the tibial and peroneal nerves
Tibial nerve	L4–L5, S1–S2	Plantar flexor of the foot and toes and invertor of the foot; innervates all intrinsic foot muscles except the extensors
Peroneal nerve	L4–L5, S1–S2	Dorsiflexor (extensor) of the foot and toes and evertor of the foot; innervates long and intrinsic extensors of the toes
Pudendal nerve	S2–S4	Innervates the urogenital diaphragm and voluntary bowel and bladder sphincters; is afferent from the external genitalia
Pelvic splanchnic nerve	S2–S4	Afferent from and efferent to the bladder wall and involuntary sphincters; vasomotor for erection

   (b) Four for the **arm**, the **musculocutaneous, radial, median**, and **ulnar nerves**
   (3) In order to remember the plan of the plexus, notice that root **C7** forms an "**axis of symmetry**" (Fig. 5-19).
      (a) Of the five spinal nerves that form the plexus, two (C5 and C6) are **rostral** to C7 and two (C8 and T1) are **caudal** to C7.
      (b) C7 runs directly into its cord (although spoiling the purity of its symmetry by branching to the upper cord), whereas C5 and C6 unite and C8 and T1 unite (see Fig. 5-19).

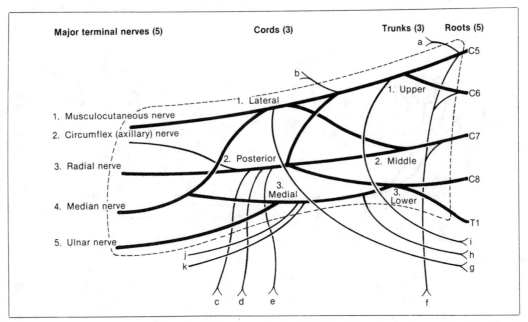

Figure 5-17. Frontal view of the right brachial plexus. The *dashed line* encloses the major roots and the largest branches. The trunks are the nerve fibers before they enter the plexus; cords are redistribution of fibers in the plexus; terminal nerves are the way out of the plexus. *a* = Dorsal scapular nerve to rhomboid muscle; *b* = supra-scapular nerve to supra- and infraspinatus muscles; *c* = inferior subscapular nerve to teres major muscle; *d* = thoracodorsal nerve to latissimus dorsi muscle; *e* = superior subscapular nerve to subscapular muscle; *f* = long thoracic nerve to serratus anterior muscle; *g* = lateral pectoral nerve to pectoralis muscle; *h* = medial pectoral nerve to pectoralis muscle; *i* = subclavian nerve to subclavius muscle; *j* = medial cutaneous nerve of the forearm; *k* = medial cutaneous nerve of the arm.

(c) After receiving communications from the united trunks of C5 and C6 and C8 and T1, C7 forms the **posterior** cord, on the **back** of the plexus.
  (i) The posterior cord **radiates** in a straight course **down the back of the arm** as the **radial nerve.**
  (ii) Its only major proximal branch is the **axillary (circumflex) nerve.**
(d) Ultimately, the C7 dermatomal fibers reach the "**digit of symmetry**," the third digit, which has the same relation to the other digits (two on one side and two on the other) as root C7 does to roots C5 and C6 and C8 and T1.
(4) Hence, to remember both the dermatomal pattern of the arm and the plan of the brachial plexus, learn the course and distribution of C7.

3. Lumbosacral plexus
  a. Anatomical pattern (Fig. 5-20)
  b. Segmental origin: L1–S4
  c. Distribution (see Table 5-4)
    (1) Like the brachial plexus, the lumbosacral plexus gives off a number of short nerves, in this case, to paravertebral and pelvic girdle muscles, before terminating in the major terminal branches.
    (2) For descriptive purposes, consider the lumbosacral plexus as **two plexuses**, a **lumbar** (L1–L4) and a **sacral** (L4–S4). One major anastomosis from L4–L5 (the lumbosacral anastomotic trunk of Furcle) connects the two plexuses (see Fig. 5-20).
      (a) The **lumbar plexus** provides two major sensorimotor nerves, the **femoral** and **obturator nerves**, and one purely sensory nerve, the **lateral femoral cutaneous nerve.**
        (i) The two major **sensorimotor nerves** innervate the extensor muscles of the knee and the adductor muscles of the thigh, respectively (Fig. 5-21).
        (ii) Innervation of the skin of the thigh
            The **femoral nerve** innervates the front of the thigh by the anterior (ventral) femoral cutaneous nerve (see Fig. 5-14).
            The **obturator nerve** innervates a small area of skin of the thigh medially (see Fig. 5-14).

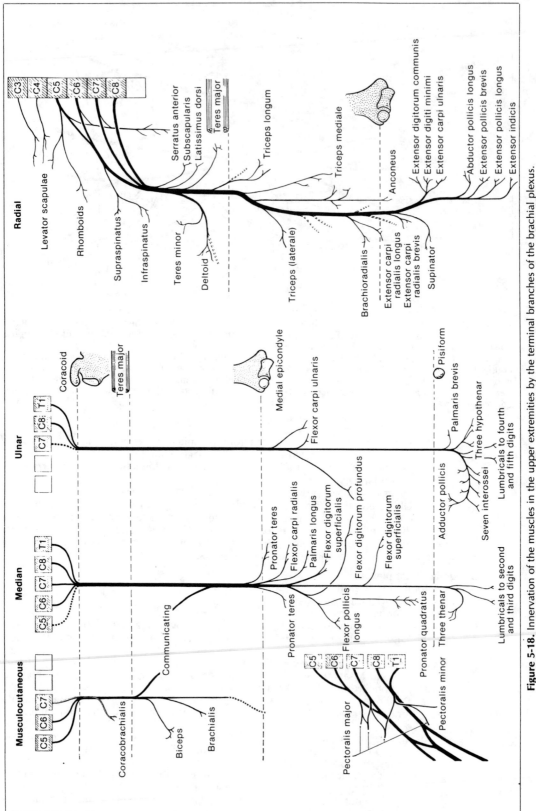

Figure 5-18. Innervation of the muscles in the upper extremities by the terminal branches of the brachial plexus. (Adapted with permission from Grant JCB: *An Atlas of Anatomy*, 5th ed. Baltimore, Williams and Wilkins, 1962.)

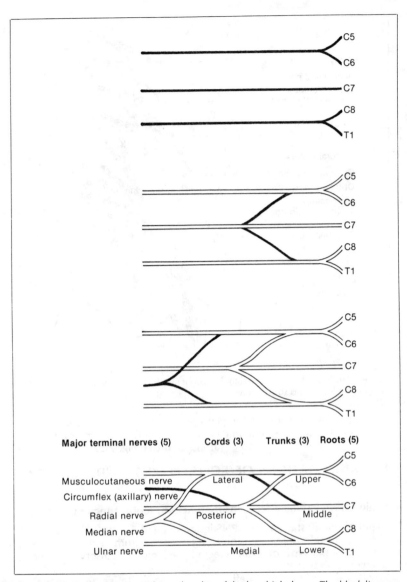

Major terminal nerves (5)   Cords (3)   Trunks (3)   Roots (5)

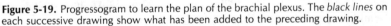

Figure 5-19. Progressogram to learn the plan of the brachial plexus. The *black lines* on each successive drawing show what has been added to the preceding drawing.

(iii) The **lateral femoral cutaneous nerve,** the one **purely sensory nerve** of the lumbar plexus, innervates the anterolateral aspect of the thigh (see Fig. 5-14). This nerve may become entrapped where it passes under the inguinal ligament. The patient complains of pain and dysesthesia on the anterolateral aspect of the thigh.

(b) The **sacral plexus** provides the **sciatic, pudendal,** and **pelvic splanchnic nerves** (see Figs. 5-20, 5-21, and 7-22).

(i) The **sciatic nerve is the largest peripheral nerve of the body** (see Fig. 5-21). It innervates the hamstring muscles of the thigh and all of the leg and foot muscles by its **tibial and peroneal branches.**

Thus, consider the sciatic nerve in its proximal portion as three nerves, the **hamstring, tibial,** and **peroneal,** bound by one epineurium.

(ii) The **pudendal** nerve (see Figs. 5-20 and 7-22) is sensorimotor. It is **motor** to the external anal and urethral sphincters and related pelvic and perineal muscles.

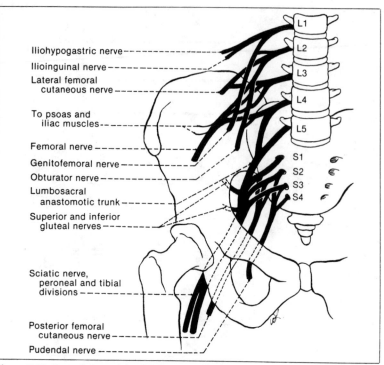

Figure 5-20. Frontal view of the right lumbosacral plexus, showing its origin in relation to vertebral levels and to the pelvis.

Labels in figure:
- Iliohypogastric nerve
- Ilioinguinal nerve
- Lateral femoral cutaneous nerve
- To psoas and iliac muscles
- Femoral nerve
- Genitofemoral nerve
- Obturator nerve
- Lumbosacral anastomotic trunk
- Superior and inferior gluteal nerves
- Sciatic nerve, peroneal and tibial divisions
- Posterior femoral cutaneous nerve
- Pudendal nerve

Vertebral levels: L1, L2, L3, L4, L5, S1, S2, S3, S4

It is **sensory** to the glans penis, clitoris, and urethra.

(iii) The **pelvic splanchnic nerve** (nervus erigens) is motor and sensory to the bladder and is vasomotor for erection (see Fig. 7-22).

VIII. CLINICAL MANIFESTATIONS OF ROOT, PLEXUS, AND PERIPHERAL NERVE LESIONS

A. Introduction. PNS lesions affect sensory function, motor function, or both.

1. The **clinical manifestations** of a PNS lesion depend on:
   a. The **anatomical site** of the lesion along the nerve from nerve root to terminal distribution
   b. The **functional type of axon** affected (i.e., motor, sensory, somatic, or visceral) [see Chapter 3, section VI C]
   c. Whether the lesion causes **deficit phenomena, irritative phenomena, or both**

2. **Definition of deficit and irritative phenomena**
   a. **Deficit phenomena are negative signs or symptoms**, indicating the reduction or loss of a function such as strength or sensation. Deficit phenomena result from interruption of the flow of nerve impulses.
   (1) Deficit phenomena from interruption of **somatic motor axons** are:
      (a) Weakness or paralysis of skeletal muscle, depending on the number of axons affected
      (b) Atrophy of the denervated muscle fibers
   (2) Deficit phenomena from interruption of **autonomic motor axons** are:
      (a) Atony of visceral walls with lack of peristalsis and failure of propulsion or emptying
      (b) Vasomotor paralysis with vasodilation
      (c) Anhidrosis
      (d) Trophic changes with loss of hair, thinning of the skin, and dystrophy of the nails
   (3) Deficit phenomena from interruption of **sensory axons** consist of numbness or anesthesia.
   b. **Irritative phenomena are positive signs or symptoms**, indicating excessive sensation or the overactivity of a muscle or gland.
   (1) Irritative phenomena result from either:
      (a) Destabilization of the axonal membrane, causing excessive impulse flow

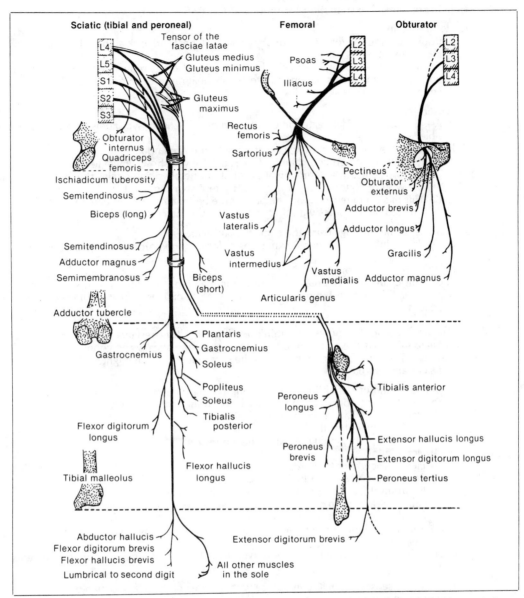

Figure 5-21. Innervation of the muscles in the lower extremities by the terminal nerves of the lumbosacral plexus. (Adapted with permission from Grant JCB: *An Atlas of Anatomy*, 5th ed. Baltimore, Williams and Wilkins, 1962.)

        (b) An imbalance in afferent input, which enhances motor activity or a certain sensation

    (2) Irritative phenomena **in the somatic nerves** consist of twitches of muscle, either myoclonic **jerks** or **fasciculations**.

        (a) A **myoclonic jerk** is a twitch of all or most of a muscle, as if an electric current had stimulated its nerve.

        (b) A **fasciculation** is a much smaller twitch of a motor unit [see Chapter 7, section IV B 3 c (2)].

    (3) Irritative phenomena of the **autonomic axons** include hyperhidrosis and vasoconstriction.

    (4) Irritative phenomena in the **sensory system** include pain, tingling (paresthesias or dysesthesias), and hyperesthesia.

  c. Sometimes **mixtures of irritative and deficit phenomena** occur, as in a dysautonomia called **causalgia**, which may cause varying degrees of vasomotor paralysis, dyshidrosis, and trophic changes, accompanied by severe pain.

B. Methods of clinical examination for lesions of the PNS

1. Motor system
   a. Inspect the muscle for atrophy or abnormal twitches, and look at the skin for excessive or absent sweating.
   b. Formally test the strength of neck, shoulder, and extremity movements by manual opposition, using movements designed to test individual muscles wherever possible.
   c. Formally list any weak muscles.

2. Sensory system
   a. Ask the patient to delineate the distribution of the sensory symptoms as carefully as possible.
   b. Formally test for sensory deficits according to the Appendix.
      (1) Review of the dermatomal map (see Fig. 5-13) will show why in testing for the level of sensory deficit in a dermatomal distribution the physician **circles the extremities** with the wisp of cotton or a pin but goes **up or down the chest**.
      (2) This pattern of testing gives the patient the best chance to compare the stimulus in the affected dermatomes with that in the adjacent intact dermatomes.

3. Analysis of the findings from the clinical examination
   a. Outline in ink on the patient's skin or on a drawing the borders of any sensory deficit discovered.
   b. Write down a list of the weak muscles.
   c. Consult charts of segmental innervation (dermatomes, myotomes, and sclerotomes) and peripheral nerve distributions to determine the site of a lesion that would account for the deficits found.

C. The neuroanatomical process of "thinking through" the nervous system. Knowledge of neuroanatomy allows the clinician to think through systematically the connections of the nervous system. The clinician can then identify the sites where a lesion might explain the constellation of signs and symptoms.

1. To analyze a **motor deficit** in the PNS, think through the motor pathway.
   a. Follow along the course of impulse flow according to the neuron doctrine:
      (1) Neuronal perikaryon in the ventral horn
      (2) Central segment of the root (intra-axial course)
      (3) Ventral root (beginning of extra-axial course)
      (4) Nerve trunk
      (5) Plexus (roots, trunks, cords)
      (6) Peripheral nerve (main trunk and branches)
      (7) Neuromyal junction [include the neuromyal junction in the analysis of weakness because diseases such as myasthenia gravis (a defect in cholinergic transmission) may affect that site]
      (8) Muscle (include the muscle itself because of the many myopathies that can cause weakness)
   b. Thus, in thinking through a motor nerve, travel from nerve cell to synapse to the effector itself.

2. To analyze a **sensory deficit**, commence with the area of the deficit drawn on the skin of the patient or on a sketch.
   a. Initially, assume that the lesion could be at any site along the sensory pathway. Commence with the skin itself because some diseases, such as leprosy, characteristically involve the nerves of the skin. Including the skin is analogous to including the muscles in thinking through the motor system.
   b. In thinking through the sensory pathway consider:
      (1) Skin and receptor endings
      (2) Peripheral nerve (main trunk and branches)
      (3) Plexus (cords, trunks)
      (4) Roots
      (5) Central termination (dorsal horn or, via a spinal cord pathway, up to and including the sensory receptive area of the cerebral cortex)

D. Clinical example of application of segmental and peripheral nerve charts

1. Patient #1
   a. Clinical history. A patient complains of pain and numbness down the leg and into the lateral side and bottom of the foot and pain in the lower back and hip.

b. Examination discloses mild weakness in foot movements and a mild decrease in pinprick perception on the lateral side of the foot.

c. Analysis

(1) Detecting the nerves or nerve root involved

(a) The sensory loss involving the lateral side of the foot suggests an S1 dermatomal distribution and thus an S1 nerve root lesion (see Fig. 5-13).

(b) Since the S1 sclerotome contributes to the shaft and the proximal end of the femur, the hip pain might also come from irritation of the S1 dorsal root (see Fig. 5-12).

(c) The myotomes of S1 contribute to several of the muscles that move the foot. Weakness of the foot is consistent with involvement of the S1 motor root (see Table 5-2).

(d) The clinical findings thus suggest a segmental distribution of sensory and motor loss affecting the dorsal and ventral roots of S1.

(2) Identifying the cause

(a) Statistically, the most common cause of such a syndrome would be herniation of the L5–S1 intervertebral disk, impinging on the dorsal and ventral S1 nerve roots as they join to exit the vertebral canal.

(b) The pain in the back might come from rupture of the longitudinal ligament and the effects of the herniated disk on intervertebral joints and adjacent tissue. The sinuvertebral nerve of Luschka and the direct branches from the primary posterior rami of dorsal roots mediate the back pain.

2. Patient #2

a. Clinical history. A woman who sits long hours at a desk complains of persistent numbness over the top of her right foot, worsened by prolonged sitting with one knee crossed over the other. She has no backache.

b. Examination. The patient has a decrease in light touch and pain sensation over the dorsum of her foot. Sensation of the toes is normal. She also has mild weakness of dorsiflexion of the foot but strong plantar-flexion.

c. Analysis

(1) The sensory complaint could be due to an L5 root or peroneal nerve lesion.

(a) The lack of symptoms in the great toe and the lack of a sensory deficit there would tend to exclude a radicular lesion.

(b) The distribution of sensory loss best matches that of the superficial peroneal nerve (see Fig. 5-14).

(c) The weakness of the anterior tibial muscle might implicate an L4 or L5 motor root lesion, but that would not explain the sensory loss.

(2) By tracing back along the sensory branch of the peroneal nerve to its union with the motor branch, we find that the union occurs just distal to where the common peroneal nerve passes around the head of the fibula (see Fig. 5-21).

(3) Compression of the common peroneal nerve at the fibular head would explain both the motor and sensory findings.

(a) The history of sitting long hours, often with the legs crossed, suggests compression of one common peroneal nerve by the opposite knee, hence, producing an entrapment or compression neuropathy.

(b) The treatment is merely to advise the patient not to sit with crossed legs.

(4) Complete interruption of the common peroneal nerve at the fibular crossing results in complete footdrop and anesthesia in a triangular patch on the dorsum of the foot, extending somewhat up the leg. In this patient, the interruption is partial, and the chance of regeneration with restoration of function is excellent.

STUDY QUESTIONS

Directions: Each question below contains five suggested answers. Choose the **one best** response to each question.

1. After fetal growth, the caudal tip of the spinal cord is at the level of the

(A) caudal thoracic vertebrae
(B) rostral lumbar vertebrae
(C) caudal lumbar vertebrae
(D) rostral sacral vertebrae
(E) caudal sacral vertebrae

2. A patient complaining of tingling and pain down a leg into the little toe would most likely have a lesion of which sensory nerve root?

(A) L2
(B) L3
(C) L4
(D) L5
(E) S1

3. A patient has weakness of his left leg. Your examination shows no muscle stretch reflex at the ankle, severe atrophy of the calf muscles, and loss of sensation over the back of the calf, sole, and lateral aspect of the foot. Most likely he has

(A) an upper motoneuron (UMN) lesion
(B) a lower motoneuron (LMN) lesion at the anterior horn cells
(C) a cerebellar lesion
(D) a primary lesion of muscle
(E) a peripheral nerve lesion

4. The dorsal root frequently missing in normal individuals is

(A) C1
(B) C3
(C) T1
(D) L5
(E) S1

5. The phrenic nerve typically originates from

(A) C1–C3
(B) C2–C3
(C) C3–C5
(D) C5–C8
(E) C6–T1

6. The "axis of symmetry" for the brachial plexus is

(A) C3
(B) C4
(C) C5
(D) C6
(E) C7

7. Histologically, peripheral nerves contain all of the following structures EXCEPT

(A) fibrous connective tissue
(B) blood vessels
(C) myelinated axons
(D) astrocytes a glia
(E) cells with basal laminae

8. The following are true statements about nerve sheaths EXCEPT

(A) the epineurium undergoes proliferation after loss of nerve fibers
(B) perineural fibers tend to orient circumferentially
(C) perineural cells and fiber sheaths divide the nerve into fascicles
(D) endoneurial fibers tend to run longitudinally
(E) the epineurium is continuous with the dura mater

9. The spinal cord region that has one more nerve than the number of vertebrae is the

(A) sacral
(B) thoracic
(C) lumbar
(D) cervical
(E) none of the above

10. A patient with a stab wound over the clavicle is unable to abduct his arm or to flex it at the elbow. The lesion most likely affects

(A) the upper trunk of the brachial plexus
(B) the C7 nerve root
(C) the radial nerve
(D) C8–T1 nerve roots
(E) the posterior cord

11. The reason that a patient with a herniated lumbar disk may feel severe pain in the hip, rather than or in addition to pain in the foot, is that

(A) the hip is often injured when the disk ruptures
(B) immobility of the leg causes a "frozen" hip joint, similar to the shoulder–hand syndrome
(C) the back spasm associated with disk pain alters the gait
(D) the piriform muscle goes into spasm, compressing the sciatic nerve
(E) the same somites contribute dermatomes to the feet and sclerotomes to the femur

12. In "thinking through" to localize the site of a lesion along the course of the motor pathway to the periphery, the clinician should commence at the

(A) neuromuscular synapse
(B) effector
(C) plexus
(D) ventral root
(E) motoneurons

Directions: Each question below contains four suggested answers of which **one or more** is correct. Choose the answer

A   if **1, 2, and 3** are correct
B   if **1 and 3** are correct
C   if **2 and 4** are correct
D   if **4** is correct
E   if **1, 2, 3, and 4** are correct

13. Correct statements about Schwann cells include which of the following?

(1) They are absent from autonomic nerves
(2) Degeneration of one Schwann cell causes degeneration of the neighboring Schwann cells
(3) The nuclei orient circumferentially
(4) Each internode has one Schwann cell nucleus

14. As nerve roots cross the subarachnoid space they have which of the following anatomical features?

(1) They are strengthened by an astrocytic framework
(2) They have a strong fascicular arrangement
(3) They lose their Schwann cells
(4) They lack an epineurium

15. The innervation of the longitudinal ligament and annulus fibrosus of the vertebrae is featured by

(1) direct branches from each ventral root
(2) special rami from the sympathetic ganglia
(3) direct branches from dorsal roots
(4) recurrent branches from the spinal nerve trunks

16. Correct statements about intercostal nerves include which of the following?

(1) They contain GSE, GSA, GVE, and GVA fibers
(2) They receive numbers instead of names
(3) They have simpler distributions than plexus nerves
(4) They extend downward onto the ventral part of the abdomen

17. Major sensorimotor somatic nerves of the lumbar plexus include which of the following?

(1) Lateral femoral cutaneous nerve
(2) Femoral nerve
(3) Pelvic splanchnic nerve
(4) Obturator nerve

18. Deficit phenomena after peripheral nerve lesions as contrasted to irritative phenomena include

(1) muscle atrophy
(2) vasodilation
(3) anesthesia
(4) fasciculations

ANSWERS AND EXPLANATIONS

1. The answer is B. (*V E 2; Figure 5-11*) Early in embryogenesis, the tip of the spinal cord is opposite the sacral vertebrae, but the vertebral column elongates during fetal growth more than the spinal cord itself. The greater elongation of the vertebral column causes the tip of the cord to rise relative to the vertebral level. Since the cord ends at about L1–L2, the physician can insert a needle into the lower lumbar region to sample spinal fluid for diagnostic analysis without injuring the cord.

2. The answer is E. (*VIII D 1*) The patient who complains of tingling and pain into the little toe would most likely have a lesion of the S1 nerve root. The L5 nerve root typically innervates the big toe. The most common cause would be compression of the nerve root by a herniated intervertebral disk. Thus, the clinical localization of the complaint implicates the nerve root that is involved by the lesion.

3. The answer is E. (*VIII A 1, B, C, D 2; Figure 5-13*) Loss of sensation over a restricted region of skin in association with severe atrophy of the muscles in the region generally suggests a lesion of a peripheral sensorimotor nerve. Lesions of any of the other components of the motor system listed would not cause loss of sensation. A primary lesion or disease of muscle would not cause a sensory loss.

4. The answer is A. [*V E 1 b; VI B 3 a (1)*] Because of rearrangement of somites at the base of the skull at the transition point from the first cervical vertebra to the occipital bone, the first cervical dorsal root may undergo regression and disappear. Since the front half of the head is innervated by CN V, the back half of the head is then innervated by C2.

5. The answer is C. [*VII B 1 c (1) (c) (i)*] The most important spinal nerve of the body, the phrenic nerve, which causes the diaphragm to contract in breathing, originates typically from C3–C5. The nerve may originate a segment or two higher or lower, thus from C2–C5 or from C4–C6 in some individuals. Interruption of the spinal cord caudal to the phrenic origin causes paralysis of the intercostal muscles, but the patient can maintain breathing by diaphragmatic action alone.

6. The answer is E. (*VII B 2 c; Figure 5-19*) In order to remember the plan of the brachial plexus, think of it as having an axis of symmetry around C7. The brachial plexus arises from two segments above C7, C5 and C6, and continues for two segments below C7, C8 and T1. The two nerve segments rostral to C7 (C5 and C6) unite into a trunk, as do those caudal to C7 (C8 and T1). C7 is located symmetrically between the two unions.

7. The answer is D. [*I A 1, 2, 3 b, 4 a (1) (b)*] The peripheral nerves contain the peripheral type of connective tissue, which is fibrous, rather than the central type of connective tissue consisting of astrocytes and other glia.

8. The answer is A. [*I A 4 a (1), (3) (a); IV A 1*] The sheaths of the peripheral nerves have different orientations of their fibers and different reactions to disease. The endoneurium, which consists of connective tissue fibers, which have essentially a longitudinal orientation, undergoes proliferation after loss of nerve fibers, a feature that is very evident in the histologic examination of injured peripheral nerve.

9. The answer is D. (*V E 1; Figure 5-11*) The cervical region has seven vertebrae but eight spinal nerves. The reason for the discrepancy is that the first cervical nerve runs rostral to the first vertebra and the eighth cervical nerve runs caudal to the seventh cervical vertebra. The nerve immediately caudal to a cervical vertebra has a number that is one greater than the vertebra itself; thus, the nerve root that issues caudal to vertebra C7 is numbered C8. The number given to thoracic, lumbar, and sacral roots corresponds to the vertebral number.

10. The answer is A. (*VII B 2 c; Table 5-4; Figure 5-18*) A patient who is unable to abduct his arm or to flex it at the elbow would have paralysis of the deltoid and biceps muscles. These muscles receive their innervation from the C5 and C6 nerve roots, which unite to form the upper trunk of the brachial plexus.

11. The answer is E. (*VIII B 3, C 1, 2, D 1*) A patient with a herniated lumbar disk compressing a nerve root may feel discomfort in all of the structures derived from the somite innervated by that nerve root. Since each somite produces a sclerotome and a dermatome, the patient feels discomfort in either one or both of the somite derivatives innervated by that particular root. L5, for example, contributes a sclerotome to the femur and a dermatome to the foot. Root compression may cause pain referred to either site. Some patients will feel pain mostly in the hip, femur, or thigh and relatively little in the dermatomal distribution in the foot, suggesting a primary disease of the hip such as arthritis rather than the correct diagnosis of a disk herniation.

12. The answer is E. (*VIII C 1*) In "thinking through" to localize a motor lesion in the PNS, the clinician should commence at the motoneurons and visualize the axon course through ventral root, nerve trunk, plexus if it is a plexus nerve, the course of the peripheral nerve along bone and through muscle and fascial compartments, and its terminal distribution into the muscle itself. In this way, the clinician will systematically consider the alternative sites for the lesion.

13. The answer is D (4). (*I B 2 b; Figure 5-4*) Each internode has one Schwann cell nucleus, which is longitudinally oriented. Degeneration of one Schwann cell does not by itself cause degeneration of neighboring Schwann cells since the cells are completely independent and separated at the nodal points. Although Schwann cells are much less numerous in autonomic nerves, they still provide the myelin sheaths for those autonomic fibers that are myelinated.

14. The answer is D (4). (*IV B*) As the axons cross the subarachnoid space in the nerve roots, they still retain peripheral supporting tissue and Schwann cells. They lack the distinct connective tissue sheaths that divide the peripheral nerve into fascicles. The fascicular pattern and epineurium commence when the roots unite at the intervertebral foramina to form the nerve trunks.

15. The answer is D (4). (*IV D; Figure 5-10*) The vertebrae and their longitudinal ligaments receive their major innervation from recurrent branches of the spinal nerve trunks. They do not receive any direct branches from the dorsal roots since the dorsal roots themselves enter the cord from the dorsal root ganglia. Because the vertebral nerves depart from the nerve trunks and curve back in through the intervertebral foramen to reach their terminations, they are called recurrent nerves (sinu-vertebral nerves of Luschka).

16. The answer is E (all). (*III A, B; VII A 3 b; Figures 5-5 and 5-14*) The intercostal nerves are the simplest of the nerves because their somites remain at their level of origin and their nerves extend directly laterally into them without going through a plexus. They are the prototype of the single spinal nerve–single somite relationship. The lowermost intercostal spinal nerves (T12) extend down onto the lower part of the abdomen, where they border on the lumbar distribution.

17. The answer is C (2, 4). [*VII B 3 c (2) (a)*] The major sensorimotor somatic nerves of the lumbar plexus include the femoral nerve and the obturator nerve. These nerves both convey considerable numbers of sensory and motor fibers to somatic structures. The lateral femoral cutaneous nerve is purely sensory; therefore, lesions of the former two nerves cause both loss of sensation and motor function, whereas damage to the lateral femoral cutaneous nerve causes only sensory disturbances. The pelvic splanchnic nerve, while sensorimotor, innervates the bladder; thus, it is visceral, not somatic. The pudendal nerve innervates the voluntary skeletal muscle sphincters of the bladder and anus.

18. The answer is A (1, 2, 3). (*VIII A 2 a*) Nerve lesions cause both deficit phenomena and irritative phenomena. Deficit phenomena include muscle atrophy, anesthesia, and vasodilation. Vasodilation is the result of interruption of sympathetic vasoconstrictor fibers. Irritative phenomena include hyperesthesia or paresthesias, pain, and fasciculations. Some lesions cause a severe, burning type of pain called causalgia.

6

Autonomic (Visceral) Nervous System

I. RATIONALE FOR SOMATIC AND VISCERAL SUBDIVISIONS OF THE NERVOUS SYSTEM. We will define the **function of the somatic and visceral systems** in the simplest possible way, by the **action of the effectors**, not by results or by epiphenomena.

A. **Somatic effectors: skeletal muscles**
  1. The **function of the skeletal muscle fibers is** either **to contract** (shorten) or **to relax**. In so doing, they activate a skeletomuscular lever or change the diameter of an external orifice (i.e., sphincter action); however, these are epiphenomena to the contraction or relaxation of the muscle fibers.
  2. Skeletal muscles, being fast acting, tend to respond quickly to stimuli that impinge on the skin surface, eyes, or ears and that generally command conscious appreciation. In turn, the skeletal muscles act mainly under the direction of the voluntary motor system of the cerebrum.

B. **Visceral effectors: smooth and cardiac muscles and glands**
  1. The **function of smooth and cardiac muscles is to contract or relax.**
    a. Because of their general radial or circumferential orientation, the visceral muscles change the diameter of an internal organ or internal orifice.
    b. The change in diameter usually moves something along, as in peristalsis or pumping blood (the pupil being an exception).
    c. An organ like the heart functions solely to change its diameter. Blood in the chambers of the heart is moved along, but that is an epiphenomenon to the basic action of a change in the heart's diameter when its muscle fibers contract or relax.
  2. The **function of glands is secretion**, either to lubricate, digest, control temperature, or change the internal chemistry of the body. If food happens to be in the gastrointestinal tract, the process of changing diameter and secreting will move the food along and digest it, but these again are epiphenomena to the basic actions of the effectors.
  3. The visceral system, with its slow-acting smooth muscles, tends to respond slowly to internal stimuli, which generally do not command conscious appreciation, except for distension and pain. In turn, the **viscera are controlled mainly by an autonomic or visceral motor system.**

II. DEFINITIONS AND NOMENCLATURE OF THE AUTONOMIC NERVOUS SYSTEM

A. The terms **visceral, vegetative**, and **autonomic nervous system (ANS) are synonyms**, but the term **sympathetic nervous system is not** synonymous.

  1. The terms **visceral** and **vegetative** signify the **essential internal homeostatic activities mediated by the ANS.**

  2. The term **autonomic** comes from **auto** (meaning self) and **nomos** (meaning law); it is the **self-lawed nervous system** because it runs on by itself, largely unconsciously, and according to its own internal laws.

  3. The term **sympathetic** comes from the ancient notion that the body contains some mechanism that mediates the obvious sympathy between the body parts—the swelling of the breasts in sympathy with the gravid uterus or the speeding up of the heart and breathing in sympathy with exercise. The ancient physicians speculated that the pre- and paravertebral ganglia and their interconnections were the mechanism of this sympathy between the parts; these are still called the sympathetic nervous system.

B. **Definition of the ANS.** If we eschew theory and ancient notions, we can eliminate all ambiguities by defining the ANS operationally, by its effectors. In so doing, we may properly define visceral afferent fibers as part of the system because they return from the territory of the effectors.

1. **Definition.** The ANS is that part of the nervous system that sends pre- or postganglionic efferent axons to glands and to smooth and cardiac muscle and that returns afferent axons from them. [The perikarya of preganglionic neurons are located inside the central nervous system (CNS); those of postganglionic neurons are located outside the CNS. The perikarya of the afferent axons are in dorsal root ganglia.]

2. The ANS is subdivided on the basis of the level of origin of the efferent axons, and it consists of two parts (Figure 6-1):

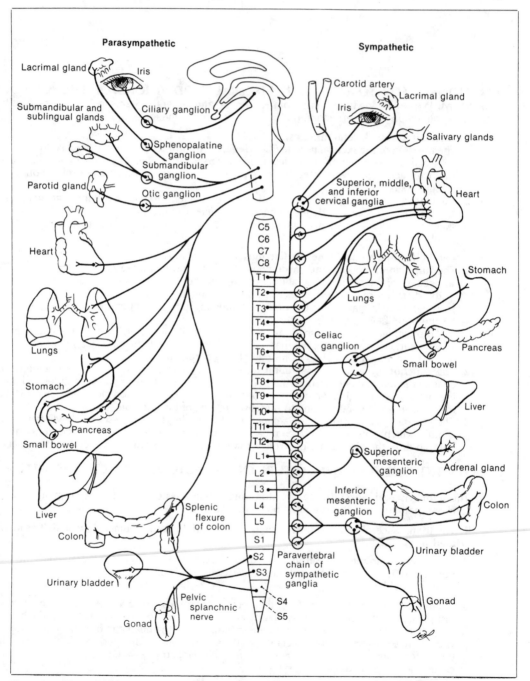

Figure 6-1. Diagram of the autonomic nervous system (ANS). The parasympathetic division (*left*) arises from CN III, CN VII, CN IX, and CN X and from spinal cord segments S2 to S4. The sympathetic division (*right*) arises from spinal cord segments T1 to L2.

     a. The **craniosacral**, or **parasympathetic**, nervous system, arising from the brainstem and sacral levels of the spinal cord

     b. The **thoracolumbar**, or **sympathetic**, nervous system, arising from the thoracic and lumbar levels of the spinal cord

C. Location of the effectors of the ANS

1. Since we have defined the ANS by its effectors (i.e., by smooth and cardiac muscles and glands), locate them by tracing around the periphery of Figure 6-1.

2. Location of smooth muscle
  a. Iris
  b. All blood vessels
  c. Pulmonary tree
  d. Walls of the gastrointestinal tract from the lower portion of the esophagus to the internal anal sphincter
  e. Walls and tubes of the genitourinary tract
  f. Piloerector muscles
  g. Splenic capsule

3. Location and types of glands
  a. Mucosal surfaces
    (1) Salivary glands
    (2) Tear glands
    (3) Mucous glands
  b. Skin
    (1) Sweat glands
    (2) Sebaceous glands
  c. Body cavities
    (1) Adrenal glands
    (2) Pancreas
    (3) Thymus and lymphoid glands and spleen
    (4) Liver
    (5) Pineal gland

4. Location of cardiac muscle: heart

III. PARASYMPATHETIC OR CRANIOSACRAL AUTONOMIC NERVOUS SYSTEM

A. Cranial division: level of origin and distribution of preganglionic axons. Of the twelve pairs of **cranial nerves**, four nerves, CN III, CN VII, CN IX, and CN X, contain preganglionic parasympathetic efferent axons.

B. Sacral division: level of origin and distribution

1. The sacral parasympathetic preganglionic axons arise from the sacral region of the spinal cord, segments S2–S4. They exit through the ventral roots, forming the **sacral plexus**, and then enter the **pelvic splanchnic nerves** [nervi erigentes] (see Fig. 7-22).

2. The pelvic splanchnic nerves form a plexus with the pelvic sympathetic axons and run to postganglionic neurons located in the walls of the bladder, the genitalia, the descending colon (from the splenic fixture distally), and the rectum (see Fig. 7-22). (For further details, see Chapter 7, section VIII C).

IV. SYMPATHETIC OR THORACOLUMBAR AUTONOMIC NERVOUS SYSTEM

A. Level of origin and preganglionic distribution

1. Preganglionic sympathetic axons arise in the intermediolateral column of the spinal cord and exit with the ventral roots of spinal nerves T1–L2 (Fig. 6-2).

2. The axons enter the nerve trunk and take one of three courses.
  a. They may form a white ramus to synapse with a paravertebral postganglionic neuron at the level of the nerve trunk (see Fig. 6-2).
  b. They may run rostrally or caudally to synapse on neighboring ganglia, forming a sympathetic chain (see Fig. 6-2).
  c. They may bypass the paravertebral chain to synapse on a prevertebral ganglion (see the celiac, superior mesenteric, and inferior mesenteric ganglia in Fig. 6-1).

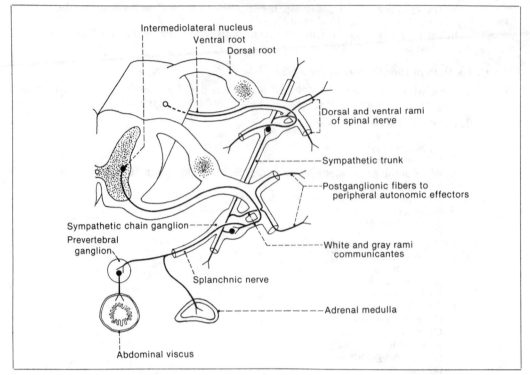

Figure 6-2. Formation of the sympathetic chain by ascending and descending axons between the sympathetic ganglia.

B. Distribution of postganglionic axons from the para- and prevertebral ganglia

1. From a **paravertebral ganglion**, an axon rejoins an adjacent nerve trunk by way of a gray ramus or travels rostrally or caudally in the sympathetic chain to another nerve trunk.

2. Typically, the axon then travels distally through a peripheral nerve or along the wall of a blood vessel to its effector (Fig. 6-3).

3. In the cervical region, the one-to-one correspondence of paravertebral ganglia with somites is lost and the ganglia fuse. The rostral-most of these fused sympathetic ganglia, the superior cervical ganglion, contains the postganglionic neurons for the head (Fig. 6-4).

V. COMPARISON OF THE SYMPATHETIC AND PARASYMPATHETIC NERVOUS SYSTEMS

A. Function. Both components of the ANS act to maintain homeostasis with the body at rest or in action.

1. The **sympathetic nervous system** dominates during **action**. It prepares us for fight, flight, or fright. It is catabolic, energy expending, since it:
   a. Increases heart rate and breathing
   b. Dilates blood vessels in skeletal and cardiac muscles and constricts them in the gastrointestinal tract
   c. Dilates the bronchial passages
   d. Dilates the pupils
   e. Erects the hairs for protection and display
   f. Increases sweat secretion
   g. Mobilizes glucose

2. The **parasympathetic nervous system** dominates during rest. It prepares us to go to sleep and to digest. It is anabolic, energy conserving, since it:
   a. Constricts the pupils
   b. Decreases the heart rate

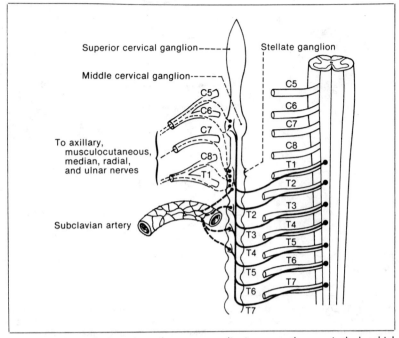

Figure 6-3. Sympathetic pathway from a preganglionic axon to the arm via the brachial plexus and the subclavian artery.

    c. Increases gastrointestinal peristalsis and secretion
    d. Expels wastes

  B. Location of sympathetic and parasympathetic ganglia. The ganglia of the sympathetic and parasympathetic nervous systems typically differ in their locations (Fig. 6-5).

    1. Sympathetic ganglia are usually proximally located in the paravertebral or prevertebral region, in orderly chains.

    2. Parasympathetic ganglia are generally more distally located, near or within the organ they innervate.

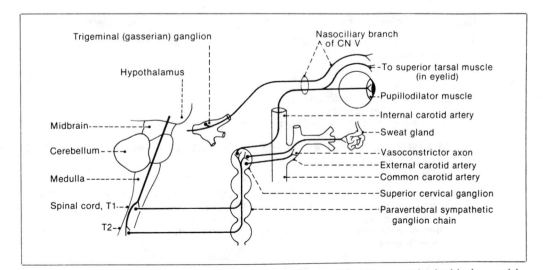

Figure 6-4. Sympathetic pathway to the pupillodilator and superior tarsal muscles, sweat glands of the face, and the smooth muscle of the carotid arteries.

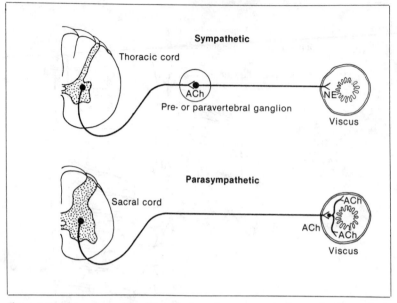

Figure 6-5. Comparison of the sympathetic and parasympathetic ganglia. Sympathetic ganglia are paravertebral or prevertebral in location, while parasympathetic ganglia are in or near the organs they innervate. The neurotransmitters of the postganglionic sympathetic neurons are adrenergic, except those for sweat glands and piloerector muscles, which are cholinergic. By contrast, all postganglionic parasympathetic neurons are cholinergic. *ACh* = acetylcholine; *NE* = norepinephrine.

C. Neurotransmitters of the ANS

1. **Cholinergic axons** include:
   a. All preganglionic axons of the ANS, both parasympathetic and sympathetic
   b. All postganglionic neurons of the parasympathetic nervous system
   c. Only the postganglionic axons of the sympathetic nervous system to the sweat glands and piloerector muscles

2. **Adrenergic axons** include the postganglionic sympathetic axons to most of the remaining smooth muscles and glands (see Fig. 6-5).

D. Oppositional action of the sympathetic and parasympathetic nervous systems

1. The actions of the sympathetic and parasympathetic nervous systems typically are directly antagonistic (Table 6-1).

2. Some excitatory effects of the sympathetic nervous system lack parasympathetic opposition, including:
   a. Splenic capsule contraction
   b. Sweating and piloerection
   c. Elevation of the upper eyelid by the superior tarsal muscle

VI. GENERAL VISCERAL AFFERENT FIBERS OF THE AUTONOMIC NERVOUS SYSTEM

A. Functional considerations

1. The general visceral afferent (GVA) fibers as a group do not mediate sensations such as touch, position and vibration, which are adequate stimuli for skin afferents. The adequate stimuli for consciously appreciated visceral sensation are distension and pain.
   a. Distension or stretch of a viscus—the bladder, bowel, ureter, or bile duct—produces intense discomfort and pain.
   b. Conversely, constriction of a portion of the wall of a viscus, causing tension or stretch on the wall, produces cramping pain.

2. Similar or allied mechanisms may produce pain from blood vessel walls.

Table 6-1. Oppositional Actions of the Sympathetic and Parasympathetic Nervous Systems

Functions Affected	Sympathetic	Parasympathetic
Pupillary size	↑	↓
Heart rate	↑	↓
Blood pressure	↑	↓
Bronchial size	↑	↓
Constriction of smooth muscle sphincters	↑	↓
Constriction of bladder wall	↓	↑
Gastrointestinal peristalsis	↓	↑

↑ = Increased; ↓ = Decreased.

B. Anatomical routes for GVA fibers to the CNS. In general, afferent fibers that mediate visceral sensation travel to the CNS by three routes:

  1. Parasympathetic nerves

  2. Sympathetic nerves

  3. Some somatic nerve trunks

C. GVA fibers in parasympathetic nerves

  1. GVA fibers travel to the CNS in CN IX and CN X and in the pelvic splanchnic nerves.
    a. CN IX conveys GVA fibers from the carotid body and carotid sinus, which influence breathing and blood pressure, and from the pharyngeal mucosa.
    b. CN X conveys GVA fibers from the laryngeal mucosa and trachea and from thoracicoabdominal viscera as far distal as the splenic flexure of the colon.
    c. The **pelvic splanchnic nerves** convey GVA fibers from the colon distal to the splenic flexure, the rectum, and the bladder.

  2. Thus, the afferent and efferent fibers of the cranial division of the parasympathetic nervous system, carried by CN X, reach the splenic flexure of the colon, whereas fibers from the sacral division, carried by the pelvic splanchnic nerves, replace them to innervate the distal colon and bladder.

D. GVA fibers in sympathetic nerves

  1. The nerves that leave the sympathetic chains and pre- and paravertebral ganglia convey GVA fibers back from the viscera and blood vessel walls.

  2. These fibers reach the dorsal roots via the communicating rami of the sympathetic ganglia.

E. GVA fibers in somatic nerves. Some GVA fibers go directly to the nerve trunk and dorsal root ganglia without passing through the sympathetic chain, and some may join branches of somatic nerves.

F. Visceral pain and referred pain

  1. Most pain fibers from the viscera run in autonomic nerves (Fig. 6-6).

  2. Some visceral pain has a fairly accurate localization. For example, we feel a full bladder at the site of the bladder. In general, pain mediated through the parasympathetic nerves (as depicted in Fig. 6-6) is better localized than pain traveling through the sympathetic fibers.

  3. Pain of some visceral structures, notably those innervated by sympathetic nerves, tends to be experienced at a site distant from its site of origin, a phenomenon called **referred pain** (Fig. 6-7).

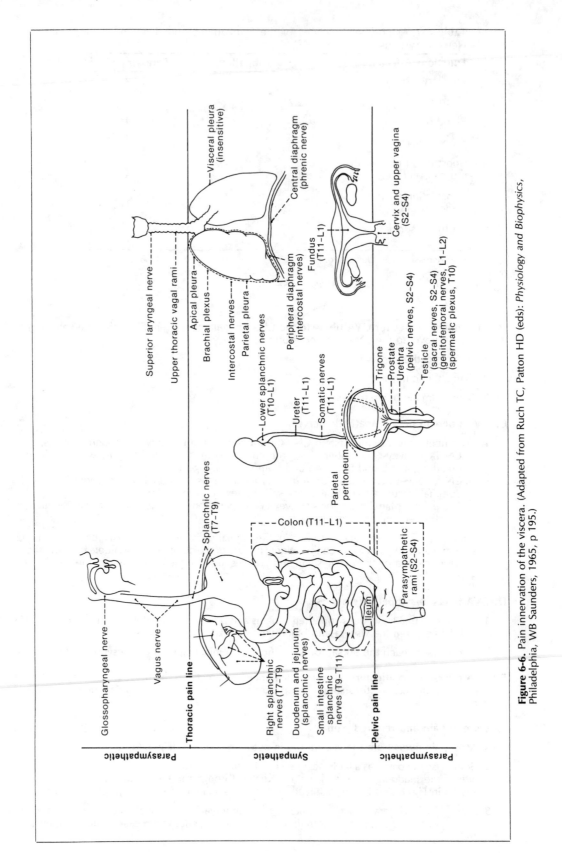

Figure 6-6. Pain innervation of the viscera. (Adapted from Ruch TC, Patton HD (eds): *Physiology and Biophysics,* Philadelphia, WB Saunders, 1965, p 195.)

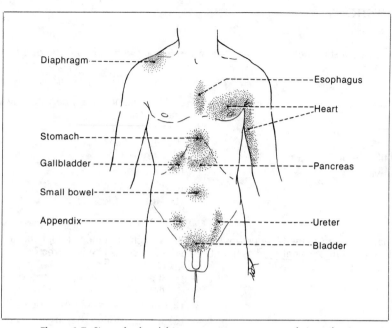

Figure 6-7. Sites of referral for some common sources of visceral pain.

    a. The patient feels the pain from a subdiaphragmatic abscess in the shoulder region. The diaphragm originates at and receives its innervation from C3–C5. The pain is referred to the distribution of dermatomes C3 and C4, over the cape area of the neck and shoulders.

    b. The patient feels the pain due to coronary artery disease in the left side of the chest and down the inner aspect of the left arm. The heart receives its autonomic innervation from T1–T5; hence, the pain is referred to these dermatomal areas.

4. The mechanism of referred pain is in dispute. In principle, the pain is usually referred to the dermatomes corresponding to the segments of the sympathetic nervous system that innervate the diseased viscus.

STUDY QUESTIONS

Directions: Each question below contains five suggested answers. Choose the **one best** response to each question.

1. The parasympathetic innervation by CN X extends to the

(A) bladder neck
(B) splenic flexure of the colon
(C) iliocecal valve
(D) ileum
(E) ureter

2. Parasympathetic fibers to the bladder would be interrupted by a lesion of spinal cord segments

(A) C1–S5
(B) T1–L2
(C) L1–S5
(D) L2–L5
(E) S2–S4

3. Sweat glands are innervated by what kind of endings?

(A) Cholinergic
(B) Adrenergic
(C) Dopaminergic
(D) Histaminergic
(E) None of these

4. Which statement about the autonomic nervous system (ANS) is correct?

(A) It makes quick adjustments of the postural reflexes
(B) It innervates smooth muscles
(C) It acts through the largest myelinated axons
(D) It conveys the pain afferents from the skin
(E) It sends axons directly to end organs without synapsing in peripheral ganglia

Directions: Each question below contains four suggested answers of which **one or more** is correct. Choose the answer

A	if **1, 2, and 3** are correct
B	if **1 and 3** are correct
C	if **2 and 4** are correct
D	if **4** is correct
E	if **1, 2, 3, and 4** are correct

5. True statements concerning transmitters in the autonomic nervous system (ANS) include which of the following?

(1) Preganglionic axons are cholinergic
(2) Postganglionic sympathetic axons are cholinergic and adrenergic
(3) Pre- and postganglionic parasympathetic neurons are cholinergic
(4) Axons that stimulate epinephrine secretion by the adrenal cortex are cholinergic

6. Cranial nerves that convey parasympathetic axons from the CNS to effectors include

(1) CN III
(2) CN VII
(3) CN IX
(4) CN XI

7. In comparison to somatic pain, visceral pain

(1) generally is poorly localized
(2) frequently is referred to a distant site
(3) generally is caused by distension of a viscus or traction on it
(4) has a more varied route through the PNS and the CNS

8. Catabolic, fright or flight, reactions mediated by the sympathetic nervous system include

(1) cardiac acceleration
(2) bronchodilation
(3) sweating
(4) pupilloconstriction

ANSWERS AND EXPLANATIONS

1. The answer is B. (*VI C 1 b*) CN X, the vagus nerve, provides parasympathetic innervation to the gut from the pharynx down to the splenic flexure of the colon. This extensive field of innervation is by far the longest of any nerve in the body.

2. The answer is E. (*III B 1, 2; Figure 6-1*) The parasympathetic axons for the distal colon and bladder arise from sacral segments S2–S4 and reach their terminal fields by the pelvic splanchnic nerve. A lesion of either the sacral cord or that nerve would interrupt the parasympathetic innervation to pelvic viscera.

3. The answer is A. (*V C 1*) The end organs of the autonomic nervous system (ANS) are generally innervated by cholinergic or catecholaminergic nerve fibers. The sweat glands receive their innervation from the cholinergic system. The salivary glands and lacrimal glands also receive cholinergic innervation.

4. The answer is B. (*I A, B 1*) The autonomic nervous system (ANS) provides all of the innervation for the smooth muscles. These muscles and the autonomic reflexes in general react slowly, in contrast to skeletal muscles and their reflexes, such as the postural reflexes, which react quickly.

5. The answer is E (all). (*V C*) The peripheral part of the autonomic nervous system (ANS) has well-defined neurotransmitters. All preganglionic axons are cholinergic. Postganglionic sympathetic axons are either cholinergic or adrenergic, with the cholinergic fibers innervating the sweat glands. The pre- and postganglionic parasympathetic neurons are cholinergic. Since the adrenal medulla corresponds to a sympathetic ganglion, its innervation corresponds to the preganglionic cholinergic fibers.

6. The answer is A (1, 2, 3). (*III A*) Parasympathetic axons travel from the brainstem through CN III, CN VII, CN IX, and CN X. CN III is the only somite cranial nerve to convey parasympathetic axons. Of the five branchial cranial nerves (CN V, CN VII, CN IX, CN X, and CN XI), neither CN V nor CN XI convey sympathetic axons in their nerve roots.

7. The answer is E (all). (*VI A 1, F*) Visceral pain in comparison to somatic pain is poorly localized and often is referred to a distant site. Thus, gallbladder pain may be referred to the anterior chest region. Generally, the pain is caused by distension of a viscus or traction on it. Both in the PNS and CNS, the pathways are more diffuse for visceral than somatic pain.

8. The answer is A (1, 2, 3). (*V A 1*) A generalized discharge of impulses from the sympathetic nervous system prepares for the energy expenditure necessary for fright or flight, when the individual faces an overwhelming stress. Included in the reaction are tachycardia, bronchodilation, sweating, and pupillo-dilation. The blood vessels to the muscles and heart will dilate, whereas those to the gut will constrict, thus shunting the blood to the muscles for action and reducing the digestive, anabolic processes of the body.

I. GROSS ANATOMY OF THE SPINAL CORD

A. Extent of the spinal cord

1. The spinal cord is a cylindrical elongated part of the central nervous system (CNS). It extends from the level of the foramen magnum to the body of the first lumbar vertebra, an average length of 43 cm (Fig. 7-1; see Fig. 1-3).

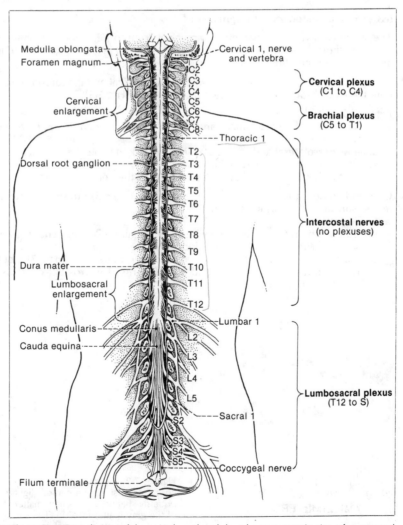

Figure 7-1. Dorsal view of the spinal cord and dorsal nerve roots in situ, after removal of the neural arches of the vertebrae.

2. Rostral and caudal limits

a. Rostrally, the spinal cord continues uninterruptedly into the medulla oblongata. The level of the foramen magnum arbitrarily divides the medulla and the cord.

b. Caudally, the spinal cord ends at the **conus medullaris** (see Fig. 7-1).

c. The tip of the conus medullaris extends to the sacrum as a thin strand, the **filum terminale**, composed only of glia.

(1) The filum terminale stretches out during the ascensus of the cord in prenatal development.

(2) After the ascensus, dorsal and ventral spinal nerve roots angle downward on either side of the filum terminale, extending from the lumbosacral cord to their original intervertebral foramina. This group of roots is called the **cauda equina** (which is Latin for "horse's tail").

B. Gross levels of the spinal cord. The spinal cord has five levels, with a total of 31 to 32 pairs of spinal nerves (see Fig. 7-1):

1. Cervical, with **8 pairs** of spinal nerves

2. Thoracic, with **12 pairs** of spinal nerves

3. Lumbar, with **5 pairs** of spinal nerves

4. Sacral, with **5 pairs** of spinal nerves

5. Coccygeal, with **1 to 2 pairs** of vestigial spinal nerves

C. Gross sectional anatomy of the spinal cord

1. The spinal cord varies in **diameter** from about 1 cm to 1.5 cm and in **shape** from round to oval. The thoracic region is the narrowest (Fig. 7-2). All in all, the spinal cord is about the diameter of your little finger.

2. The spinal cord has two gross **enlargements**, the **cervical** and the **lumbosacral**, to accommodate the extra neurons that innervate the limbs (see Fig. 7-1).

3. External longitudinal grooves

a. A shallow **dorsal median sulcus** and a deep **ventral median fissure** mark the exact sagittal plane of the spinal cord (Fig. 7-3).

b. Shallow **dorsolateral** and **ventrolateral sulci** mark the line of attachment of the dorsal and ventral nerve roots (see Fig. 7-3).

c. A shallow **dorsal intermediate sulcus** occurs in the cervical region.

4. Gray and white matter. Any transverse section of the spinal cord shows a central core of gray matter surrounded by white matter.

a. Gray matter

(1) **Composition.** Gray matter consists of neuronal perikarya, dendrites with their synapses, glial supporting cells, and blood vessels.

(2) **Shape.** The gray matter is H-shaped or, better, butterfly-shaped. The butterfly projects **dorsal horns**, **ventral horns**, and **lateral horns**. The crossbar contains a tiny **central canal** (see Fig. 7-3).

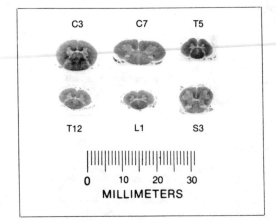

C3 C7 T5

T12 L1 S3

0   10   20   30

MILLIMETERS

Figure 7-2. Cross sections of myelin-stained spinal cord, actual size. The central, lighter unstained H, or butterfly-shaped area, is gray matter. The ventral horns of the gray matter face up. The surrounding area consists of darkly stained myelinated nerve fibers.

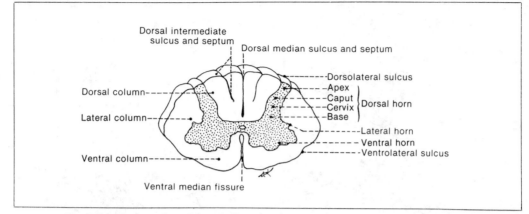

Figure 7-3. Cross section of the spinal cord with nomenclature for crevices and regions.

b. White matter
  (1) **Composition.** The white matter consists of bundles of nerve fibers, glia, and blood vessels. The nerve fibers run rostrally and caudally along the gray matter and, to some extent, through it.
  (2) **Columns of white matter.** The gray H and the external longitudinal sulci demarcate three **columns**, or **funiculi**, of white matter, the **dorsal, lateral**, and **ventral columns**, which extend the length of the cord (see Fig. 7-3).

II. GRAY MATTER OF THE SPINAL CORD: ANATOMICAL AND FUNCTIONAL SUBDIVISIONS

  A. Anatomical organization. The gray matter of the spinal cord is organized into **nuclei** and **laminae**.

  1. **Nuclei.** The neuronal perikarya of the spinal gray matter differ greatly in size, shape, and connections. Perikarya of similar size, shape, and function assemble into cell columns, called **nuclei** (Fig. 7-4; see Fig. 7-4A).
    a. Figure 7-5A shows some of the typical neurons of selected nuclei.
    b. Figure 7-6 shows the longitudinal extent of the nuclei in the spinal cord (Table 7-1).

  2. **Laminae.** Rexed mapped out the perikaryal columns into segments called **laminae** (see Fig. 7-4B), which extend the length of the cord. The laminae correspond closely, but not completely, to the nuclei (see Table 7-1 and Fig. 7-4).

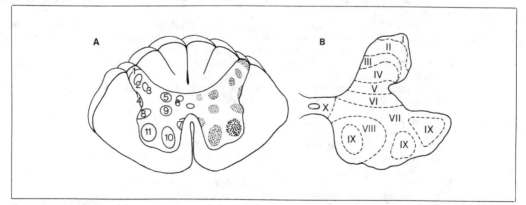

Figure 7-4. Nuclear and laminar patterns of the spinal cord gray matter. (A) Conventional nomenclature of the nuclei: *1* = dorsomarginal nucleus; *2* = substantia gelatinosa; *3* = nucleus proprius; *4* = reticular nucleus; *5* = nucleus dorsalis of Clarke; *6* = dorsal commissural nucleus; *7* = ventral commissural nucleus; *8* = intermediolateral nucleus; *9* = intermediomedial nucleus; *10* = medial motoneuron nucleus; *11* = lateral motoneuron nucleus. (B) Laminae of Rexed.

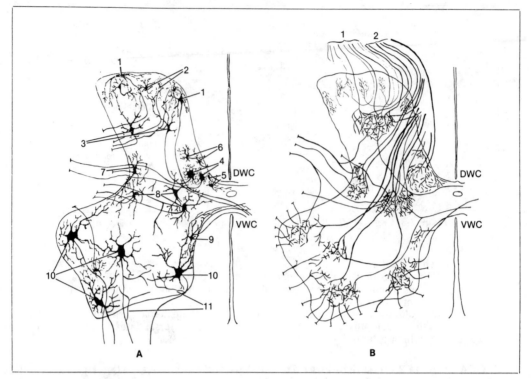

Figure 7-5. Cross sections of the gray matter of the right half of the spinal cord. (A) Typical neurons of some of the spinal cord nuclei (Golgi impregnation): *1* = dorsomarginal nucleus; *2* = substantia gelatinosa; *3* = nucleus proprius; *4* = nucleus dorsalis of Clarke; *5* = dorsal commissural nucleus; *6* = medial basal nucleus; *7* = lateral basal nucleus; *8* = intermediomedial and intermediolateral nuclei; *9* = ventral commissural nucleus; *10* = medial and lateral motoneuron nuclei; *11* = recurrent collaterals from axons of ventral motoneurons. *DWC* = Dorsal white commissure; *VWC* = ventral white commissure. (B) Typical distribution of dorsal root afferent axons (silver impregnation). Compare with the distribution of axonal terminals with the nuclear groups upon which they end, as shown in Figure 7-5A. *1* = Lateral division of dorsal root (small unmyelinated axons, group C fibers); *2* = medial division of dorsal root (large myelinated axons, group A or class I fibers).

B. Functional organization

1. **Internal organization.** The organization of the spinal cord gray matter corresponds to the division of the peripheral nervous system (PNS) into dorsal (sensory) and ventral (motor) roots (the **law of Bell and Magendie**) and into somatic and visceral nerve fibers (the **theory of nerve components**).
   a. The **dorsal horn**, like the dorsal roots, is **sensory** in function. It receives the general somatic afferent (GSA) and general visceral afferent (GVA) fibers and originates sensory pathways, but dorsal root afferents also extend into the ventral horns.
   b. The **ventral horn**, like the ventral roots, is **motor** in function, sending general somatic efferent (GSE) axons into the ventral roots.
   c. The **lateral horn** is **motor**, sending general visceral efferent (GVE) axons of the autonomic nervous system (ANS) into the ventral roots.

2. **Afferents to spinal gray matter**
   a. The nuclei of any one segment of the cord receive afferents from:
      (1) Dorsal roots of the same segment or from other segments
      (2) Interneurons in the same segment or in rostral or caudal segments
      (3) Descending axons from the brainstem and cerebrum
   b. Therefore, the nuclei of any one spinal cord segment receive:
      (1) **Intrasegmental** afferents from the same segment
      (2) **Intersegmental** afferents from caudal and rostral segments
      (3) **Suprasegmental** afferents from the brainstem and cerebrum

3. Table 7-1 summarizes the spinal cord gray matter nuclei, their location in the spinal cord, and their connections or functions.

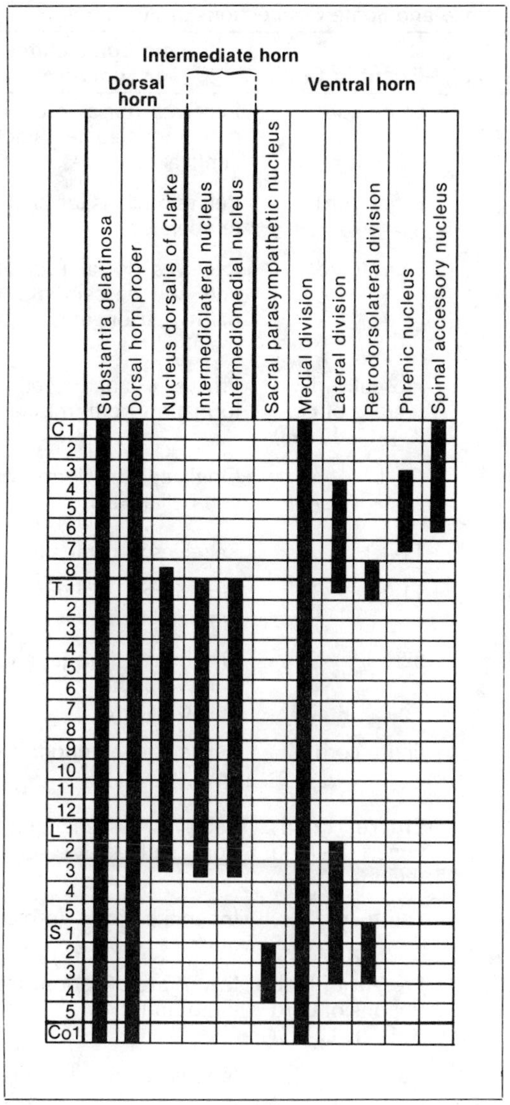

Figure 7-6. Longitudinal extent of the nuclei in the spinal cord.

III. CONNECTIONS OF THE DORSAL HORN AND DISPERSION OF THE DORSAL ROOTS

A. **Nuclear groupings of the dorsal horns.** The dorsal horns contain several nuclei or laminae that are directly in the path of the entering dorsal root axons. These include the:

1. **Dorsomarginal nucleus**

2. **Substantia gelatinosa**

3. **Nucleus proprius**

4. **Nucleus dorsalis of Clarke**

B. **Dispersion of dorsal root axons**

1. As the dorsal root axons pierce the spinal cord at the dorsolateral sulcus, the **small** axons segregate into a **lateral** bundle and the **large** axons segregate into a **medial** bundle (see Fig. 7-5B).

2. Each dorsal root axon in either the lateral or the medial bundle typically bifurcates into ascending and descending branches, which in turn produce horizontal collaterals (Fig. 7-7).

Table 7-1. Spinal Cord Nuclei Collated with Laminae and Some Connections or Functions

Horn	Nuclear Column	Lamina	Extent in Cord	Some Connections or Functions
Dorsal	Dorsomarginal n.	I	Entire cord	Receives dorsal root afferents; sends some spinothalamic axons
	Substantia gelatinosa of Rolando	II, III	Entire cord	Relays nucleus for pain and temperature
	N. proprius of the dorsal horn	IV, V	Entire cord	Receives dorsal root afferents and descending brain pathways; originates spinothalamic tracts
	. . .	VI	Present in limb regions of cord (C4–T1; L2–S3)	Processes proprioceptive information from muscles
	N. dorsalis of Clarke	VII	C8–L3	Originates the dorsal spinocerebellar tract
Intermediate zone	Intermediomedial n.	VII	T1–L3	Receives visceral afferents
	Intermediolateral n.	VII	T1–L3	Originates preganglionic sympathetic axons
	Sacral parasympathetic n. of Onufrowicz	VII	S2–S4	Originates preganglionic parasympathetic axons for pelvic viscera
	Periependymal gray matter	X	Entire cord	Related to autonomic nervous system
Ventral	. . .	VIII	Entire cord, largest in limb regions	Receives descending axons from the brain
	Medial motoneuron n.	IX	Entire cord	Innervates axial (proximal) muscles
	Lateral motoneuron n.	IX	Present in limb regions of cord (C4–T1; L2–S3)	Innervates appendicular (limb) muscles
	Phrenic n.	IX	C3–C5	Innervates the diaphragm
	Spinal lateral n.	IX	C1–C6	Innervates sternocleidomastoid and trapezius muscles

N., n. = nucleus.

    a. Thus, the fiber may synapse at its level of entry or travel varying distances up and down the cord.

    b. Most branches end in the ipsilateral spinal gray matter, but a few cross to the contralateral gray matter.

3. Dispersion of the lateral division of the dorsal roots

    a. Composition. The lateral bundle of primary sensory afferents consists of the **smaller, mostly unmyelinated C fibers** of peripheral nerve (see Table 5-1).

    b. Function. The lateral afferents mediate **pain and temperature** sensation.

    c. Route

        (1) The pain and temperature axons of the lateral bundle branch up and down in the typical manner, but most synapse at the segment of entry or after traveling up or down only a segment or two.

        (2) As these fibers accumulate at the apex of the dorsal horn, they form the **dorsolateral tract of Lissauer** (see Fig. 7-11).

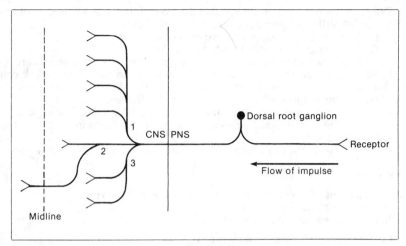

Figure 7-7. Typical branching of an entering dorsal root axon. *1* = ascending branch; *2* = horizontal branch; *3* = descending branch.

(a) The primary axons of the dorsolateral tract enter the dorsal horn to synapse on the posteromarginal nucleus, the substantia gelatinosa, and the nucleus proprius (laminae I–V of Rexed).

(b) By means of complicated interconnections that remain in some doubt, the neurons of these secondary sensory nuclei synapse on neurons in laminae VI, VII, and VIII.

(c) The neurons of laminae VI–VIII send axons up the contralateral white matter in the **lateral spinothalamic tract**. The axons cross in the ventral white commissure.

4. **Dispersion of the medial division of the dorsal roots**

   a. **Composition.** The medial bundle of primary sensory afferents consists of the **larger, heavily myelinated A fibers** of peripheral nerve (see Table 5-1).

   b. **Function.** These large fibers, in both the PNS and CNS, mediate discriminative **sensory modalities** consisting of touch, perception of texture, perception of form, and a modality termed **proprioception**, which gives a sense of where our body parts are (position sense) and of the tension on joints and muscles.

   c. **Route**

   (1) The **ascending branches** of the large fibers terminate as follows:

   (a) Some terminate at various segmental and intersegmental levels as described below for descending fibers and collaterals.

   (b) Many travel up the dorsal white columns to terminate at the cervicomedullary level.

   (2) The **descending branches** and the **collaterals of both the ascending and descending branches** distribute as follows:

   (a) Some branches go to the **substantia gelatinosa** (lamina II).

   (b) Some go to laminae III and IV (the **nucleus proprius**).

   (c) Some go to the **nucleus dorsalis of Clarke** and other parts of laminae VII and VIII.

   (d) Some synapse directly on the GSE motoneurons of the ventral horns to mediate monosynaptic muscle stretch reflexes (MSRs).

IV. CONNECTIONS OF THE VENTRAL HORN AND DISPERSION OF THE VENTRAL ROOTS

A. **Nuclei and laminae of the ventral horn**

1. **Visceral nuclei.** The most dorsal part of the ventral horn, the **intermediate zone**, contains the **intermediomedial** and **intermediolateral nuclei** and, in the sacral region, the **nucleus of Onufrowicz**, all of which belong to lamina VII of Rexed.

   a. The **intermediomedial nucleus** is presumed to receive GVA fibers from the dorsal roots and to relay fibers to the intermediolateral nucleus.

   b. The **intermediolateral nucleus** originates the sympathetic preganglionic GVE axons for the ventral roots. It extends from T1–L3 (see Table 7-1).

   c. The **nucleus of Onufrowicz** in the sacral region is the homologue of the intermediolateral nucleus in the thoracolumbar region. It sends parasympathetic preganglionic GVE axons into the sacral ventral roots.

2. The more ventral parts of the ventral horn contain laminae VIII and IX of Rexed.

    a. Lamina VIII is a heterogeneous interneuronal pool.

        (1) It receives suprasegmental and dorsal root fibers.

        (2) It connects with ventral horn motoneurons.

        (3) It originates spinothalamic tracts that mediate pain and temperature.

    b. Somatic nuclei. Lamina IX contains the **medial and lateral motor cell columns** (see Fig. 7-4). These nuclei provide the GSE axons for the skeletal muscles.

        (1) The **medial motor cell column** innervates the **axial** muscles.

        (2) The **lateral motor cell column** innervates the **appendicular** muscles.

            (a) The most dorsolateral neurons of the ventral horns in the cervical region innervate the hands.

            (b) The motor cell columns of the lumbosacral region have a similar topography.

B. Motoneurons of the ventral horn

    1. Motoneurons of the ventral horn belong to one of two **types**:

        a. Large, or **alpha**, **motoneurons**

        b. Small, or **gamma**, **motoneurons**

    2. Characteristics of alpha motoneurons

        a. The medial and lateral motor cell columns contain many neurons with very large, multipolar perikarya. They are the largest in the spinal cord and among the largest in the nervous system (see Fig. 7-5A).

        b. In general, large perikarya have large dendritic trees, large axons, or both.

        c. Since the large motor axons of peripheral nerves are classified as alpha axons (see Table 5-1), the large motoneurons are called **alpha motoneurons**. Synonyms for alpha motoneurons are:

            (1) Ventral motoneurons

            (2) GSE neurons in the spinal cord and brainstem

            (3) Special visceral efferent (SVE) neurons of the brainstem

            (4) Lamina IX of Rexed

            (5) Lower motoneurons (LMNs)

            (6) Final common pathway

        d. The alpha motoneurons innervate the regular skeletal muscle fibers that activate skeletomuscular levers or external sphincters. They do so in the form of **motor units**.

    3. Concept of motor units

        a. Definition. A **motor unit** is an alpha motoneuron, its axon, and all of the muscle fibers it innervates (Fig. 7-8).

        (1) A motoneuron, in the brainstem or spinal cord, may innervate as few as one or as many as hundreds of muscle fibers.

            (a) In the smaller, finer muscles such as the extraocular muscles, the ratio may be nearly one to one; that is, one neuron per muscle fiber.

            (b) In the larger muscles such as the quadriceps muscle of the thigh, the ratio may be one neuron to hundreds of muscle fibers.

        (2) Each muscle fiber receives only one axonal terminal.

        b. A motor unit is the smallest **unit of behavior** because the neuron responds on an all-or-none principle, the axon conducts on an all-or-none principle, and a muscle fiber responds all-or-none.

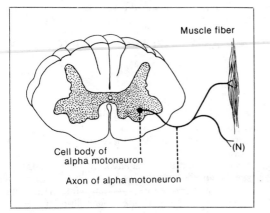

Muscle fiber

Cell body of
alpha motoneuron

Axon of alpha motoneuron

(N)

Figure 7-8. Motor unit consisting of an alpha motoneuron, its axon, and all of the muscle fibers it innervates. N = any number of additional muscle fibers up to several hundred.

    (1) Once an impulse starts down the main trunk of an axon, it will propagate to all of the axonal terminals.

    (2) Hence, to graduate the strength of contraction, the nervous system has to increase the number of motor units that are firing and the frequency with which they fire.

  c. Pathologic reactions of motor units

    (1) Death of a motoneuron or interruption of its axon results in paralysis of all of the muscle fibers of that motor unit.

      (a) If the axon does not regenerate, the muscle fibers will ultimately die because they receive no stimulation.

      (b) If the axon regenerates, the motor unit can be reestablished.

      (c) If one axon dies but an adjacent one remains, the remaining axon may sprout new collaterals to innervate the denervated muscle fibers. This enlarges the size of the motor unit.

    (2) Motor unit fasciculations

      (a) Diseases may destabilize the membrane of the alpha motoneuron or its axon, causing impulses to arise spontaneously, rather than in response to normal synaptic excitation.

      (b) In this case, all of the muscle fibers attached to the affected axon will contract, producing a visible ripple or twitch of a part of a muscle. The twitch, evident on clinical inspection and recordable by electromyography, is called a **fasciculation**.

  d. Thus, the motor unit is the anatomical, functional, pathologic, and regenerative unit of the neuromuscular system, in support of the neuron doctrine (see Chapter 2, section IV A).

4. Gamma motoneurons

  a. The smaller **gamma motoneurons** of the ventral horn send gamma-sized axons into the peripheral nerves (see Table 5-1).

  b. The axons of gamma motoneurons end on specialized skeletal muscle fibers contained in muscle spindles.

5. Muscle spindles

  a. Muscle spindles are specialized spindle-shaped structures scattered throughout all skeletal muscles (Fig. 7-9).

  b. Since the Latin word for spindle is fusus, the muscle fibers within a spindle are called **intrafusal muscle fibers**. The regular muscle fibers innervated by alpha motoneurons are called **extrafusal fibers**.

  c. Muscle spindles mediate **MSRs**.

6. Muscle stretch reflexes

  a. The **monosynaptic reflex arc** (see Fig. 2-7) links an afferent (receptor) neuron with an efferent (motor) neuron to activate an effector.

  b. The simplest reflex arc of skeletal muscles is the **MSR**, in which the muscle responds to stretch by contracting.

    (1) The **receptor** for the MSR is the **muscle spindle** (see Fig. 7-9).

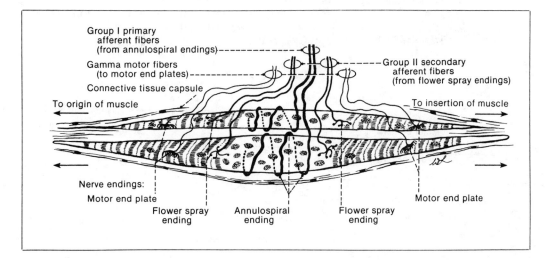

Figure 7-9. Muscle spindle and its innervation by gamma motoneuron efferents and type I afferents.

(2) Stretch of the muscle spindle from a pull on the muscle (usually via its tendon) activates receptor endings in the muscle spindle, which send a volley of **impulses** through **large myelinated afferents**.

(3) The afferents traverse the **medial bundle** of the **dorsal root** to form a **direct (monosynaptic) synapse** on the **alpha motoneuron**.

(4) Firing of the alpha motoneuron contracts all of the **extrafusal fibers** that it innervates, with a resultant **twitch** of that part of the **muscle**.

c. Contraction of the intrafusal muscle fibers as influenced by the **gamma motoneurons** sets the tension in the muscle spindles and their sensitivity to stretch.

d. The MSR is an important postural reflex. It maintains muscle tone as a foundation for voluntary movements.

e. The sum total of excitatory and inhibitory influences from peripheral afferents, spinal neurons, and suprasegmental pathways affects the activity of alpha and gamma motoneurons.

(1) Hence, a lesion of CNS pathways may increase or decrease the magnitude of the MSR.

(2) A lesion of the reflex arc itself, affecting either the afferent or the efferent axons, will generally reduce or abolish the MSR, as may disease of the muscle itself.

7. Renshaw cells

a. The alpha motoneuron sends a collateral axon to an interneuron, the **Renshaw cell**, which sends an inhibitory synapse back to the alpha motoneuron (see Fig. 7-5, no. 11).

b. Afferents from elsewhere in the nervous system affect the discharge of Renshaw neurons in much the same way that alpha and gamma motoneurons are affected. Physiological or pathological changes in the balance of excitatory and inhibitory impulses playing on the Renshaw cells and alpha motoneurons may cause the MSRs to be hyperactive or hypoactive, which can be detected when the clinican elicits the MSRs.

8. Alpha motoneurons as the final common pathway

a. The discharge of alpha motoneurons depends on the algebraic sum of excitatory and inhibitory impulses from all the pathways that converge upon them, including (Fig. 7-10):

(1) Dorsal roots, mainly the medial divisions of the segment where the motoneuron originates

(2) Intrasegmental neurons of the spinal cord, including Renshaw cells

(3) Intersegmental sensory afferent neurons and interneurons

(4) Descending tracts from the brain

b. The alpha motoneuron is considered the **final common pathway out of the nervous system** because of the following:

(1) The alpha motoneurons provide the only axons to skeletal muscle.

(2) All reflex and voluntary behavior expressed through skeletal muscles requires activation of the alpha motoneurons.

(3) The rest of the CNS is regarded as a huge multicircuited interneuronal pool that ultimately expresses itself in skeletal muscle activity through the alpha motoneurons.

9. Alpha motoneurons as lower motoneurons

a. The large GSE motoneurons of the medial and lateral nuclei of the ventral horns and corresponding brainstem neurons receive yet another name, **lower motoneurons (LMNs)**.

b. The LMNs contrast with the upper motoneurons (UMNs), which descend from the brain (see section VII B 5).

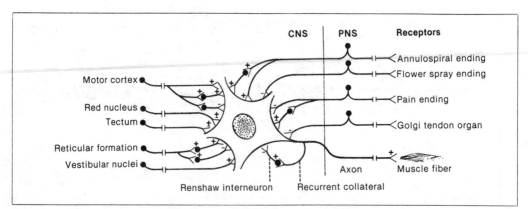

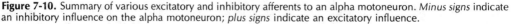

Figure 7-10. Summary of various excitatory and inhibitory afferents to an alpha motoneuron. *Minus signs* indicate an inhibitory influence on the alpha motoneuron; *plus signs* indicate an excitatory influence.

V. WHITE MATTER OF THE SPINAL CORD: OVERVIEW OF ASCENDING AND DE-
SCENDING PATHWAYS. Table 7-2 lists the ascending and descending spinal tracts, and Figure 7-11 shows the location of the major tracts on a cross section of the spinal cord.

A. Origin of pathways in the spinal white matter. Clinically testable pathways in the spinal cord arise from four sources:

1. Dorsal roots

2. Sensory neurons and interneurons of the spinal cord gray matter

3. Brainstem tegmentum

4. Cerebral cortex

B. Arrangement of the spinal pathways

1. Certain morphologic laws aid in remembering the origin, course, location, and termination of spinal pathways:
  a. Law of the peripheral position of long fibers
  b. Law of lamination by phylogeny
  c. Law of lamination by level of entry or body topography
  d. Law of separation of sensory pathways by sensory modalities

---

Table 7-2. Tracts of the Spinal Cord

Ascending tracts
    Primary (first-order) axons (from dorsal root ganglia)
        Fasciculus gracilis (Goll's column)
        Fasciculus cuneatus (Burdach's column)
    Secondary (second-order) axons (from interneurons)
        Ventral spinothalamic tract
        Lateral spinothalamic tract
        Ventral spinocerebellar tract
        Dorsal spinocerebellar tract
        Spino-olivary tract
        Spinovestibular tract
        Spinotectal tract
        Spinoreticular tract
        Spinocervical tract (importance in humans is questionable)

Descending tracts (ultimately acting on the motoneurons)
    Supraspinal in origin*
        Ventral corticospinal tract
        Lateral corticospinal tract
        Tectospinal tract
        Rubrospinal tract
        Reticulospinal tract
        Cerulospinal tract
        Vestibulospinal tract
        Olivospinal tract
    Spinal in origin
        In dorsal columns
            Interfascicular fasciculus (Schultze's comma tract or semilunar tract)
            Septomarginal fasciculus
        In ventral columns
            Sulcomarginal fasciculus

Mixed ascending and descending tracts
    Dorsolateral tract of Lissauer (primary axons from dorsal roots plus axons
        of intrinsic spinal neurons)
    Fasciculi proprii (ground bundles) [secondary axons from interneurons of
        gray matter] and branches from dorsal roots

---

*Notice that no descending tracts of clinical significance arise from the cerebellum, diencephalon, or basal ganglia or from the cerebral cortex apart from the region around the central sulcus (sensorimotor cortex).

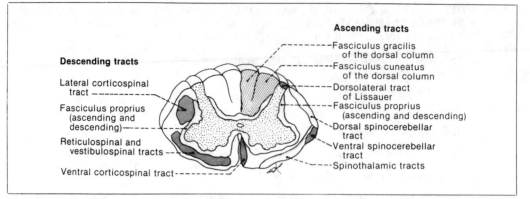

Figure 7-11. Cross section of the spinal cord showing the location of the major ascending and descending tracts.

2. Concentric arrangement of the spinal pathways (law of the peripheral position of long fibers)
   a. The fundamental plan of the spinal cord calls for three concentric zones (Fig. 7-12):
   (1) The **central** H-shaped core of gray matter
   (2) A **proximal** sleeve of short-running fibers called **fasciculi proprii**, or **ground bundles**
   (3) A **peripheral** sleeve of long-running fibers
   b. The **short-running ground bundles**, which are phylogenetically old, ascend and descend adjacent to the gray matter.
   (1) The ground bundles arise from:
      (a) Interneurons of the spinal cord gray matter
      (b) Dorsal root collaterals
   (2) The individual axons of the ground bundles extend only a few spinal cord segments at most. Thus, they mediate intrasegmental spinal reflexes (e.g., MSRs) and short-running intersegmental reflexes.
   c. The **long-running fibers** surround the ground bundles. They occupy the white matter between the ground bundles and the surface of the cord (see Fig. 7-12).
   (1) Ascending long fibers come from:
      (a) Interneurons of spinal cord gray matter, which send axons to the brain
      (b) Dorsal roots
   (2) Most **descending long fibers** come from the brain. Some descending fibers in the dorsal column come from descending branches of dorsal root axons (see Fig. 7-7).

C. Demonstration of the ground bundles

   1. To demonstrate the ground bundles, a segment of the spinal cord is isolated by transecting the cord in two places (Fig. 7-13; see Fig. 7-13A).
   a. The **rostral cut** interrupts all **long descending axons** that arise rostral to it.
   b. The **caudal cut** interrupts all **long ascending axons** that arise caudal to it.
   c. Only the short-running axons whose perikarya lie in dorsal root ganglia or spinal cord gray matter remain between the two cuts.

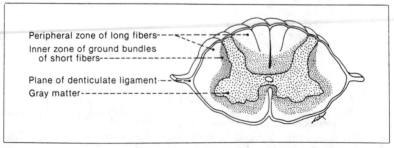

Figure 7-12. Cross section of the spinal cord showing the ground bundles of short fibers (*stippled*) immediately surrounding the gray matter and the zone of long fibers (*white*) on the periphery.

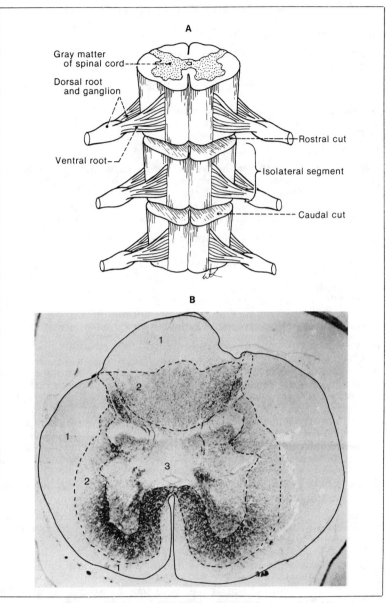

Figure 7-13. (*A*) Surgical isolation of a thoracic segment of cat spinal cord by transverse cuts rostral and caudal to the segment. (*B*) Myelin-stained transverse section of the isolated spinal cord segment (ventral horns, down). All long ascending and descending axons on the periphery of the cord (*zone 1*) have degenerated, leaving only the zone of ground bundles (*zone 2*), which arise in the segment, intact around the gray matter (*zone 3*). Compare with Figure 7-12. (Adapted with permission from Anderson FD: The structure of a chronically isolated segment of the cat spinal cord. *J Comp Neur* 120:297–316, 1963.)

2. The two transections have the following effects:
    a. All interrupted ascending and descending axons undergo wallerian degeneration.
    b. Interruption of all descending motor axons causes paralysis of all movements directed by the brain or by spinal gray matter rostral to the cut.
    c. Intrasegmental reflexes (e.g., MSRs) of the isolated segment remain.
    d. Interruption of all ascending sensory axons causes anesthesia caudal to the rostral cut.

VI. ASCENDING PATHWAYS OF THE SPINAL WHITE MATTER

A. Features of the ascending pathways

1. Ascending pathways run in each of the three **columns** of white matter, the **dorsal**, **lateral**, and **ventral**.

2. The ascending long pathways all transmit information derived from sensory receptors and destined to:
   a. Produce conscious sensation, somatic or visceral
   b. Mediate reflexes, somatic or visceral
   c. Guide the motor centers in the cerebellum, brainstem, diencephalon, basal ganglia, and cortex

3. Ascending somatosensory **pathways that mediate conscious sensation** include the:
   a. Lateral spinothalamic tract (pain and temperature)
   b. Ventral spinothalamic tract (touch)
   c. Fasciculus gracilis and fasciculus cuneatus of the **dorsal columns** [discriminative modalities: touch, form, texture, position sense (see section VI C 1 b)]

4. Ascending somatosensory **pathways that mediate unconscious sensory functions** include the following.
   a. Spinocerebellar pathways provide information to the cerebellum for the coordination of volitional movements.
   b. Spinoreticular pathways provide information to the brainstem tegmentum and reticular formation to mediate somatic and visceral reflexes.

B. Common plan of the somatosensory pathways for conscious sensation

1. Each somatosensory pathway for conscious sensation runs from a peripheral receptor to the cerebral cortex.
   a. The pathway begins in a **receptor** in the skin (Fig. 7-14) or the skeletomuscular system. Some sensory modalities arise in specific sensory receptors and have discrete central pathways, but both peripheral receptors and central pathways tend to overlap for other modalities.
   b. The **primary**, or **first-order**, **neuron** in the pathway has its perikaryon in a dorsal root ganglion (Fig. 7-15).
   c. The **secondary**, or **second-order**, **neuron** is in the spinal cord or brainstem. Its axon decussates and ascends to the brainstem, where all pathways join in the medial lemniscus to synapse on tertiary neurons in the contralateral thalamus.
   d. The **tertiary**, or **third-order**, **neuron** runs from the thalamus to the somatosensory area of the cerebral cortex, the postcentral gyrus.

2. The clinician ''thinks through'' this circuitry in analyzing any sensory loss that could result from a lesion of a sensory pathway. To think it through, the clinician must know the
   a. Receptor location
   b. Route through the PNS
   c. Location of primary, secondary, and tertiary neuronal perikarya
   d. Site or level of decussation for the second-order neuron
   e. Column of the cord—dorsal, lateral, or ventral—by which the pathway ascends
   f. Brainstem course via the medial lemniscus
   g. Thalamic relay nucleus
   h. White matter between thalamus and cortex
   i. Cortical receptive area

C. Dorsal columns and dorsal column sensory modalities

1. **Function**
   a. The dorsal columns convey axons that mediate touch localization, form, texture, position sense, pressure, vibration, and allied sensations.
   b. The sensations mediated by the dorsal columns are very specific as to stimulus, location, and spatial and temporal discrimination. Hence, they are sometimes called **discriminative modalities**.

2. **Peripheral course**
   a. The **receptors** for the dorsal column modalities are located in the skin and the skeletomuscular system.
   (1) Receptors in the skin include **Meissner's** and **pacinian corpuscles** (see Fig. 7-14). The axons from these receptors are in the medium to large (A fiber) range (see Table 5-1).

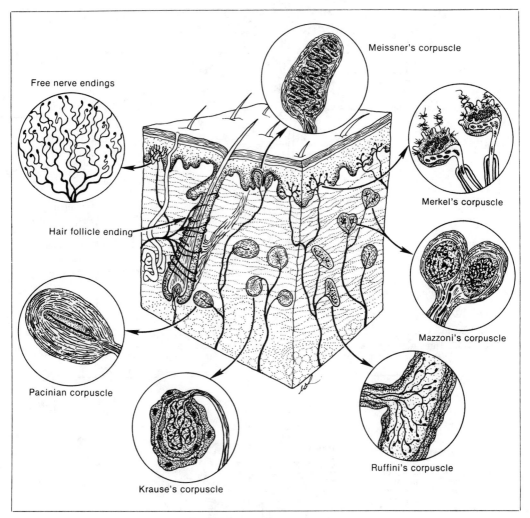

Figure 7-14. Skin receptors.

    (2) Receptors in the skeletomuscular apparatus include **muscle spindles** and **Golgi tendon organs**. The axons from these receptors are in the large (1α and 1β) range (see Fig. 7-9 and Table 5-1).
   b. The **peripheral axons** arise from dorsal root ganglia and enter the spinal cord through the dorsal roots (Fig. 7-16).

3. Central course
   a. After coursing through the medial division of the root and dividing, the **ascending axonal branch** runs up the **ipsilateral** dorsal column.
    (1) Hence, the dorsal columns contain primary sensory afferent axons whose cell body is outside the CNS.
    (2) The dorsolateral tract of Lissauer is the only other spinal tract so constituted.
   b. Descending branches of dorsal root axons travel caudally in the dorsal columns as the fasciculus interfascicularis and septomarginal fasciculus, but their destination and function are unknown.
   c. Both **ascending and descending axonal branches** send numerous collaterals into the spinal gray matter [see section III B 4 c (2) and Fig. 7-7].
   d. Ascending fibers
    (1) As the fibers accumulate in the dorsal columns from caudal to rostral, they illustrate the **law of lamination by level of entry** and thus reflect the body topography (Fig. 7-17; see Fig. 7-16).

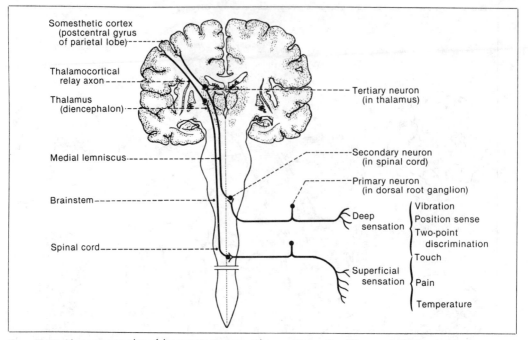

Somesthetic cortex
(postcentral gyrus
of parietal lobe)

Thalamocortical
relay axon

Thalamus
(diencephalon)

Medial lemniscus

Brainstem

Spinal cord

Tertiary neuron
(in thalamus)

Secondary neuron
(in spinal cord)

Primary neuron
(in dorsal root ganglion)

Deep
sensation

Vibration

Position sense

Two-point
discrimination

Touch

Superficial
sensation

Pain

Temperature

Figure 7-15. Three-neuron plan of the somatosensory pathways. Notice the difference in the level of decussation of the pathways for superficial and deep sensation and the dual pathways for touch.

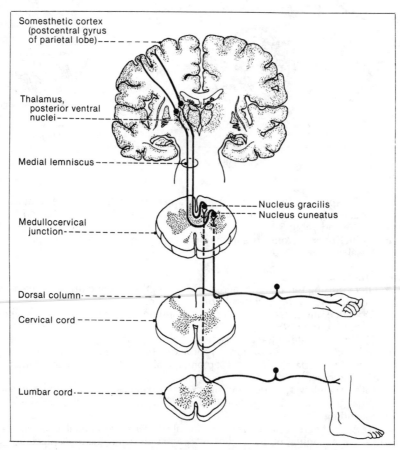

Somesthetic cortex
(postcentral gyrus
of parietal lobe)

Thalamus,
posterior ventral
nuclei

Medial lemniscus

Nucleus gracilis
Nucleus cuneatus

Medullocervical
junction

Dorsal column

Cervical cord

Lumbar cord

Figure 7-16. Somatosensory pathway for dorsal column modalities.

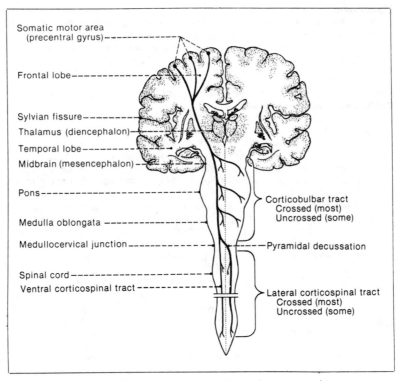

Figure 7-20. Course of the corticobulbar and corticospinal tracts.

  b. Ventral corticospinal tract. A minority of fibers continue **ipsilaterally** into the ventral column as the ventral corticospinal tract (see Fig. 7-11).

4. Termination
 a. The **lateral corticospinal tract** descends the length of the cord.
  (1) It sends axons into the gray matter at all levels. Hence, it gradually diminishes in size as it descends.
  (2) The **crossed lateral** corticospinal axons veer into the intermediate zone of the spinal gray matter to synapse on:
   (a) Neurons of laminae IV–VII (majority of terminals)
   (b) Alpha motoneurons of lamina IX (minority of terminals, estimated at 10% in humans)
  (3) The **uncrossed lateral** corticospinal axons terminate at synapses in the base of the dorsal horn, intermediate zone, and central parts of the ventral horn.
 b. The **ventral corticospinal tract** crosses in the ventral white commissure to synapse mainly in lamina VII.

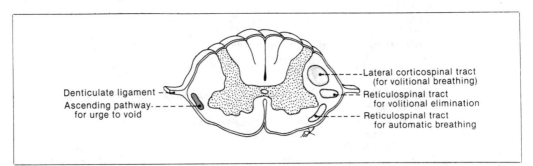

Figure 7-21. Transverse section of the spinal cord showing the location of the pathways for the control of breathing and elimination by the bladder and bowel.

5. Upper motoneurons

a. Although the term LMN applies only to the alpha motoneuron, the term **UMN** has two meanings, one general and the other restricted. Thus, UMNs may mean either:

(1) **All descending tracts** from the brain that ultimately influence the LMNs

(2) **Only the cortical efferent pathway**; that is, the **pyramidal tract**

b. The meaning should be clear from the context.

6. Clinical significance of the decussation and the lateral corticospinal tract: hemiplegia, quadriplegia, and paraplegia

a. Interruption of a pyramidal tract will paralyze voluntary movement on one side of the body, a condition called **hemiplegia**.

b. The **side of the hemiplegia** depends on whether the lesion interrupts the pyramidal tract rostral or caudal to the cervicomedullary decussation.

(1) A lesion **rostral to the decussation** causes **contralateral hemiplegia**. Certain corticobulbar movements will also be paralyzed, most notably voluntary movements of the lower part of the face.

(2) A lesion **caudal to the decussation** causes **ipsilateral hemiplegia**. The face is spared.

c. **Bilateral interruption** of the corticospinal tracts after the decussation causes **quadriplegia** if rostral to the arms and thus paralyzing all four extremities or **paraplegia** if caudal to the arms and thus paralyzing only the two legs (see Fig. 7-24A).

d. Of the three corticospinal tracts in the spinal cord, the crossed is by far the most important UMN pathway.

(1) In most individuals, interruption of the lateral tract will cause complete ipsilateral paralysis of voluntary movements caudal to the level of the lesion.

(2) Because of some variability in the number of decussating fibers in the corticospinal tracts, particularly because of some variability in the size of the ventral tract, interruption of only one lateral corticospinal tract may not cause complete paralysis in some individuals.

(3) The fibers that descend ipsilaterally in the ventral tract before crossing may account for some degree of recovery after a lateral corticospinal tract lesion.

7. Clinical signs of corticospinal tract (UMN) lesions and LMN lesions

a. Both UMN and LMN lesions cause paresis or paralysis, but the lesions differ in location and usually in type, and the clinical features differ (Table 7-3).

b. Effect of acute, severe UMN lesions

(1) Acute complete or nearly complete interruption of UMNs may result in a transient stage called **spinal shock** or **cerebral shock**, in which, in addition to total paralysis, the patient exhibits:

(a) Areflexia and hypotonia

(b) Absence of abdominal and cremasteric reflexes

(c) Absence of plantar response

(2) If the lesion transects the cord, the patient shows in addition:

(a) Hypotonic paralysis of bowel and bladder

(b) Hypotension and anhidrosis

Table 7-3. Clinical Features of UMN and LMN Lesions

UMN lesions (pyramidal syndrome)
Paralyze movements in hemiplegic, quadriplegic, or paraplegic distribution, not individual muscles
Atrophy of disuse only (late and slight)
Hyperactive MSRs
Clonus
Clasp-knife spasticity
Absent abdominal and cremasteric reflexes
Extensor toe sign (Babinski sign)

LMN lesions
Paralyze individual muscles or sets of muscles in root or peripheral nerve distribution
Atrophy of denervation (early and severe)
Fasciculations and fibrillations
Hypoactive or absent MSRs
Hypotonia

UMN = upper motoneuron; LMN = lower motoneuron; MSRs = muscle stretch reflexes.

(3) Within hours, days, or weeks, the hypotonia changes to spasticity and the MSRs become hyperactive, giving the classic UMN syndrome (see Table 7-3).
    c. The exact pathophysiologic mechanisms of the changes in reflexes and plantar responses in acute or chronic UMN lesions are not known.

C. Descending tracts from the brainstem

  1. Tectospinal, rubrospinal, cerulospinal, and **olivospinal tracts**, which are not testable clinically

  2. Vestibulospinal tract

  3. Reticulospinal tracts, which affect somatic and visceral motor functions
    a. These tracts affect skeletal muscle tone, but there are no specific clinical syndromes due to their interruption.
    b. The role of the reticulospinal tracts in the control of visceral activities is discussed in section VIII B 1 b.

VIII. ASCENDING AND DESCENDING SPINAL PATHWAYS FOR VISCERAL FUNCTIONS

A. Volitional and reflex control of visceromotor actions

  1. Ascending and descending pathways in the spinal cord control the following visceral motor functions: breathing, elimination, blood pressure and pulse, sweating and other glandular secretions, and gut motility.

  2. Some visceral functions have a dual volitional and reflex control, notably breathing and the sphincters of bladder and bowel. The remaining visceral functions are largely controlled by autonomic reflexes.

  3. Anatomically, the viscerosensory and autonomic visceromotor tracts occupy the ventrolateral quadrant of the spinal cord. They intermingle considerably with each other and with the ventral and lateral spinothalamic tracts.

B. Role of the spinal cord in breathing (see also Chapter 8, section XIII L)

  1. UMN control. Breathing is controlled by volitional and automatic UMN pathways. Both ultimately activate the same LMNs.
    a. The **lateral corticospinal tract** is the essential pathway for **volitional** control of breathing. It occupies the plane dorsal to the denticulate ligament (see Fig. 7-21).
    b. The **medullary (lateral) reticulospinal tract (bulboreticulospinal tract)** controls **automatic** breathing.
      (1) This tract runs ventral to the plane of the denticulate ligament in the ventrolateral white matter just off the tip of the ventral horn (see Fig. 7-21).
      (2) It arises in the respiratory center in the medullary reticular formation (see Chapter 8, section XIII L, and Fig. 8-44).

  2. LMN innervation for breathing
    a. Spinal segments C3–C5 innervate the diaphragm through the phrenic nerve.
    b. Spinal segments T2–T12 innervate the intercostal and abdominal muscles through the intercostal nerves.

  3. Afferent pathways for the control of breathing
    a. Afferent pathways run in CN IX and CN X (see Table 8-6).
    b. An ascending pathway of unknown origin also runs to the medullary respiratory center via the ventrolateral quadrant of the cord.

  4. Effect of spinal cord lesions on breathing (see also Chapter 8, section VIII H)
    a. Transection of the cord at or rostral to C2 paralyzes all volitional and automatic breathing. The patient dies unless given artificial respiration because the spinal cord contains no centers that can initiate or maintain breathing.
    b. Hemisection of the cord at or **rostral to C2** paralyzes both volitional and automatic breathing ipsilaterally by paralyzing the ipsilateral diaphragm and intercostal muscles.
    c. Ventrolateral quadrant lesions interrupt both the descending autonomic pathways for breathing and the ascending pathways that provide part of the drive to breathe.
      (1) Interruption of the ascending pathway in the ventrolateral quadrant reduces the ventilatory response to carbon dioxide.
      (2) Bilateral section of the ventrolateral quadrants of the cord at C2 paralyzes automatic breathing, and the patient is condemned to stay awake to breathe by utilizing pyramidal pathways, a condition called **Ondine's curse** (see Chapter 8, section VIII H 6).

d. Transection of the cord at C6 paralyzes intercostal breathing, but the diaphragm with its phrenic nerve spared can maintain adequate ventilation, at least with the patient in the resting state.

e. Transection of the dorsal roots of all intercostal nerves reduces breathing. The reason is uncertain.

C. Role of the spinal cord in micturition

1. LMN or segmental innervation of the bladder

  a. Efferents run to the bladder and its sphincters from the three motor systems (Fig. 7-22):

   (1) Sympathetic: T6–L3, via the hypogastric nerve and plexus
   (2) Parasympathetic: S2–S4, via the pelvic splanchnic nerves
   (3) Somatomotor: S2–S4, via the pudendal nerve

  b. Afferents return to the spinal cord from all three nerves.

2. Reflex emptying of the bladder

  a. Unlike breathing, micturition and ejaculation can occur reflexly after spinal cord transection.

  b. The spinal cord has a center for reflex micturition, located in the sacral segments, but brainstem and cerebral centers superimpose UMN control.

3. UMN innervation of the bladder

  a. The UMN pathway for volitional micturition is presumed to descend in the white matter midway between the lateral horn and the periphery of the cord (see Fig. 7-21). Hence, it is at or just ventral to the plane of the denticulate ligament.

  b. Bilateral interruption of the ventrolateral quadrants of the cord causes an immediate flaccid paralysis of the bladder, which will then later begin to empty reflexly.

4. Ascending pathways for bladder sensation. The major ascending pathway for the urge to void (see Fig. 7-21) apparently travels in the periphery of the cord and appears to correspond to the site of the sacral fibers in the lateral spinothalamic tract.

D. Role of the spinal cord in defecation

1. The **descending pathways** for volitional control of defecation appear to overlap those for micturition but may be a little more lateral.

2. The **ascending pathway** is presumably the same as for micturition.

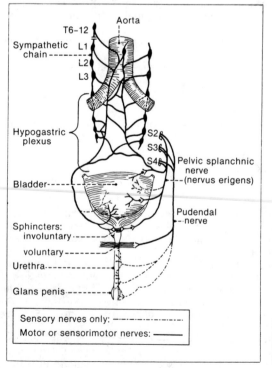

Sensory nerves only: ─·─·─·─·─·─·
Motor or sensorimotor nerves: ─────

Figure 7-22. Innervation of the bladder by the hypogastric plexus (sympathetic), pelvic splanchnic nerve (parasympathetic and visceral sensory), and pudendal nerve (somatosensorimotor).

3. Reflex bowel movement can occur after spinal cord transection, just as reflex bladder empty-ing can.

E. Vasomotor and sudomotor pathways

1. Vasomotor and sudomotor autonomic UMN pathways descend in the ventrolateral columns of white matter, intermingled with and medial to the lateral spinothalamic tract. The efferent pathway is through the intermediolateral nuclei to the sympathetic ganglia.

2. Interruption of descending UMN autonomic pathways causes loss of sweating below the level of the lesion and vasodilation with hypotension.
  a. The hypotension is orthostatic.
    (1) When the patient is elevated from a horizontal to a vertical position, the brain cannot produce reflex vasoconstriction through the interrupted descending autonomic path-way. The hydrostatic pressure from the pull of gravity causes the blood to pool in the dilated vessels and blood flow to stagnate.
    (2) Since insufficient blood returns to the heart, the heart cannot maintain the intracranial circulation, and the patient faints.
  b. In the **Shy-Drager syndrome**, the patient has orthostatic hypotension and fainting because the neurons in the autonomic ganglia selectively degenerate.

IX. CLINICO-ANATOMICAL SYNDROMES OF THE SPINAL CORD (Fig. 7-23)

A. Motoneuron diseases

1. Diseases of LMNs (see Fig. 7-23*A*). Two diseases may destroy alpha motoneurons relatively selectively.
  a. Progressive muscular atrophy is a heredofamilial degenerative disease, which in pure form affects only the ventral motoneurons. The patient gradually becomes weaker and dies.
  b. Poliomyelitis is an acute inflammatory viral infection.
    (1) The virus has a predilection for the LMNs, although it may also involve other neurons to lesser degrees.
    (2) It may affect only a segment or part of a segment of the cord or brainstem and cause only a selective atrophy of the relevant muscles or even a part of one muscle.

2. Diseases of UMNs (see Fig. 7-23*B*). In **familial spastic paraplegia**, the pyramidal tracts under-go a dying-back process. The patient first has lower extremity paralysis, then upper extremity paralysis, and finally corticobulbar paralysis, with difficulty in speaking and swallowing.

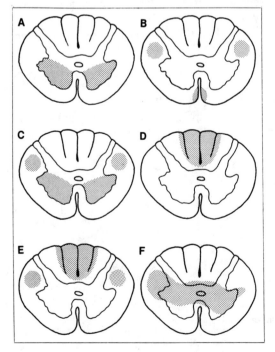

Figure 7-23. Clinical syndromes of spinal cord lesions. (*A*) Lower motoneuron (LMN) disease: progressive spinal muscular atrophy or poliomyelitis. (*B*) Upper mo-toneuron (UMN) disease: familial spastic paraplegia. (*C*) Combined UMN and LMN disease: amyotrophic lateral sclerosis. (*D*) Sensory neuron disease of dorsal roots and dorsal columns: hereditary sensory neuropathy or tabes dorsalis. (*E*) Combined degeneration of the dorsal and lateral funiculi: subacute combined degeneration or spinocerebellar degeneration. (*F*) Syringomyelia.

3. **Combined UMN and LMN disease** (see Fig. 7-23C). **Amyotrophic lateral sclerosis** ("Lou Gehrig's disease") is the prototypic disease. The patient shows a combination of UMN and LMN signs.
   a. The **amyotrophy** refers to the muscular atrophy from degeneration of the LMNs.
   b. The **lateral sclerosis** refers to the pyramidal tract degeneration, which results in astrocytic proliferation in the lateral columns, in analogy with multiple sclerosis.

B. **Sensory neuron disease of dorsal roots and dorsal columns** (see Fig. 7-23D)

   1. In **hereditary sensory neuropathy**, the dorsal roots selectively degenerate, causing loss of sensation.

   2. In **tabes dorsalis**, a form of **syphilis**, the dorsal columns degenerate. The patient loses dorsal column modalities but retains pain sensation and often has lancinating pains in the extremities. Lower extremities are more affected than upper, and leg fibers of the dorsal column are more severely degenerated than arm fibers (see Fig. 7-23D).

C. **Combined degeneration of dorsal and lateral columns** (see Fig. 7-23E)

   1. **Diseases**
      a. **Subacute combined degeneration of the dorsal and lateral columns**, or **posterolateral sclerosis**, is caused by a deficiency of vitamin B_{12}. The patient has a combination of UMN signs and dorsal column sensory loss.
      b. **Spinocerebellar degenerative diseases** involve the dorsal columns and spinocerebellar tracts, and, to varying degrees, the pyramidal tracts.

   2. **Effects**
      a. Patients with dorsal and lateral column diseases may show hyperreflexia or hyporeflexia, depending on which column shows the most advanced lesion.
      b. With severe dorsal column involvement, the MSRs ultimately disappear because of interruption of the afferent arc, in spite of the corticospinal tract lesion.

D. **Syringomyelia syndrome** (see Fig. 7-23F). In syringomyelia, a cavitating process causes destruction of tissue around the central canal. The destruction then spreads irregularly from the central gray matter into the white matter. The lesion is most common in the cervical cord or medulla.

   1. The first fibers affected are the pain and temperature fibers that decussate in the ventral white commissure to turn upward into the lateral spinothalamic tract.

   2. The patient loses pain and temperature sensation and may suffer burns of the fingers because of loss of the protective sensory modalities.

   3. The lesion may expand out to involve one or both corticospinal tracts, or the alpha motoneurons, causing UMN and LMN signs in addition to the sensory loss.

E. **Syndromes of partial or complete transection of the spinal cord.** These syndromes are most commonly caused by trauma, neoplasms, vascular occlusion, or multiple sclerosis. The lesion may partially or completely interrupt the spinal cord (Fig. 7-24).

   1. **Complete transection** (see Fig. 7-24A) causes quadriplegia if above the arms or paraplegia if caudal to the arms. Caudal to the level of the lesion the patient shows:
      a. Paralysis of all voluntary movements, with UMN signs
      b. Anesthesia

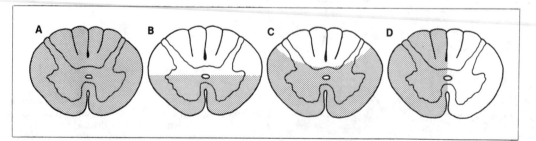

Figure 7-24. Syndromes of partial or complete interruption of the spinal cord at the cervical level. (A) Complete transection of the spinal cord. (B) Transection of the ventrolateral quadrants of the spinal cord. (C) Transection of the ventral two-thirds of the spinal cord. (D) Hemitransection (hemisection) of the spinal cord.

      c. Loss of bladder and bowel control (although reflex emptying may occur)

      d. Anhidrosis and loss of vasomotor tone

      e. Paralysis of volitional and automatic breathing if the lesion is in the rostral part of the cervical cord

  2. Ventrolateral quadrant transection (see Fig. 7-24*B*)

    a. Transection of the ventrolateral quadrants **in the cervical region** results in:

      (1) Paralysis of automatic breathing and decreased sensitivity to carbon dioxide

      (2) Loss of voluntary bladder and bowel control, with preservation of reflex emptying

      (3) Loss of the urge to urinate

      (4) Anhidrosis

      (5) Hypotension

      (6) Loss of pain and temperature sensation

    b. The patient retains voluntary control of the skeletal muscles and retains other sensations.

  3. Transection of the ventral two-thirds of the cord (see Fig. 7-24*C*)

    a. Occlusion of the ventral spinal artery (see Chapter 15, section II A) results in infarction of the ventral two-thirds of the spinal cord.

    b. The patient shows paralysis of voluntary movements in addition to the signs of ventrolateral quadrant transection listed in section IX E 2 a.

  4. Hemisection of the spinal cord (Brown-Séquard syndrome) [Table 7-4; see Fig. 7-24*D*]. This classic syndrome is the testing ground for knowledge of clinical spinal cord anatomy.

F. Conus medullaris–cauda equina syndrome. Compressive or expanding lesions of the distal cord or cauda equina, frequently neoplasms or large herniated disks, interrupt bladder and bowel function and cause pain, paresthesia, numbness, and loss of MSRs in the lower extremities.

Table 7-4. Clinical Features of the Brown-Séquard Syndrome (Spinal Cord Hemisection)

Clinical Findings	Anatomical Basis
Contralateral effects	
Loss of pain and temperature sensation caudal to lesion	Interruption of spinothalamic tract
Ipsilateral effects	
Paralysis of voluntary movements caudal to level of lesion; hyperreflexia, spasticity, and extensor toe sign	Interruption of lateral corticospinal tract
Loss of vibration, position sense, form perception, and two-point discrimination	Interruption of dorsal columns
Segmental weakness and atrophy	Destruction of ventral motoneurons at level of lesion
Segmental anesthesia	Destruction of dorsal rootlets at level of lesion
Loss of sweating caudal to level of lesion, and, if lesion is cervical, ipsilateral Horner's syndrome (pupilloconstriction, ptosis, and hemifacial anhidrosis)	Interruption of descending autonomic fibers in ventral column

STUDY QUESTIONS

Directions: Each question below contains five suggested answers. Choose the **one best** response to each question.

1. Axons for the distal limb muscles derive from

(A) the intermediolateral cell column
(B) the nucleus dorsalis of Clarke
(C) the medial motor cell column of the ventral horn
(D) the lateral motor cell column of the ventral horn
(E) none of the above

2. The sacral fibers of the spinothalamic tract, which conveys pain and temperature impulses, are located

(A) close to the sagittal plane of the spinal cord
(B) deep in the dorsal median sulcus
(C) just ventral to the plane of the denticulate ligament
(D) halfway between the ventral median fissure and the ventral root
(E) diffusely scattered in the spinothalamic tract

3. Which of the following statements about the diameter of the spinal cord is true?

(A) The thoracic cord has the greatest diameter
(B) The transverse diameter at C8–T1 exceeds the anteroposterior diameter
(C) The diameter of the pyramidal tract area is smaller in the cervical than in the thoracic region
(D) The diameter of the substantia gelatinosa is smallest in the rostral cervical region
(E) None of the above

4. The ventral corticospinal tract in humans has which one of the following characteristics?

(A) It is located along the ventral median fissure
(B) It is larger than the lateral corticospinal tract
(C) It is composed of decussated axons
(D) It is composed of very small, unmyelinated axons
(E) None of the above

5. A neurosurgeon wishing to eliminate pain in a particular dermatome without causing loss of the sense of touch would make a cut at which one of the following sites?

(A) Where the lateral fibers of the dorsal root attach to the cord
(B) In the midportion of the root as it crosses the subarachnoid space
(C) Just after the dorsal root enters the subarachnoid space from the intervertebral foramen
(D) Just at the distal edge of the dorsal root ganglion
(E) In the nerve trunk about 1 cm distal to the ganglion

6. If an experimenter wanted to demonstrate the lateral corticospinal tracts selectively by means of wallerian degeneration, he could

(A) section the medullary pyramids transversely
(B) transect the sacral region of the spinal cord
(C) section the dorsal columns high in the cervical region
(D) transect the ventral columns in the cervical region
(E) make a 1-cm midsagittal cut through the ventral column near the cervicomedullary junction

7. The pyramidal tract has its main decussation at the junction of the

(A) spinal cord and medulla
(B) medulla and pons
(C) pons and midbrain
(D) midbrain and diencephalon
(E) none of the above

8. The afferent axons for the muscle stretch reflexes (MSRs) synapse on the

(A) substantia gelatinosa
(B) lamina I of Rexed
(C) ventral motoneuron
(D) nucleus reticularis
(E) dorsal root ganglion

9. A patient shows weakness of all arm and hand movements, slight atrophy of the arm muscles, hyperreflexia, and slight clasp-knife spasticity. The most likely cause is

(A) an upper motoneuron (UMN) lesion
(B) a cerebellar lesion
(C) a primary lesion of muscle
(D) a peripheral nerve lesion
(E) a basal ganglia lesion

10. Recognition of a coin felt in your pocket, but not seen, depends on the

(A) dorsal column pathway
(B) spinocerebellar tract
(C) spinoreticular tracts
(D) ground bundles
(E) none of the above

Directions: Each question below contains four suggested answers of which **one or more** is correct. Choose the answer

A	if **1, 2, and 3** are correct
B	if **1 and 3** are correct
C	if **2 and 4** are correct
D	if **4** is correct
E	if **1, 2, 3, and 4** are correct

11. The dorsal columns contain which of the following axons?

(1) Axons from dorsal root ganglia neurons
(2) Some corticospinal axons
(3) Some descending axons
(4) Many vestibulospinal axons

12. Nuclei or cell columns that extend along the entire spinal cord include which of the following?

(1) Medial motor cell column of the ventral horn
(2) Nucleus dorsalis of Clarke
(3) Substantia gelatinosa
(4) Intermediolateral nucleus

13. The large fibers entering from the dorsal roots synapse on the

(1) ventral motoneurons
(2) nucleus dorsalis of Clarke
(3) nucleus gracilis
(4) intermediolateral cell column

14. True statements about the long tracts of the spinal cord include which of the following?

(1) They almost all arise in the cerebrum
(2) They almost all are sensory pathways
(3) They enter the brainstem without a synapse in the spinal cord
(4) They tend to run on the periphery

15. True statements about the nucleus gracilis include which of the following?

(1) It is caudomedial to the nucleus cuneatus
(2) It is visible macroscopically on cut sections
(3) It is the origin of the medial lemniscus
(4) It conveys the dorsal column pathway from the legs

16. Clinical effects seen immediately after interruption of the pyramidal tracts in the spinal cord, but not seen later, include which of the following?

(1) Loss of voluntary control of bladder and bowel
(2) Paralysis of volitional extremity movements caudal to the lesion
(3) Loss of vasomotor reflexes (leading to orthostatic hypotension)
(4) Hypotonia and areflexia

17. Operations that reduce breathing include which of the following?

(1) Transection of the ventrolateral quadrants of the spinal cord at T1
(2) Section of the lumbar dorsal roots
(3) Hemisection (dorsal column, lateral column, and ventral column) of the spinal cord at C2
(4) Transection of both dorsal columns at C2

SUMMARY OF DIRECTIONS

A	B	C	D	E
1, 2, 3 only	1, 3 only	2, 4 only	4 only	All are correct

CVR → all spinal tracts are smaller

18. After complete spinal cord transection at C2, which of the following functions can take place automatically through local spinal reflexes?

(1) Micturition and defecation
(2) Ejaculation
(3) Intestinal peristalsis
(4) Breathing

A

19. After spinal cord hemisection at C1 (i.e., section of the dorsal, lateral, and ventral columns on one side), the patient would show which of the following clinical deficits caudal to the lesion?

(1) Nearly complete ipsilateral loss of touch
(2) Contralateral loss of pain and temperature sensation
(3) Contralateral diaphragmatic paralysis
(4) Paralysis of the ipsilateral arm and leg

C

20. Tracts that are smaller in size in the lumbosacral than in the cervical region include the

(1) corticospinal
(2) vestibulospinal
(3) reticulospinal
(4) spinothalamic

A

21. True statements about the denticulate ligaments include which of the following?

(1) Transection of the spinal cord dorsal to the plane of the ligaments will cause weakness or paralysis of volitional movements
(2) The denticulate ligaments are composed of glia
(3) The denticulate ligaments attach to the lateral aspects of the spinal cord
(4) The denticulate ligaments travel along the ventral roots

D

ANSWERS AND EXPLANATIONS

1. The answer is D. (*IV A 2 b*) The motor cell columns of the ventral horn have a topographic arrangement, with the medial motor cell column (the medial nuclear group of motoneurons) supplying the axial muscles and the lateral motor cell column (the lateral nuclear group) supplying the appendicular muscles. Thus, axons for the distal limb muscles would come from the lateral—actually the laterodorsal—group of ventral motoneurons.

2. The answer is C. (*VI D 2; Figure 7-17*) The lateral spinothalamic pain and temperature tracts in the spinal cord have a distinct lamination, following the law of lamination by level of entry. Thus, the sacral fibers are most dorsolateral, followed, going ventromedially, by the leg, trunk, and arm fibers. The topography extends through the brainstem and thalamic sensory nucleus to the postcentral gyrus.

3. The answer is B. (*I C 1; Figure 7-2*) The spinal cord changes in diameter and shape at the various levels. It has the smallest diameter in the thoracic region. In the C8–T1 region, the transverse diameter exceeds the anteroposterior diameter because of the lateral expansion of the gray matter to accommodate the greater number of neurons needed for the arms.

4. The answer is A. (*VII B 3 c; Figure 7-12*) The ventral corticospinal tract, which borders on the ventral median fissure, is often rather sizeable, but it is not as large as the lateral corticospinal tract. The ventral corticospinal tract consists of myelinated axons of various sizes. The axons run straight down from the medullary pyramids without decussating at the cervicomedullary junction. However, many of these axons are thought to decussate before terminating in the ventral horns.

5. The answer is A. (*III B; VI D, E 2*) The dorsal roots divide into medial and lateral bundles. The lateral bundle, which consists of small, poorly myelinated fibers, mediates pain and temperature. Neurosurgeons have attempted to treat some types of chronic pain by selective section of these roots just where they attach to the cord, leaving the larger, heavily myelinated touch and proprioceptive fibers of the medial division of the root intact. Elsewhere in the nerve root and trunk, the fibers intermingle too much to permit selective sectioning.

6. The answer is E. (*V C 2*) Demonstrating a tract by wallerian degeneration requires cutting the axons prior to their entering the field of study. To demonstrate only the lateral corticospinal tracts by wallerian degeneration, leaving the ventral corticospinal tracts intact, the experimenter would make a midsagittal cut through the pyramidal decussation near the cervicomedullary junction (see Fig. 8-25). The crossed axons of the lateral tract would be severed, and the resulting degeneration would demonstrate their route in the lateral columns.

7. The answer is A. (*VII B 2*) The most important motor decussation in the CNS occurs at the junction of the spinal cord and medulla where the pyramidal tract crosses. This voluntary motor pathway, which originates in one hemisphere, is the ultimate pathway in man for the control of movements on the opposite side of the body.

8. The answer is C. (*IV B 1, 2 c, 6*) The muscle stretch reflexes (MSRs) are monosynaptic. The afferent axons that elicit the reflex synapse directly on the ventral motoneurons, which return the motor axons to the muscle fibers.

9. The answer is A. (*VIII B 7 b; IX A 2; Table 7-3*) Lesions of each of the components of the motor system cause a different clinical syndrome. The upper motoneuron (UMN) syndrome consists of hyperreflexia, spasticity, weakness of all movements, and slight disuse atrophy of the muscles. This characteristic syndrome is not produced by lesions in the other motor circuits or in the PNS.

10. The answer is A. (*VI A 3 c, C 1*) Recognition of an object felt but not seen requires superficial and deep sensation. The superficial sensation gives information as to temperature, whereas the deep sensation, which travels through dorsal column pathways, provides a sense of form or stereognosis. The brain integrates these pieces of information to identify an object felt by the fingers.

11. The answer is B (1, 3). [*III B 4 c (1) (b); VI C 2 b, 3 a*] The dorsal columns consist of direct axons from the dorsal root ganglia, which ultimately synapse on the nucleus gracilis and nucleus cuneatus at the cervicomedullary junction. The dorsal columns do contain some descending axons but not descending motor tracts from the cerebrum or brainstem.

12. The answer is B (1, 3). (*Table 7-1; Figure 7-6*) The nuclear groups or cell columns of the spinal cord vary in their longitudinal extent. Some extend throughout the length of the cord, such as the medial motor cell column, which innervates the axial muscles, and the substantia gelatinosa, which mediates pain and temperature sensations from the entire body. Other nuclear groups have a more restricted longitudinal extent; an example is the intermediolateral nucleus, which provides preganglionic sympathetic axons to roots T1–L3. The extent of the nucleus dorsalis (Clarke's column) approximates that of the intermediolateral nucleus.

13. The answer is A (1, 2, 3). [*III A 2, B 4 c (2); VI C 3 d (2)*] The large fibers that enter along the medial divisions of the dorsal roots synapse on motoneurons of the ventral horns and on the nucleus dorsalis of Clarke, the nucleus gracilis, and the nucleus cuneatus. In addition, they synapse on many interneurons of the dorsal and ventral horns.

14. The answer is D (4). [*V B 1 a, 2 a (3), c*] The long tracts of the spinal cord tend to run on the periphery. Thus, they surround the ground bundles, which are the short, inter- and intrasegmental connecting pathways. The long pathways consist of both motor and sensory fibers. All of the primary sensory fibers synapse before entering the brainstem, except for dorsal root proprioceptive fibers from the arm and neck, which reach the lateral cuneate nucleus. This tract corresponds to the dorsal spinocerebellar tract of the remainder of the cord.

15. The answer is E (all). [*VI C 3 d (1)–(3); Figure 7-11*] The nucleus gracilis, which can be seen on gross section, is located at the cervicomedullary junction, caudal and medial to the nucleus cuneatus. The nucleus gracilis receives the dorsal column pathways from the leg and contains perikarya of origin of the medial lemniscus.

16. The answer is D (4). (*VII B 7; Table 7-3*) Immediately after interruption of the corticospinal (pyramidal) tracts in the cord, the patient will have a stage of spinal shock, with hypotonia and areflexia. This immediate, acute stage differs from the usual upper motoneuron (UMN) syndrome seen in the chronic stage, in which the patient has spasticity and hyperreflexia. In both stages, the patient loses voluntary control of the bladder, the bowel, and the extremities caudal to the lesion.

17. The answer is B (1, 3). (*VIII B 4; IX E*) Transection of the ventrolateral quadrants of the spinal cord at T1 interrupts reticulospinal tracts and would paralyze the intercostal muscles during automatic breathing. Hemisection of the cord at C2 would reduce both automatic and voluntary breathing. After interruption of one corticospinal tract, the corresponding hemidiaphragm may be paralyzed in some individuals. Section of thoracic dorsal roots may reduce breathing, but section of only the lumbar dorsal roots or dorsal column has little effect.

18. The answer is A (1, 2, 3). (*VIII C 2; IX E*) After spinal cord transection, all voluntary movements distal to the lesion are lost but a number of visceral reflexes remain. The patient will not be able to breathe, however, because the spinal cord does not have its own intrinsic neural mechanisms for breathing. Retained reflex actions include micturition, defecation, intestinal peristalsis, and even ejaculation. Thus, a quadriplegic male can still have a reflex erection and ejaculate in response to penile stimulation, although he may have no sensation of the sexual act.

19. The answer is C (2, 4). (*IX E 4; Figure 7-24; Table 7-4*) Hemisection of the spinal cord at C1 would cause a Brown-Séquard syndrome. The patient loses pain and temperature sensation contralaterally because the lesion interrupts the crossed spinothalamic tract in the ventrolateral quadrant of the cord, which conveys these modalities to the thalamus. The ipsilateral arm and leg would be paralyzed because of interruption of the descending pyramidal tract fibers in the lateral columns, which cross at the level of the medullary decussation. Touch sensation might be mildly impaired, but since the touch pathways ascend by crossed and uncrossed tracts through the cord, the sensation of touch is not greatly affected.

20. The answer is A (1, 2, 3). (*VIII C 4 a*) The general rule is that in the spinal cord the motor tracts decrease in size as they descend and the sensory tracts increase in size as they ascend. Since the descending tracts end at all levels of the cord, only a few axons destined for the distal part of the cord will remain at the distal end of the descending tract. The ascending tracts, essentially the sensory tracts like the spinothalamic, increase in size as they go up the cord because they continue to receive additional fibers as they ascend to the brainstem or thalamus.

21. The answer is D (4). (*VII B 3; Figures 7-12 and 7-21*) The denticulate ligaments attach to the lateral aspect of the spinal cord midway between the dorsal and ventral roots. They extend from the pia to the dura and are composed of fibrous connective tissue. A transverse line connecting the denticulate ligaments on each side separates the dorsal half of the lateral white column, which contains the bulk of the corticospinal axons, from the ventral half, which conveys axons for the control of automatic breathing, bladder, and bowel function.

8

Brainstem and Cranial Nerves

I. GENERAL PLAN OF THE BRAINSTEM. The basic somite plan of the spinal cord continues into the brainstem, but major new components, not present in the spinal cord, are added:

A. A special column of motoneurons and a set of peripheral nerves for the branchial arches

B. Nuclei and pathways for the special senses of taste, hearing, and equilibrium

C. Pathways for the control of eye movements

D. Reticular formation

E. Supplementary motor nuclei

F. Quadrigeminal plate

G. Cerebellum

II. GROSS ANATOMY OF THE BRAINSTEM (MIDBRAIN, PONS, AND MEDULLA)

A. Three transverse subdivisions of the brainstem

　1. The brainstem consists of three transverse subdivisions, the **midbrain, pons,** and **medulla oblongata,** in rostrocaudal order (Figs. 8-1, 8-2, and 8-3).

　2. Although the midbrain, pons, and medulla differ somewhat in cross-sectional contour, a single, generalized outline represents all three (Fig. 8-4).

B. Three longitudinal subdivisions of the brainstem

　1. Three continuous longitudinal laminae, the **tectum, tegmentum,** and **basis,** extend through the midbrain, pons, and medulla, as does the original neural canal (Fig. 8-5).

　2. The midbrain, pons, and medulla all have a similar plan of internal organization, based on the concept of a tectum, tegmentum, and basis.

C. Composition of the tectum

　1. Definition. The tectum is the plate of brainstem tissue dorsal to the plane of the aqueduct (tectum means roof).

　2. The tectum consists in rostrocaudal order of the:
　　a. Quadrigeminal plate over the midbrain
　　b. Anterior medullary velum over the pons
　　c. Posterior medullary velum over the medulla

　3. In Figure 8-6, note that:
　　a. The **rostral** part of the tectum, the quadrigeminal plate of the midbrain, roofs the aqueductal part of the original neural canal.
　　b. The **caudal** part of the tectum, the anterior and posterior medullary vela, roofs the fourth ventricular part of the original neural canal. The vela meet at the peak of the fourth ventricle, which is called the **fastigium.**

　4. The tectum contains no cranial nerve nuclei, no reticular formation, and no longitudinally coursing long motor or sensory pathways.

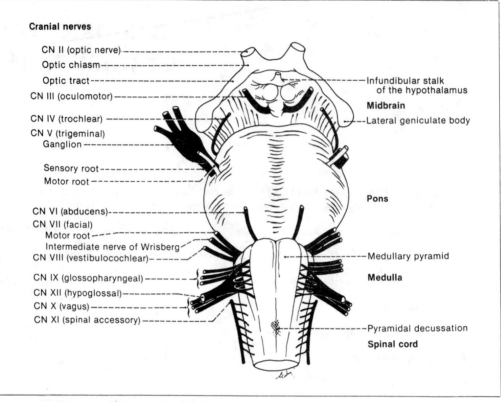

Figure 8-1. Ventral view of the brainstem and cranial nerves.

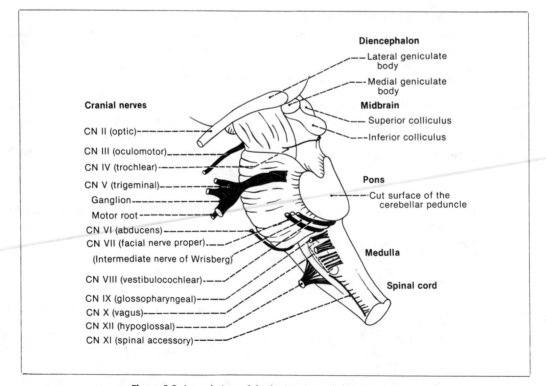

Figure 8-2. Lateral view of the brainstem and cranial nerves.

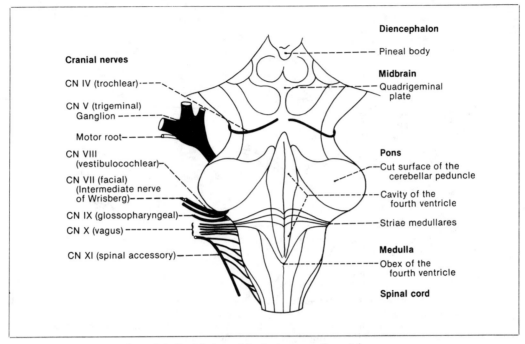

Figure 8-3. Dorsal view of the brainstem and cranial nerves.

D. Composition of the basis

1. The brainstem basis consists of descending cortical motor tracts intermingled with nuclei in the basis pontis. The motor tracts consist of the:
   a. **Pyramidal tracts**
      (1) **Corticobulbar tract**
      (2) **Corticospinal tract**
   b. **Corticopontine tracts** of the corticopontocerebellar pathway

2. **Differences in the bases of the midbrain, pons, and medulla**
   a. The **midbrain basis** conveys the corticobulbar, corticospinal, and corticopontine tracts into the pontine basis. It has no nuclei.

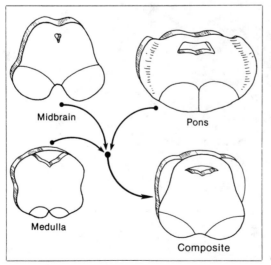

Figure 8-4. Composite of the cross-sectional contours of the midbrain, pons, and medulla.

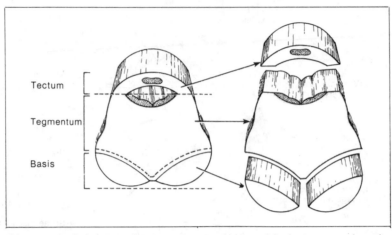

Figure 8-5. Exploded view of a composite cross section of the brainstem to show the three longitudinal subdivisions into tectum, tegmentum, and basis.

b. The **pontine basis** is the largest basis because it contains the cortical efferent tracts plus numerous nuclei.

(1) The nuclei all receive the corticopontine fibers and project to the cerebellum. They are the only significant nuclei in the brainstem basis.

(2) All corticospinal and some remaining corticobulbar fibers proceed through the pontine basis into the medullary basis.

c. The **medullary basis** is the smallest (see Fig. 8-1) because:

(1) Most corticobulbar fibers have already entered the tegmentum rostral to the medulla (see Fig. 7-20), but some proceed into the medullary basis and then into the medullary tegmentum.

(2) The corticopontine fibers have terminated on the nuclei in the basis pontis.

d. Because the corticofugal tracts in the medullary basis have an oval or pyramidal shape on cross section (see Fig. 8-27), they are called the **medullary pyramids**, and, hence, the **pyramidal tracts**.

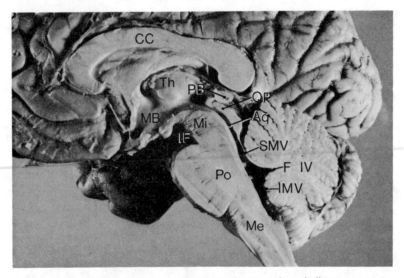

Figure 8-6. Sagittal section of the brainstem, cerebrum, and cerebellum. *Aq* = aqueduct; *CC* = corpus callosum; *F IV* = fastigium of the fourth ventricle; *IF* = interpeduncular fossa; *IMV* = inferior medullary velum; *MB* = mamillary body; *Me* = medulla; *Mi* = midbrain; *PB* = pineal body; *Po* = pons; *QP* = quadrigeminal plate; *SMV* = superior medullary velum; *Th* = thalamus.

E. Composition of the tegmentum (tegmen means covering, the covering of the basis)

   1. Definition. The tegmentum is the plate of neurons and tracts sandwiched between the tectum and basis of the brainstem.

   2. In contrast to the basis and tectum, the tegmentum is the complicated part of the brainstem. It contains gray matter and white matter.

   a. Tegmental gray matter consists of:

   (1) Motor and sensory nuclei of CN III to CN XII, with the exception of CN XI

   (2) Reticular formation, including certain chemically specified nuclei and tracts

   (3) Supplementary motor and sensory nuclei

   b. Tegmental white matter consists of:

   (1) All long sensory tracts that ascend from the spinal cord or cranial nerve nuclei to the cerebellum, brainstem, and thalamus

   (2) Medial longitudinal fasciculus, the ground bundle of the brainstem

   (3) Cerebellar afferent and efferent pathways

   (4) The **central tegmental tract**, which interconnects the tegmentum, diencephalon, and basal forebrain gray matter

   (5) Profuse unnamed pathways in the reticular formation

   3. Diagrammatic cross section of the tegmentum. Notice in Figure 8-7 that:

   a. The general somatomotor and general sensory cranial nerve nuclei cluster in the dorsal tier of the tegmentum. No cranial nerve nuclei occupy the tectum or basis.

   b. Special visceral efferent (SVE) nuclei migrate to a position ventrolateral to the general somatic efferent (GSE) motoneurons.

   c. Supplementary motor nuclei occupy the ventral tier of the tegmentum or basis of the pons.

   (1) In the medulla, these are inferior olivary nuclei.

   (2) In the pons, these are the nuclei of the basis.

   (3) In the midbrain, they include the red nucleus and substantia nigra.

   d. Sensory tracts to the thalamus called **lemnisci** run in the ventral and lateral part of the tegmentum.

   e. Reticular formation fills in the space unoccupied by cranial nerve nuclei, supplementary motor and sensory nuclei, and long tracts.

III. EMBRYOLOGY–PHYLOGENY OF THE BRAINSTEM

A. Early stages. The brainstem can be considered as a phylogenetic elaboration of the basic plan of the spinal cord.

   1. The neural tube closes around a neural canal.

   2. Roof and floor plates and paired basal and alar plates develop.

   3. The neural tube wall shows the ependymal, mantle, and marginal layers.

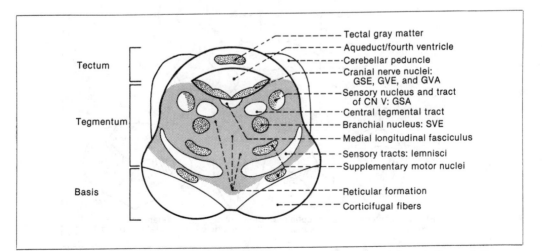

Figure 8-7. Diagrammatic cross section of the brainstem tegmentum. *GSE* = general somatic efferent; *GVE* = general visceral efferent; *GVA* = general visceral afferent; *GSA* = general somatic afferent; *SVE* = special visceral efferent.

B. Rhombencephalic roof plate and the rhomboid fossa

1. In the hindbrain, or rhombencephalon, the dorsal lips of the alar plates remain separated by a broad rhombencephalic roof plate, which becomes the anterior and posterior medullary vela (Fig. 8-8).

2. The hindbrain and forebrain roof plates, although completing the closure of the neural tube, consist only of a two-layered membrane.
a. Ependyma forms the inside of the membrane.
b. Pia mater forms the outside of the membrane, covering the external surface of the ependyma.

3. Perforations of the rhombencephalic roof plate
a. On about the fiftieth day of gestation, the posterior medullary velum perforates to form the median **foramen of Magendie**.
b. Similar perforations occur in the pia–ependymal roof plate membrane at the lateral recesses, forming lateral **foramina of Luschka**.
c. These perforations allow cerebrospinal fluid (CSF) to escape from the neural canal into the subarachnoid space.

4. The expanded, rhomboid-shaped floor of the fourth ventricle, the **rhomboid fossa**, justifies the term **rhombencephalon** for the hindbrain (see Figs. 8-3 and 8-8).

5. Extent of the fourth ventricle
a. Rostrally, the fourth ventricle gradually narrows into the aqueduct of the midbrain (see Fig. 1-7).
b. Caudally, the fourth ventricle abruptly narrows into the central canal of the spinal cord.
c. Laterally, the fourth ventricle has its widest diameter at the **lateral recesses** of the rhomboid fossa (see Fig. 8-3).
(1) The plane across the lateral recesses marks the plane of the pontomedullary junction.
(2) This plane also marks the peak of the fourth ventricle, the fastigium, where the anterior and posterior medullary vela meet (see Fig. 8-6).

C. Derivatives of the alar plates and rhombic lips

1. Neuroblasts proliferate prodigiously in the rhombic lips of the alar plates; some remain more or less in situ dorsally, but others migrate ventrally into the expanding mantle zone and tegmentum.
a. The neuroblasts that remain more or less in situ dorsally form the:
(1) Cerebellum from the pontine rhombic lips
(2) Auditory (cochlear) and vestibular nuclei, the special somatic afferent (SSA) nuclei

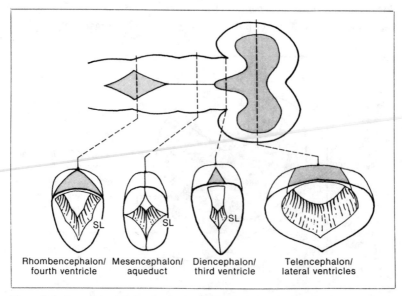

| Rhombencephalon/ fourth ventricle | Mesencephalon/ aqueduct | Diencephalon/ third ventricle | Telencephalon/ lateral ventricles |

Figure 8-8. Dorsal view of the developing brain (*above*) and corresponding cross sections (*below*). The membranous portions of the roof plate are shaded. *SL* = sulcus limitans.

   b. The neuroblasts that migrate ventrally form:
- **(1)** Inferior olivary nuclei of the medullary tegmentum for the olivocerebellar motor pathways
- **(2)** Nuclei of the pontine basis for the corticopontocerebellar motor pathway
- **(3)** Superior olivary nuclei of the pontine tegmentum for the auditory sensory pathways

2. Surface protrusions
   a. Three of these new rhombic lip derivatives form protrusions visible on the external surface of the brainstem:
- **(1)** Cerebellum
- **(2)** Inferior olivary complex (see the olivary eminence in the medulla in Figs. 8-22 and 8-23C)
- **(3)** Bulk of the basis pontis

   b. Massive circuitry links these three structures of common embryologic origin into a system that coordinates skeletal muscle contraction during voluntary movement.

D. Brainstem somites

1. Somite plan and somite neuronal columns
   a. The somite plan of the embryonic spinal cord continues to the rostral end of the midbrain, where the rostral-most motor cranial nerve, CN III, exits.
   b. Correspondingly, both spinal cord and brainstem develop nuclear groups in basal (motor) and alar (sensory) plates, separated by a sulcus limitans (see Fig. 8-8).

2. Fate of the rostral, intermediate, and caudal groups of cranial somites
   a. The **rostral** group of cranial somites, opposite the midbrain, produce extraocular muscles that rotate the eyeballs. CN III, CN IV, and CN VI innervate these muscles.
   b. The **caudal** group of cranial somites, opposite the medulla, produce the tongue muscles. CN XII, the hypoglossal nerve, a composite nerve formed by ventral rootlets of several somites, innervates the tongue muscles.
   c. The **intermediate** group of cranial somites, opposite the pons, mostly disappears, as do the tegmental nuclei, which would have formed their cranial nerves. Only the nucleus of CN VI, which innervates an extraocular muscle, remains in the GSE column in the pons. The GSE column, which is continuous through the entire spinal cord and caudal medulla, thus becomes discontinuous through the pontine tegmentum. (See the motor nuclei of CN III, CN IV, CN VI, and CN XI in Figure 8-11.)

3. The dorsal roots of many of the somites remain and adapt to serve the general and special sensory functions of the brainstem.

E. Branchial arches

1. Plan of the branchial arches
   a. The branchial or gill arches of water-dwelling vertebrates are incorporated in land-dwellers into the:
- **(1)** Cheeks, jaws, and ears
- **(2)** Pharynx, larynx, and upper esophagus

   b. Branchial arches resemble somites in:
- **(1)** Having a serial order (Fig. 8-9)
- **(2)** Receiving a single nerve
- **(3)** Receiving a single artery
- **(4)** Differentiating into skin, muscle, and bone
- **(5)** Retaining their original innervation as they undergo phylogenetic adaptation

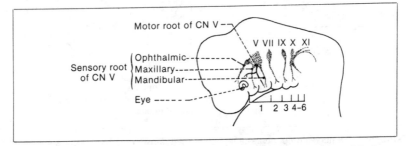

Figure 8-9. Lateral view of the head of an embryo showing the innervation of the branchial arches (*Arabic numerals*) by branchial cranial nerves (*Roman numerals*).

2. Innervation of branchial arches

    a. The five rostral-most branchial arches each receive and retain one nerve, CN V, CN VII, CN IX, CN X, and CN XI (see Fig. 9-9).

    b. The branchiomotor nuclei form from neuroblasts that migrate from the periventricular matrix zone of the basal plate to a ventrolateral site in the tegmentum (see Figs. 8-7, 8-10, and 8-27).

    c. Skeletal muscles move the branchial arches. The motor nuclei of CN V, CN VII, CN IX, CN X, and CN XI, which innervate these muscles, consist of alpha motoneurons similar to the somatomotor neurons. Nevertheless, they are classed as **SVE** in the theory of nerve components because the branchial arches, or gills, originally served a visceral function, oxygenation of the blood.

F. Theory of nerve components as applied to the cranial nerves

1. Various cranial nerves may contain the four components found in the spinal nerves: GSE, general visceral afferent (GVA), general visceral efferent (GVE), and general somatic afferent (GSA) axons. In addition, they may contain one or more special components, including:

    a. SVE axons of the branchiomotor system

    b. Special visceral afferent (SVA) axons of the special senses of taste and smell

    c. SSA axons of the special senses of hearing and equilibrium

2. These special senses require additional brainstem nuclei (Fig. 8-10; see Fig. 5-6).

G. Formation of the brainstem white matter

1. As neuroblasts expand the tegmentum, their axons commence to invade the surrounding marginal zone.

2. Finally, longitudinal axonal pathways surround the gray matter, as occurs in the spinal cord, but they do not travel longitudinally through the rhombic roof plate or quadrigeminal plate, which constitute the tectum.

3. Ground bundle of the brainstem. As occurs in the spinal cord, a ground bundle, the medial longitudinal fasciculus, interconnects somite nuclei CN III, CN IV, and CN VI. These nuclei innervate muscles that rotate the eyeball (see Fig. 8-15).

4. Long tracts. As occurs in the spinal cord, the long tracts, such as the pyramidal tracts, spinocerebellar tracts, and lemnisci, tend to accumulate on the periphery of the brainstem gray matter (not including the tectum). In the basis pontis and ventral part of the tegmentum, gray matter does intermingle with the long tracts.

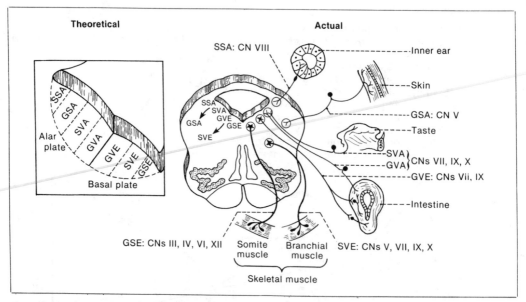

Figure 8-10. Theory of nerve components as applied to the brainstem. *SSA* = special somatic afferent; *GSA* = general somatic afferent; *SVA* = special visceral afferent; *GVA* = general visceral afferent; *GVE* = general visceral efferent; *SVE* = special visceral efferent; *GSE* = general somatic efferent.

IV. INTRODUCTION TO THE CRANIAL NERVES

A. Definition. A cranial nerve is any one of twelve paired major nerves that run through a major foramen in the base of the skull (see Fig. 8-13). The cranial nerves differ in embryologic origin, phylogeny, function, and fiber composition.

B. Numbers and names of the cranial nerves

1. The **number** tells:
   a. The rostrocaudal order in which the nerves exit from the series of foramina in the base of the skull (see Fig. 8-13)
   b. The rostrocaudal order in which the nerves attach to the brain, with the exception of CN XI, which attaches to the rostral end of the spinal cord (see Fig. 8-1)
2. The **name** tells something about the course or function of the nerve but otherwise has no systematic meaning (Table 8-1).

C. Classification of the cranial nerves. Grouping the 12 cranial nerves into three sets, special sensory, somatomotor, and branchial, based on the theory of nerve components, makes them much easier to learn (Table 8-2).

1. Solely special sensory set (SSSS): CN I, CN II, and CN VIII. The three nerves of the SSSS contain no motor fibers to muscles or glands (see Table 8-2).
   a. CN I, the **olfactory nerve**, is not quite a nerve. It consists only of axonal filaments, which synapse on the olfactory bulb.
   b. CN II, the **optic nerve**, conveys axons from the retina, but it is a stalk grown out from the diencephalon, not actually a peripheral nerve. All cranial nerves after CN I and CN II are true peripheral nerves histologically.
   c. CN VIII, the **vestibulocochlear nerve**, consists of vestibular and cochlear (auditory) divisions. CN VIII, a homologue of dorsal root ganglia, has no ventral root.
   d. Setting aside CN I, CN II, and CN VIII leaves only nine to consider, four in the GSE set and five in the SVE set.

2. Somitic or somatomotor (GSE) set: CN III, CN IV, CN VI, and CN XII. The somatomotor set contrasts directly with the SSSS because of the following.
   a. The nerves are all somitic nerves directly homologous with spinal nerves.
   b. The nerves are essentially motor (GSE) in function.

Table 8-1. Twelve Cranial Nerves

Number/Name/Derivation of Name	Brief Summary of Function
I Olfactory	Smells
II Optic	Sees
III Oculomotor	Moves eyeball and constricts pupil
IV Trochlear [tendon runs through trochlea (pulley)]	Moves eyeball
V Trigeminal (three large sensory branches)	Feels front half of head and chews
VI Abducens (leads eyeball away from sagittal plane)	Moves eyeball
VII Facial	Moves face; tears, tastes, and salivates
VIII Vestibulocochlear (to vestibule and cochlea)	Equilibriates and hears
IX Glossopharyngeal (runs to tongue and pharynx)	Tastes, salivates, and swallows and monitors carotid body and sinus
X Vagus (vagrant, wandering from pharynx to splenic flexure of colon)	Tastes, swallows, lifts palate, and phonates; sensorimotor to thoracicoabdominal viscera
XI Spinal accessory (arises in spinal cord to convey some accessory fibers from medulla to CN X)	Turns head and shrugs shoulders
XII Hypoglossal (runs under tongue)	Moves tongue

Table 8-2. Functional Components of the Three Sets of Cranial Nerves

	GSE	SVE	GVE	GVA	SVA	GSA	SSA
Solely special sensory set							
I					+		
II							+
VIII							+
Somatomotor set							
III	+		+			+*	
IV	+					+*	
VI	+					+*	
XII	+					+*	
Branchial set							
V		+				+	
VII		+	+	+	+	+	
IX		+	+	+	+	+	
X		+	+	+	+	+	
XI		+				+*	

GSE = general somatic efferent; SVE = special visceral efferent; GVE = general visceral efferent; GVA = general visceral afferent; SVA = special visceral afferent; GSA = general somatic afferent; SSA = special somatic afferent.

*Proprioceptive GSA components only; no cutaneous or special senses.

c. The nerves convey only a small GSA sensory component for proprioception and no other special or general sensation. Although the nerves convey some proprioceptive afferents from their muscles, they lack individual dorsal root ganglia. Their afferent perikarya for proprioception may be:
  (1) Scattered along the course of the nerves
  (2) Gathered into the huge ganglion of the trigeminal nerve or in its mesencephalic nucleus (the proprioceptive fibers enter the motor cranial nerves by a peripheral anastomosis with the trigeminal nerve branches)
d. Peripheral distribution
  (1) CN III, CN IV, and CN VI innervate only muscles of the eyes, thus forming an **optomotor group** (see Fig. 8-15).
  (2) Only CN III of the somatomotor group conveys autonomic axons—parasympathetic axons to the ciliary and pupilloconstrictor muscles.
  (3) CN XII innervates the tongue muscles. It conveys proprioceptive sensation but no taste, touch, or other sensations.
e. Setting aside the SSSS and the GSE or somite nerves reduces the problem to five cranial nerves.

3. Branchial arch (SVE) set: CN V, CN VII, CN IX, CN X, and CN XI (see Fig. 8-9)
  a. Each SVE nerve innervates skeletal muscles of branchial arch origin. Two of the nerves, CN V and CN XI, have no other motor components.
  b. First, set aside CN XI.
    (1) The simplest of the set, CN XI differs because it arises in the gray matter of the cervical spinal cord and enters the skull through the foramen magnum (see Fig. 8-22).
    (2) Essentially, it is a motor nerve innervating only skeletal muscles (the trapezius and sternocleidomastoid muscles) and has only a proprioceptive sensory component; therefore, it resembles the somatomotor set.
    (3) Now there are only four cranial nerves left, all sensorimotor.
  c. Next, set aside CN V.
    (1) CN V differs from CN XI and the remaining branchial nerves, CN VII, CN IX, and CN X, because it has three huge (GSA) sensory divisions in addition to its small (SVE) motor root.
    (2) CN V lacks special sensory fibers and motor fibers to glands and smooth muscle.
    (3) Setting aside CN V and CN XI, the first and last of the branchial group, leaves only CN VII, CN IX, and CN X, which, while complex, share a common plan.
  d. CN VII, CN IX, and CN X have five components in common, SVE, GVE, GVA, SVA, and GSA (Table 8-3).

Table 8-3. Nerve Components of CN VII, CN IX, and CN X and Their Peripheral Distribution

	Branchiomotor (SVE)	Visceromotor (GVE) (All Parasympathetic Nerves)	GVA	Taste (SVA)	GSA
CN VII	To all muscles of the face and facial orifices and to the stapedius muscles	To lacrimal, submandibular, and sublingual glands of the head, except the parotid gland; to the nasal mucosa	From the posterior naso-pharynx and soft palate; from the salivary glands	From the anterior two-thirds of the tongue (clinically significant)	Twig from the ear
CN IX	To the pharyngeal plexus for swallowing	To the parotid gland and the pharyngeal mucosa	From the soft palate and upper pharynx and from the carotid body and sinus	From the posterior two-thirds of the tongue (clinically insignificant)	Twig from the ear
CN X	To the pharyngeal plexus and laryngeal muscles (via the accessory branch of CN XI)	To the pharyngeal and laryngeal mucosa and to the glands and smooth muscle of the thoracicoabdominal viscera; sends inhibitory axons to the heart	From the pharynx and larynx and the thoracico-abdominal viscera; from the aortic bodies	From the region of the epiglottis (clinically insignificant)	Twig from the ear

SVE = special visceral efferent; GVE = general visceral efferent; GVA = general visceral afferent; SVA = special visceral afferent; GSA = general somatic afferent.

V. ANATOMICAL RELATIONSHIPS OF THE CRANIAL NERVES TO THE BRAINSTEM AND SKULL BASE

A. Location of the cranial nerve nuclei within the brainstem

1. The cranial nerve nuclei occupy sites in the brainstem predicted by the theory of nerve components (Fig. 8-11).

2. **Sensory nuclei are located dorsolaterally in the tegmentum** in the part derived from the alar plate (see Fig. 8-10).
   a. **Trigeminal sensory nucleus.** Notice in Figure 8-11 that the trigeminal sensory nucleus extends from the midbrain into the rostral part of the spinal cord. It is the only sensory or motor nuclear column that is continuous through the length of the brainstem.
   b. The **nucleus solitarius**, while confined to the medulla, mediates taste (SVA) and GVA sensation from CN VII, CN IX, and CN X.
   c. The **cochlear** and **vestibular** nuclei straddle the pontomedullary junction.

3. **Motor nuclei.** The motor nuclear columns of the brainstem show gaps because various nuclear groupings have disappeared during phylogenetic retrogression of their peripheral somite or branchial arch tissues.
   a. The **somatomotor (GSE) nuclei** are all located in the paramedian plane, just ventral to the floor of the fourth ventricle or aqueduct, where they are adjacent to the medial longitudinal fasciculus. On Figure 8-11, draw a colored line down through these nuclei to emphasize their paramedian location.
   b. The **branchiomotor (SVE) nuclei** all migrate into the ventrolateral part of the tegmentum (see Fig. 8-10). Draw a line of another color through these nuclei on Figure 8-11 to emphasize their location.
   c. One continuous branchiomotor or SVE nucleus, the nucleus ambiguus, serves CN IX and CN X.
   d. The **visceromotor nuclei**, the preganglionic parasympathetic nuclei, occupy in general the location predicted from their site in the spinal gray matter, although there appear to be medial and lateral groups of salivatory nuclei.

B. Anatomical segments of the cranial nerves. The clinician divides the cranial nerves into segments to think through their course to localize lesions. (Fig. 8-12).

C. Intra-axial segments of the motor divisions of the cranial nerves. The intra-axial course and sites of exit of the motor cranial nerves follow a predictable course.

1. **Somatomotor (GSE) group**
   a. Somatomotor CN III, CN VI, and CN XII drop fairly straight down (ventrally) in the paramedian plane (see CN XII in Fig. 8-27) to exit in the paramedian plane on the ventral surface of the brainstem (see Figs. 8-1 and 8-27).
   b. CN IV is an exception.

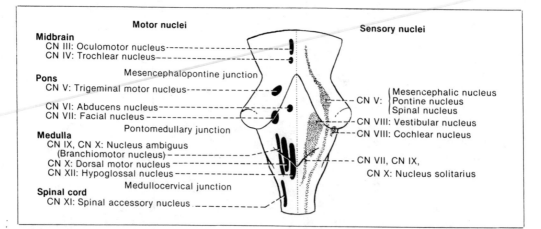

Figure 8-11. Dorsal view of the brainstem showing the location of the motor and sensory nuclei of the cranial nerves.

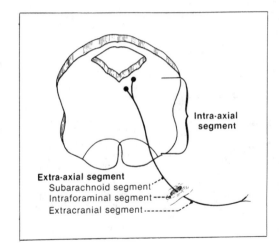

Intra-axial
segment

Extra-axial segment
Subarachnoid segment'
Intraforaminal segment---
Extracranial segment--------

Figure 8-12. Segments of cranial nerves for "thinking through" the course of nerve impulses.

      (1) It undergoes a complete internal decussation.
      (2) It **exits dorsally** through the tectum at the junction of the quadrigeminal plate with the anterior medullary velum. Again, however, being a somitic nerve, it exits in the paramedian plane.

   2. Branchial arch (SVE) group. The branchial arch nerves tend to undergo an internal loop before exiting.
     a. CN VII makes the most distinctive loop, forming an actual **genu** around the nucleus of CN VI (see Fig. 8-30).
     b. CN V is the exception in this group; it does not make a distinct internal loop.

 D. Sites of attachment of the cranial nerves to the neuraxis

   1. Three cranial nerves do not attach to the brainstem.
     a. CN I, the olfactory nerve, attaches to the olfactory bulb. It is the only nerve to attach to the cerebrum itself (see Fig. 8-14*A*).
     b. CN II, the optic nerve, attaches to the diencephalon and is the only cranial nerve to do so.
     c. CN XI attaches to the spinal cord, the only cranial nerve to do so.

   2. The remaining cranial nerves all attach to the brainstem.
     a. The **somatomotor (GSE) nerves** all attach in a line along the paramedian plane. CN III, CN VI, and CN XII attach ventrally, and CN IV attaches dorsally. Draw a colored line through them on Figure 8-1.
     b. The **branchial arch (SVE) nerves** all attach in a line **lateral to the somatomotor nerves.** Draw a line of another color through the branchial nerves on Figure 8-1.

   3. CN VI, CN VII, and CN VIII attach in numerical, **ventrodorsal order** at the pontomedullary sulcus (see Figs. 8-1 and 8-2).

 E. Sites of exit of the cranial nerves from the skull. The cranial nerves all cross the subarachnoid space to exit through foramina in the base of the skull (Fig. 8-13).

VI. PERIPHERAL DISTRIBUTION OF THE CRANIAL NERVES

 A. SSSS cranial nerves: CN I, CN II, and CN VIII

   1. CN I (olfactory nerve)
     a. The **functional component** is SVA, smell only.
     b. Primary neurons are bipolar cells in the nasal mucosa, outside the skull (Fig. 8-14; see Fig. 8-14*A*).
     c. The nerve is not a trunk but only the proximal axon filaments that pierce the cribriform plate.
     d. The **central synapse** is in the olfactory bulb.
     e. The **clinical effect of a nerve lesion** is the loss of smell (**anosmia**).

   2. CN II (optic nerve) [see Chapter 10, section III C]

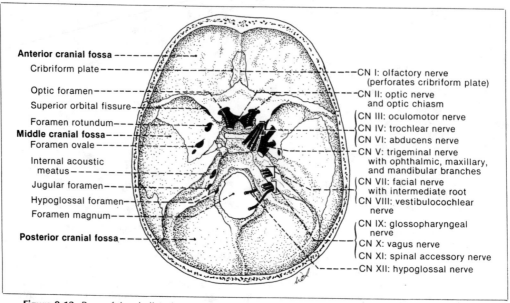

Figure 8-13. Base of the skull (calvaria removed) to show the foramina traversed by the cranial nerves.

3. **CN VIII (vestibulocochlear nerve)** [see Fig. 8-36]
   a. The **functional component** is SSA, divided into cochlear and vestibular systems.
   b. The **primary neurons are bipolar**. They are:
      (1) In the spiral ganglion of the cochlea for hearing
      (2) In the vestibular (Scarpa's) ganglion in the internal auditory meatus for the vestibular system (see Fig. 8-37)
   c. The **central synapse** (secondary neuron) is in cochlear or vestibular nuclei, respectively. Figures 8-36 and 8-37 show the pathways.
   d. For the **clinical effects of nerve lesions**, see sections X D 8 and E 11.

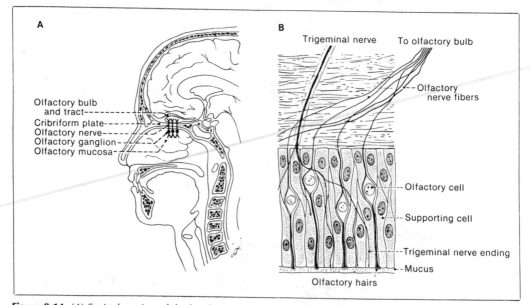

Figure 8-14. (*A*) Sagittal section of the head to show the olfactory ganglion and bulb. (*B*) Detail of the olfactory mucosa to show its dual innervation, the olfactory nerve (CN I) for smell and the trigeminal nerve (CN V) for other sensations. (Adapted with permission from Amoore JE, Johnston JW Jr, Rubin M: The stereochemical theory of odor. *Sci Am* 210:42, 1964.)

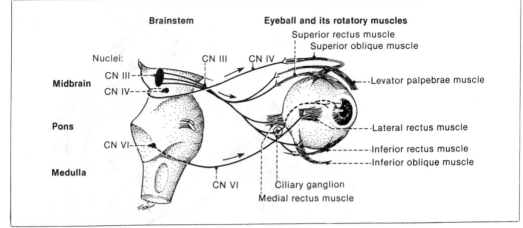

Figure 8-15. Peripheral distribution of CN III, CN IV, and CN VI.

B. GSE (somatomotor) cranial nerves: CN III, CN IV, CN VI, and CN XII

   1. CN III, CN IV, and CN VI are detailed in Chapter 10, section V B–D (Fig. 8-15).

   2. CN XII (hypoglossal nerve) [Fig. 8-16]

   a. Functional components

      (1) The **GSE** component innervates intrinsic and extrinsic tongue muscles.

      (2) The **GSA** component (proprioception only) has peripheral anastomoses with CN V.

   b. The **motor nucleus** is the hypoglossal nucleus in the caudal medullary tegmentum (see Fig. 8-11).

   c. The **major clinical effects of a nerve lesion** are paralysis of ipsilateral tongue muscles with difficulty in speaking and swallowing and clinically visible atrophy of the paralyzed half of the tongue.

C. SVE (branchial arch) cranial nerves: CN V, CN VII, CN IX, CN X, and CN XI

   1. CN V (trigeminal nerve) [Fig. 8-17]

   a. Functional components

      (1) The **SVE** component innervates the chewing muscles (as well as the tensor tympani and tensor palatini).

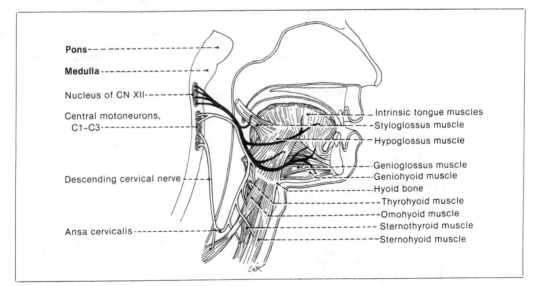

Figure 8-16. Peripheral distribution of CN XII. The hypoglossal nerve is in *black*; the cervical nerves are in *white*.

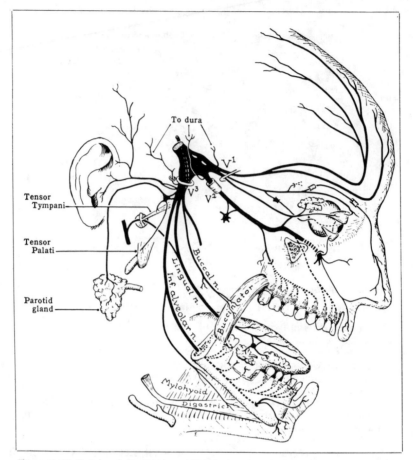

Figure 8-17. Peripheral distribution of CN V, the trigeminal nerve. *V1* = ophthalmic branch; *V2* = maxillary branch; *V3* = mandibular branch. (Reprinted with permission from Grant JCB: *An Atlas of Anatomy*, 2nd ed. Baltimore, Williams and Wilkins, 1947, p 468.)

   (2) The **GSA** component mediates touch and pain sensation from the face; the mucous membranes of the nose, sinuses, and tongue; and the dura mater as well as proprioception from most of the head muscles. Thus, CN V essentially mediates somatic sensation from the front half of the head, from the interaural line forward (see Figs. 8-17 and 8-38).
   b. The central trigeminal sensory nucleus extends from the midbrain to the spinal cord (see Fig. 8-11).
   c. The trigeminal motor nucleus is confined to the pons (see Fig. 8-11).
   d. Major clinical signs of a nerve lesion
      (1) Sensory loss or pain in one or more of the three peripheral divisions
      (2) Loss of corneal reflex
      (3) Paralysis of ipsilateral chewing muscles

2. CN VII (facial nerve) [Fig. 8-18]
   a. Functional components (see Table 8-3)
   b. Peripheral ganglia (see Fig. 8-18)
      (1) Sensory: geniculate ganglion
      (2) Parasympathetic: sphenopalatine (pterygopalatine) and submandibular ganglia
   c. The **central sensory nucleus**, which is both GVA and SVA, is the nucleus solitarius and is shared with CN IX and CN X.
   d. Motor nuclei
      (1) The **SVE** nucleus is the facial nucleus in the caudal pontine tegmentum (see Fig. 8-11).

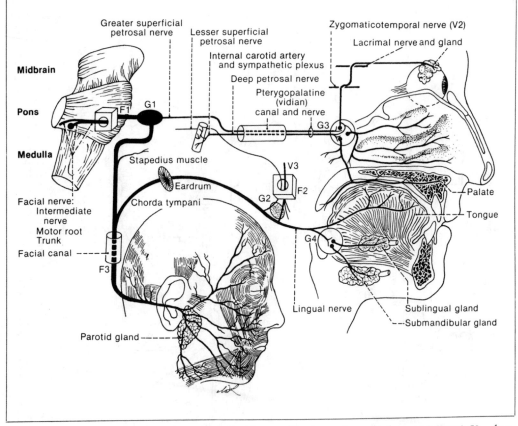

Figure 8-18. Peripheral distribution of CN VII, the facial nerve. *F1* = internal acoustic foramen (meatus); *F2* = foramen ovale; *F3* = stylomastoid foramen; *G1* = geniculate ganglion; *G2* = otic ganglion; *G3* = pterygopalatine ganglion; *G4* = submandibular ganglion; *V* = CN V branches.

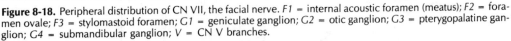

(2) The **GVE** nuclei are the salivatory nuclei in the caudal pontine tegmentum.

e. The **distribution of CN VII is simplified by considering it as two nerves**, the facial nerve proper (i.e., the motor root) and the intermediate nerve of Wrisberg.

(1) The **facial nerve proper** is the motor root (SVE). Figure 8-19 shows that the SVE motor fibers:

(a) Run through the middle ear, where they supply the stapedius muscle and separate from the chorda tympani

(b) Drop through the facial canal to emerge through the stylomastoid foramen

(c) Run through, but not to, the parotid gland to disperse to the facial muscles

(2) The **intermediate nerve of Wrisberg** is called intermediate because it is between CN VII proper and CN VIII. It is a sensorimotor nerve that conveys preganglionic parasympathetic axons (GVE) and taste axons (SVA) [see Fig. 8-19]. The taste fibers arise from unipolar, dorsal root–type neurons of the geniculate ganglion.

(3) Notice that the facial nerve proper and the intermediate root:

(a) Separate where they attach to the pontomedullary sulcus (see Fig. 8-2)

(b) Unite to run through the internal auditory meatus

(c) Separate again at the geniculate ganglion and chorda tympani nerve to reach their terminations

(4) The preganglionic parasympathetic axons of the intermediate nerve divide into two streams (see Fig. 8-19).

(a) One stream goes via the greater superficial petrosal nerve to the pterygopalatine ganglion and hence to the lacrimal gland and glands of the nasal mucosa.

(b) The other stream goes via the chorda tympani to the submandibular ganglion and hence to the submandibular and sublingual salivary glands and glands of the oral mucosa.

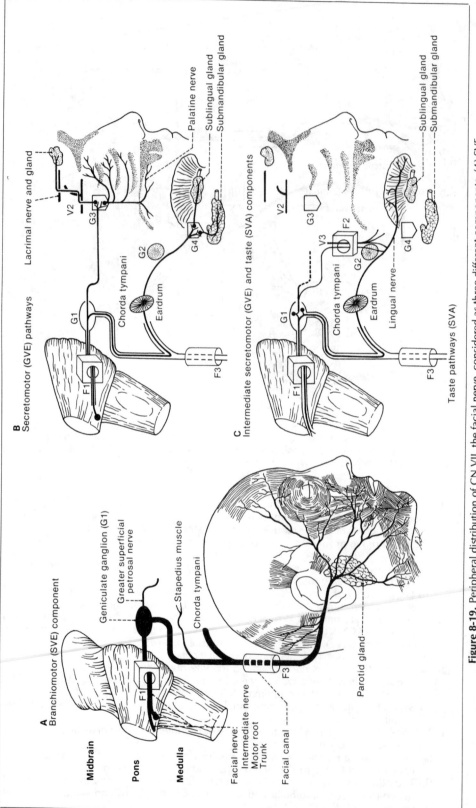

Figure 8-19. Peripheral distribution of CN VII, the facial nerve, considered as three different components. (*A*) SVE (special visceral efferent) component to facial muscles. (*B*) GVE (general visceral efferent) secretomotor component of the intermediate nerve to glands. (*C*) SVA (special visceral afferent) component of the intermediate nerve for taste on the anterior two-thirds of the tongue. *F1* = internal acoustic meatus; *F2* = foramen ovale; *F3* = stylomastoid foramen; *G1* = geniculate ganglion; *G2* = otic ganglion; *G3* = pterygopalatine ganglion; *G4* = submandibular ganglion; *V* = CN V branches.

(5) The SVA axons for taste traverse four named peripheral nerve segments, in proximo-distal order (see Fig. 8-19) the:
  (a) Intermediate nerve of Wrisberg
  (b) Trunk of CN VII
  (c) Chorda tympani
  (d) Lingual branch of the trigeminal nerve
(6) The GVE axons to the salivary glands and the SVA axons may meander from nerve to nerve at the base of the skull. Thus, the otic and submandibular ganglia do not neatly divide the parotid and the submandibular and sublingual glands. Similarly, some afferent axons for taste may detour from the chorda tympani to the greater superficial petrosal nerve. Nevertheless, the simplified diagrams given here suffice for clinical purposes.
  f. The **clinical signs of CN VII lesions** depend on the site of the lesion along the nerve and the fiber components affected. A proximal lesion affecting the main trunk of the nerve causes:
  (1) Paralysis of all the ipsilateral facial muscles
  (2) Hyperacusis due to stapedius muscle paralysis (the stapedius muscle dampens loud sounds)
  (3) Absence of lacrimation
  (4) Dry mouth from absence of salivary secretion
  (5) Loss of taste on the anterior two-thirds of the tongue (but not loss of touch, which is a CN V function)
  g. **CN VII as prototype.** CN V and CN XI are simple branchial nerves, having only SVE and GSA components. CN VII serves as the prototype of the three complicated branchial nerves, illustrating all of their common features (see Table 8-3).
3. **CN IX (glossopharyngeal nerve)** [Fig. 8-20]
  a. The **functional components** number five in all (see Table 8-3).
  b. **Peripheral ganglia**
    (1) **Sensory**: GSA superior ganglion and GVA and SVA inferior ganglion (see Fig. 8-20)
    (2) **Parasympathetic**: otic ganglion
  c. **Central sensory nuclei**
    (1) **GVA**: nucleus tractus solitarius
    (2) **SVA**: nucleus tractus solitarius for taste, shared with CN VII and CN X

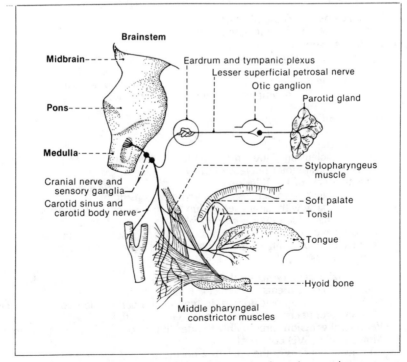

Figure 8-20. Peripheral distribution of CN IX, the glossopharyngeal nerve.

(3) GSA: trigeminal nucleus for the skin of the ear
d. **Motor nuclei** (see Fig. 8-11)
    (1) SVE: nucleus ambiguus in the medullary tegmentum
    (2) GVE: inferior salivatory nucleus in the medullary tegmentum
e. Notice in Figures 8-19 and 8-20 that the lesser superficial petrosal nerve essentially belongs to CN IX, whereas the greater superficial petrosal nerve belongs to CN VII.
f. **Overlapping central and peripheral distributions of CN IX and CN X**
    (1) Isolated lesions of either CN IX or CN X are rare for the following reasons.
        (a) CN IX and CN X share a common motor nucleus, the nucleus ambiguus, and a common sensory nucleus, the nucleus solitarius.
        (b) They cross the subarachnoid space together and both exit through the jugular foramen.
        (c) CN IX follows the course of CN X in the neck as far as CN IX goes, and both go similarly to the palate and pharynx.
    (2) CN IX shares pharyngeal and, in some individuals, palatal muscles with CN X. The one muscle that CN IX innervates exclusively, the stylopharyngeus muscle, cannot be tested clinically.
    (3) Three cranial nerves innervate palatal muscles.
        (a) CN V innervates the tensor palatini, a clinically unimportant muscle.
        (b) CN IX and, mainly, CN X innervate the levator palatini, the clinically most important muscle for palatal elevation. A lesion of CN X or, in some individuals, CN IX causes paralysis of elevation of the soft palate on the affected side.
    (4) CN IX innervates the carotid body and the carotid sinus. CN X innervates the aortic bodies and may overlap with CN IX to innervate the carotid body.
        (a) The carotid and aortic bodies stimulate breathing in response to low oxygen tension in the arterial blood.
        (b) The carotid sinus initiates reflexes that slow the heart in response to increased blood pressure.
g. **Clinical effects of CN IX nerve lesions**
    (1) Palatal palsy and loss of the gag reflex due to interruption of afferent or efferent palatal axons
    (2) Dysphagia due to paralysis of the pharyngeal constrictor muscles
    (3) Loss of carotid sinus and carotid body reflexes
    (4) Loss of taste on the posterior part of the tongue, which generally cannot be appreciated by the patient nor conveniently tested clinically

4. CN X (vagus nerve) [Fig. 8-21]
  a. Table 8-2 lists the five functional components.
  b. **Peripheral ganglia**
    (1) Sensory: superior (petrosal) ganglion for GSA and inferior (nodose) ganglion for GVA and SVA
    (2) Parasympathetic: ganglia and plexuses are in the thoracicoabdominal viscera (CN X innervates no parasympathetic ganglion in the head)
  c. **Central sensory nuclei**
    (1) SVA and GVA: nucleus solitarius
    (2) GSA (ear twig): trigeminal nucleus
  d. **Motor nuclei**
    (1) SVE: nucleus ambiguus in the medullary tegmentum (shared with CN IX)
    (2) GVE: dorsal motor nucleus of the vagus nerve
  e. **Clinical effects of CN X lesions**
    (1) Dysphagia due to paralysis of pharyngeal constrictors
    (2) Palatal palsy with nasal speech due to paralysis of the levator palatini muscle
    (3) Hoarseness due to vocal cord paralysis
    (4) Absence of vagus-mediated cardioinhibitory, respiratory, and gastrointestinal reflexes
    (5) Bilateral subdiaphragmatic vagotomy, leading to anorexia, vomiting, and progressive weight loss

5. CN XI (spinal accessory nerve) [Fig. 8-22]
  a. **Functional components**
    (1) SVE: to the sternocleidomastoid muscle and part of the trapezius muscle
    (2) GSA: proprioception from the muscles innervated
  b. **Peripheral ganglion**: presumably the dorsal root of C2 serves proprioception
  c. **Motor nuclei** (SVE) consist of:
    (1) Caudal neurons of the nucleus ambiguus
    (2) Rostral ventral horn neurons of the spinal cord (supraspinal nucleus)

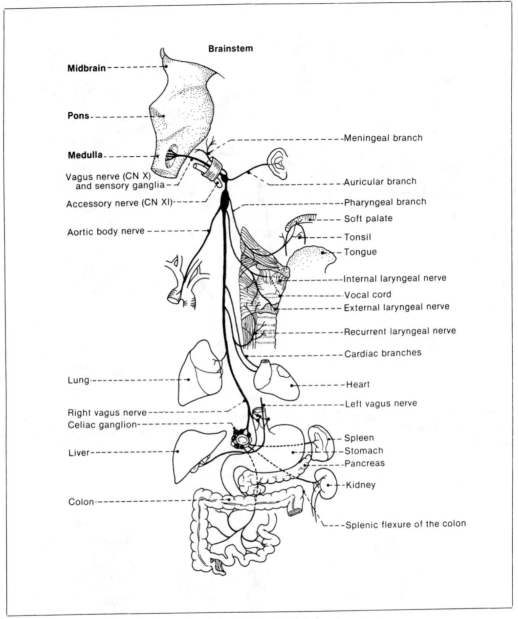

Figure 8-21. Peripheral distribution of CN X, the vagus nerve.

d. Nomenclature of the spinal accessory nerve
(1) The **spinal** part of the nerve arises in the spinal cord and innervates the sternocleido-mastoid muscle and part of the trapezius muscle.
(2) The **accessory** part merely conveys some vagal fibers, which accompany the spinal part of the nerve. These accessory fibers to the vagus nerve arise in the nucleus am-biguus and innervate the larynx (vocal cords) through the inferior (recurrent) laryngeal nerve (see Fig. 8-22).

e. Clinical signs of nerve interruption
(1) Weakness of head rotation due to sternocleidomastoid muscle paralysis
(2) Weakness of shoulder shrugging due to paralysis of the upper part of the trapezius muscle
(3) Vocal cord paralysis and hoarseness if accessory fibers are involved

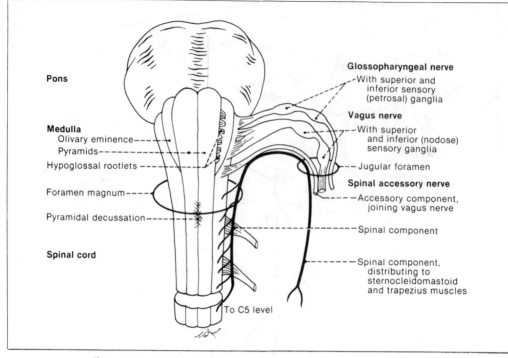

Figure 8-22. Peripheral distribution of CN XI, the spinal accessory nerve.

VII. AN ATLAS OF THE EXTERNAL AND INTERNAL ANATOMY OF THE BRAINSTEM.

Figures 8-23 through 8-35 provide an atlas, which will be referred to in sections VIII through XI, to follow.

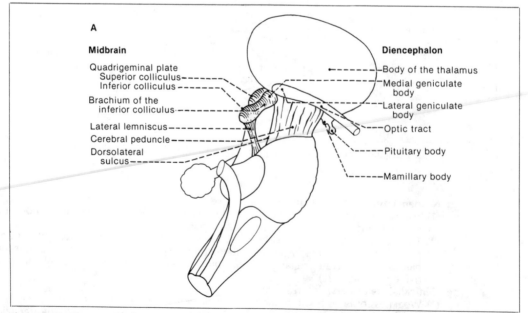

Figure 8-23. Gross external anatomy of the brainstem. (*A*) Midbrain and diencephalon. (*B*) Pons. (C) Medulla oblongata.

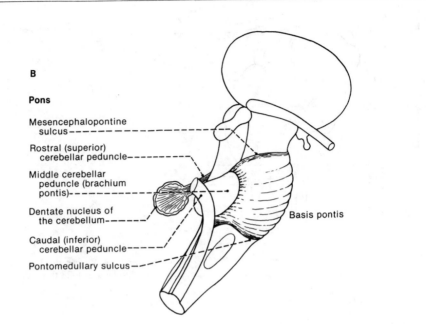

B

Pons

Mesencephalopontine sulcus

Rostral (superior) cerebellar peduncle

Middle cerebellar peduncle (brachium pontis)

Dentate nucleus of the cerebellum

Caudal (inferior) cerebellar peduncle

Pontomedullary sulcus

Basis pontis

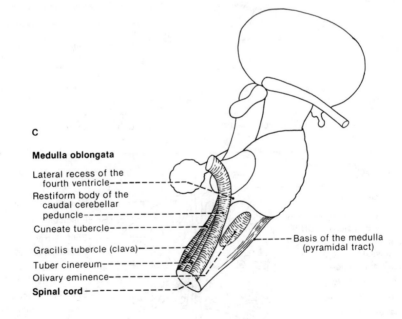

C

Medulla oblongata

Lateral recess of the fourth ventricle

Restiform body of the caudal cerebellar peduncle

Cuneate tubercle

Gracilis tubercle (clava)

Tuber cinereum

Olivary eminence

Spinal cord

Basis of the medulla (pyramidal tract)

Figure 8-23. Continued.

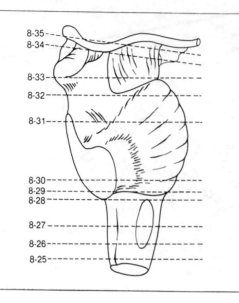

Figure 8-24. Key to the levels of the brainstem illustrated in Figures 8-25 through 8-35.

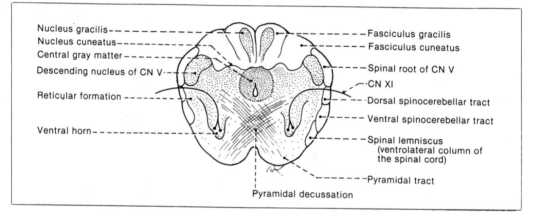

Nucleus gracilis
Nucleus cuneatus
Central gray matter
Descending nucleus of CN V
Reticular formation
Ventral horn

Fasciculus gracilis
Fasciculus cuneatus
Spinal root of CN V
CN XI
Dorsal spinocerebellar tract
Ventral spinocerebellar tract
Spinal lemniscus (ventrolateral column of the spinal cord)
Pyramidal tract

Pyramidal decussation

Figure 8-25. Transverse section of the cervicomedullary junction.

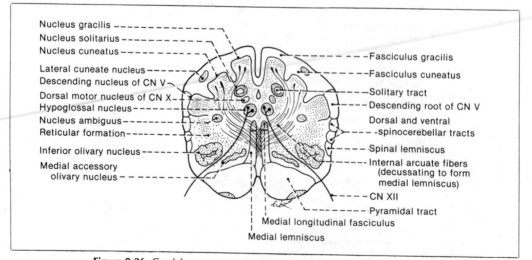

Nucleus gracilis
Nucleus solitarius
Nucleus cuneatus
Lateral cuneate nucleus
Descending nucleus of CN V
Dorsal motor nucleus of CN X
Hypoglossal nucleus
Nucleus ambiguus
Reticular formation
Inferior olivary nucleus
Medial accessory olivary nucleus

Fasciculus gracilis
Fasciculus cuneatus
Solitary tract
Descending root of CN V
Dorsal and ventral spinocerebellar tracts
Spinal lemniscus
Internal arcuate fibers (decussating to form medial lemniscus)
CN XII
Pyramidal tract

Medial longitudinal fasciculus
Medial lemniscus

Figure 8-26. Caudal-most transverse section of the medulla oblongata.

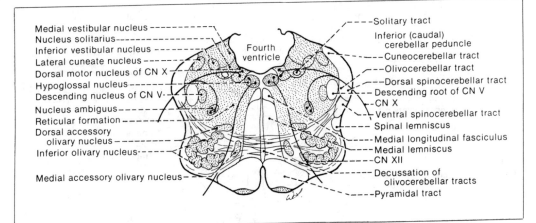

Figure 8-27. Caudal transverse section of the medulla oblongata.

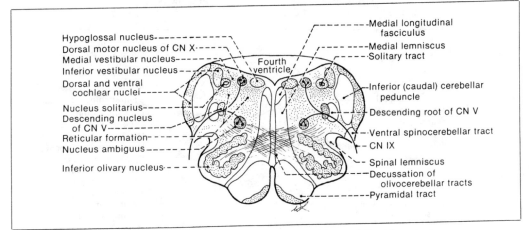

Figure 8-28. Midlevel transverse section of the medulla oblongata.

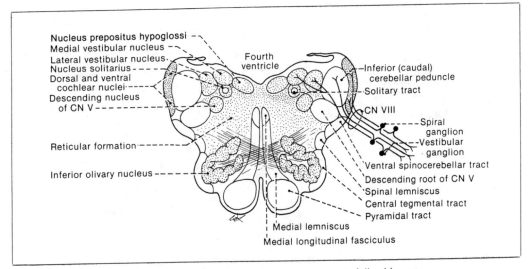

Figure 8-29. Rostral-most transverse section of the medulla oblongata.

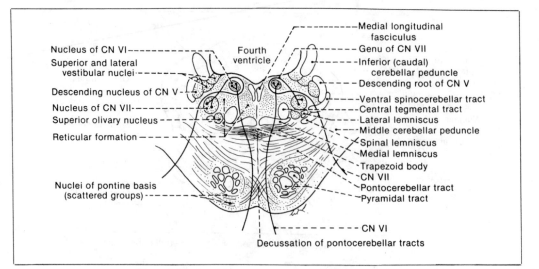

Figure 8-30. Caudal transverse section of the pons.

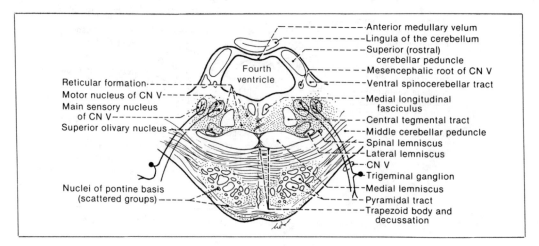

Figure 8-31. Rostral transverse section of the pons.

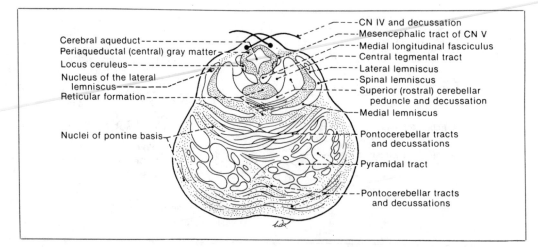
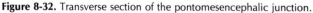

Figure 8-32. Transverse section of the pontomesencephalic junction.

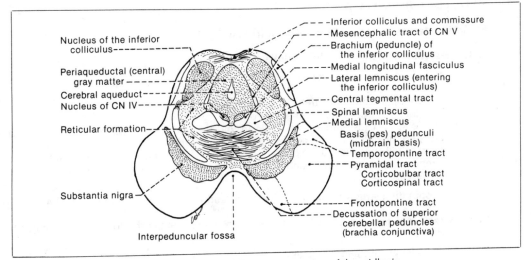

Figure 8-33. Caudal transverse section of the midbrain.

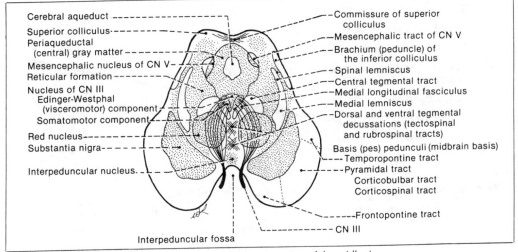

Figure 8-34. Rostral transverse section of the midbrain.

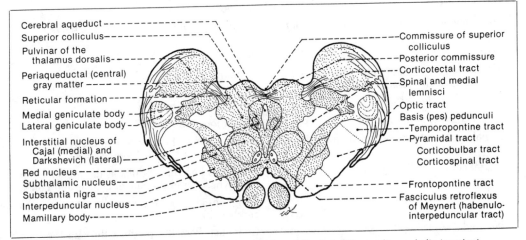

Figure 8-35. Rostral-most transverse section of the midbrain (midbrain–diencephalic junction).

VIII. MEDULLA OBLONGATA

A. Gross external anatomy of the medulla (review Fig. 8-23C)

B. Cross-sectional anatomy of the medulla

1. The medulla is an elaborated spinal cord.
   a. The alar and basal plates angle outward (see Fig. 8-8).
   b. The roof plate (tectum) stretches out.
   c. The gray matter (tegmentum) thickens.
   d. The long tracts assemble, as a shell, around the periphery of the gray matter. In Figure 8-27, commence with the cerebellar peduncle (upper right) and trace around the white matter shell consisting of the descending root of CN V, ventral spinocerebellar tract, spinal lemniscus, pyramidal tract, and dorsal to it, the medial longitudinal fasciculus and medial lemniscus.

2. **Corresponding structures of the spinal cord and medulla** are listed in Table 8-4.

C. Gray matter at the cervicomedullary transition zone. Identify the following in Figures 8-25 through 8-29.

1. GSA nuclei gracilis and cuneatus

2. GSA spinal nucleus and the tract of CN V (pain and temperature component), which merge with the substantia gelatinosa and the dorsolateral fasciculus of Lissauer

3. SVE nucleus of CN XI

4. GSE nucleus of CN XII

5. SVE nucleus ambiguus for CN IX and CN X

6. GVE dorsal motor nucleus of CN X (the nucleus ambiguus is the ventral motor nucleus of CN X)

7. GVA and SVA nuclei and the solitary tract for CN VII, CN IX, and CN X

8. SSA vestibular nuclei

9. Inferior olivary complex

Table 8-4. Corresponding Structures of the Spinal Cord and Medulla

Spinal Cord Structure	Medullary Structure
Central canal	Fourth ventricle
Roof plate	Posterior medullary velum
Ventral motoneurons	Nucleus of CN XII
Motoneurons of CN XI	Nucleus ambiguus
Preganglionic parasympathetic neurons of the sacral cord	Dorsal motor nucleus of the vagus nerve
Reticular nucleus	Reticular formation
Substantia gelatinosa of Rolando and dorsolateral fasciculus of Lissauer	Spinal nucleus and tract of CN V
Nucleus dorsalis of Clarke	Lateral cuneate nucleus
Intersegmental ground bundles	Medial longitudinal fasciculus
Spinal lemniscus (lateral and ventral spinothalamic tracts)	Continues into the medial lemniscus, which is also joined by the trigeminal lemniscus
Dorsal column pathway	Continues into the medulla as the medial lemniscus after synapsing in the nuclei gracilis and cuneatus
Spinocerebellar tracts	Continues through the medulla into the pons and cerebellum
Pyramidal tract	Continues from the medulla through the length of the spinal cord

D. Decussations at the cervicomedullary junction. Five clinically important decussations occur at the cervicomedullary transition. They are listed in dorsoventral order.

  1. Reticulospinal respiratory pathways for automatic breathing, just ventral to the obex of the fourth ventricle (see Fig. 8-43)

  2. Internal arcuate fibers, which consist of the:
    a. Trigeminal lemniscus, from the spinal nucleus of CN V (see Fig. 8-38)
    b. Medial lemniscus, from the nuclei gracilis and cuneatus (see Fig. 8-28)
    c. Olivocerebellar tracts from inferior olivary nuclei (see Figs. 8-26 and 8-27)

  3. Pyramidal tract decussation (see Fig. 8-25)

IX. MEDIAL LEMNISCUS

  A. Origin. The medial lemniscus originates from the nuclei gracilis and cuneatus, relay stations in the dorsal column pathway.

  1. As these axons sweep ventromedially to decussate, they form most of the caudal part of the internal arcuate decussation (see Fig. 8-26).

  2. The decussation of the olivocerebellar tracts forms most of the rostral part (see Fig. 8-27).

  B. Course of the medial lemniscus

  1. At its origin and through the medulla, the medial lemniscus runs in the paramedian zone (see Figs. 8-26 through 8-29).

  2. As the medial lemniscus ascends, two changes occur.
    a. Its location shifts.
    b. Other fiber systems join it.

  3. As it ascends into the pons, the lemniscus flattens out (see Figs. 8-30 and 8-31). In the midbrain, it shifts dorsolaterally to contact the lateral lemniscus (see Fig. 8-32).

  C. Additional fiber systems in the medial lemniscus

  1. As the medial lemniscus ascends into the pons, two other ascending sensory pathways join it:
    a. The **trigeminal lemniscus**, which originates in the spinal nucleus of CN V and has decussated
    b. The **spinal lemniscus**, consisting of lateral and ventral spinothalamic tracts, which have both decussated in the spinal cord

  2. Some **corticobulbar fibers** depart from the corticobulbar tract in the midbrain to **descend** in the medial lemniscus.

  3. Thus, the composition and position of the medial lemniscus varies depending on the brainstem level.

  D. Termination of the medial lemniscus

  1. By definition, all lemnisci end in a specific thalamic sensory relay nucleus. The medial lemniscus ends in the posteromedial and lateral ventral nuclei, which relay to the somatosensory receptive area in the postcentral gyrus of the parietal lobe.

  2. The ascending pain and temperature fibers of the spinal lemniscus send collaterals into the reticular formation along the way to the thalamus, but the medial lemniscal fibers continuing the dorsal column pathway probably do not.

X. PONS

  A. Gross external anatomy (see Fig. 8-23B)

  B. The pons consists of longitudinal, peduncular, motor cranial nerve nuclei, and sensory cranial nerve nuclei triads.

  1. Longitudinal triads
    a. The **tectum** consists of the anterior medullary velum.
    b. The **tegmentum** is a relatively thin plate of gray matter bounded ventrally by the medial lemniscus.
    c. The **basis**, a bulging belly, consists of longitudinally coursing cortical efferent fibers and nuclear masses, which relay the corticopontocerebellar pathway.

2. Peduncular triads. Three paired peduncles, **caudal**, **middle**, and **rostral**, attach the cerebellum to the pons. They consist solely of afferent and efferent cerebellar tracts (see Fig. 8-23B).

3. Motor cranial nerve triad: CN V, CN VI, and CN VII
   a. The three motor nuclei, CN V, CN VI (GSE), and CN VII (SVE), occupy the positions expected from the theory of nerve components (see Fig. 8-11).
   b. The one major peculiarity is the internal loop of CN VII over the nucleus of CN VI (see Fig. 8-30).

4. Sensory cranial nerve triads
   a. The pons contains parts of three sensory nuclei: rostral continuations of the **cochlear and vestibular nuclei of CN VIII** and part of the **sensory nucleus of CN V**.
   b. The sensory nucleus of CN V has three divisions (see Fig. 8-11), the:
      (1) Mesencephalic nucleus (GSA for proprioception)
      (2) Main sensory nucleus in the pons itself (GSA for touch)
      (3) Spinal nucleus in the medulla and rostral cervical cord (GSA for pain and temperature) [see Fig. 8-38]
   c. The trigeminal ganglion has three main peripheral sensory branches (see Figs. 8-17 and 8-38):
      (1) Ophthalmic (V1)
      (2) Mandibular (V2)
      (3) Maxillary (V3)

C. Anatomical features of the pontomedullary junction. Like the cervicomedullary junction, the pontomedullary junction is critical to know because of these facts.

1. CN VI, CN VII, and CN VIII attach in ventrodorsal order to the pontomedullary sulcus (see Fig. 8-1). You can organize a great deal of information around this fact.
   a. The somite nerve, CN VI, attaches most ventrally in the paramedian plane, as is typical of somite nerves.
   b. The branchiomotor nerve, CN VII, attaches laterally, as is typical of branchiomotor nerves.
   c. The sensory nerve, CN VIII, attaches most dorsolaterally, as is typical of sensory roots.
   d. If CN VI, CN VII, and CN VIII attach in the transverse line at the pontomedullary sulcus, then CN I through CN V must attach **rostral** to that plane and CN IX through CN XII must attach **caudal** to it.

2. The nuclei of CN VI and CN VII and the internal genu of CN VII lie just rostral to the plane of the pontomedullary junction.

3. CN V commences the transition from the pontine nucleus to the spinal nucleus, which mediates pain and temperature.

4. Salivatory nuclei are located in the dorsal tegmentum at the pontomedullary junction.

5. The cochlear and vestibular nuclei straddle the plane.

6. The pontomedullary plane separates the superior olivary complex and trapezoid body of the pons (the auditory relay system) from the inferior olivary complex of the medulla (the olivo-cerebellar component of the somatomotor system).

7. The **tallest point of the fourth ventricle**, the **fastigium**, and the **widest point**, the **lateral recesses**, are in the plane of the pontomedullary junction.

8. The cerebellum with its deep nuclei lies over the fastigium.

9. The caudal cerebellar peduncle conveying the dorsal spinocerebellar tract turns dorsally into the cerebellum just rostral to the plane.

10. The medial lemniscus begins to migrate laterally from its paramedian location in the medulla. It flattens out into a fillet as the other ascending lemnisci join it.

11. Ventrally, the pyramidal tracts emerge from the basis pontis into the medullary basis.

12. Ventrally, the vertebral arteries unite to form the basilar artery (see Fig. 15-9).

D. CN VIII, vestibular component (Fig. 8-36)

1. Phylogenetic relation of the vestibular and cochlear systems
   a. Phylogenetically, the vestibular system antedates the cochlear. The vestibular system is found in all vertebrates, while the cochlear system is found first in amphibians. In accordance with the law of lamination by phylogenesis, the cochlear nuclei are piled on dorsolateral or peripheral to the vestibular nuclei (see Fig. 8-29).

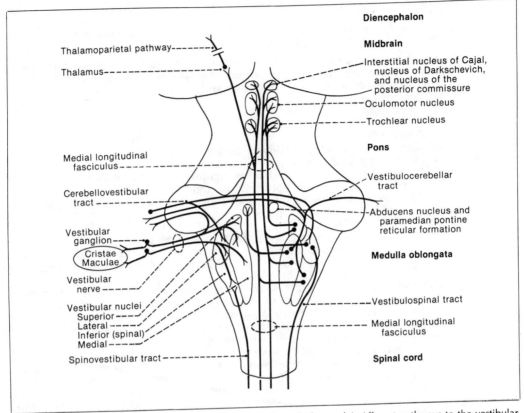

Figure 8-36. Pathways of the vestibulocochlear nerve and vestibular nuclei. Afferent pathways to the vestibular nuclei are on the left; efferents are on the right. The profuse to-and-fro connections with the reticular formation are not shown.

    b. The peripheral axons of the two systems travel in a common nerve to the brainstem, but they have different central pathways and different end organs.

2. Vestibular receptors
    a. The vestibular receptors respond to head movements and to the pull of gravity.
    b. Two vestibular receptors
        (1) Cristae of the ampullae of the semicircular canals detect rotational or angular acceleration.
        (2) Maculae of the utricle and saccule detect linear acceleration and the pull of gravity.

3. Vestibular ganglion
    a. The ganglion sits at the distal end of the internal auditory meatus, near the receptors.
    b. Its bipolar neurons have **distal and central processes**, the latter combining into the vestibular nerve.

4. Extra-axial course of the vestibular nerve
    a. The vestibular nerve, joined by the cochlear nerve, forms CN VIII. CN VIII travels centrally in the internal auditory canal along with the two components of CN VII, the motor root and the intermediate nerve (see Fig. 8-13).
    b. After crossing the subarachnoid space, CN VIII attaches to the pontomedullary junction near the lateral recess of the fourth ventricle.

5. Intra-axial connections of vestibular afferent fibers
    a. The caudal cerebellar peduncle splits the two entering groups of CN VIII fibers (see Fig. 8-29).
        (1) The **vestibular** fibers split away **ventrally** to reach the vestibular nuclei.
        (2) The **cochlear** fibers split away **dorsally** to enter the cochlear nuclei.
    b. The primary vestibular fibers terminate in:
        (1) Vestibular nuclei

(2) Cerebellum (flocculonodular lobe)
(3) Reticular formation
c. No primary vestibular fibers go directly to the spinal cord, other cranial nerve nuclei, the diencephalon, or the cerebrum.

6. **Vestibular nuclei.** The four vestibular nuclei straddle the pontomedullary junction. They contain the secondary neurons of the vestibular pathways (see Fig. 8-36).
   a. **Afferent connections of the vestibular nuclei**
      (1) Vestibular portion of CN VIII
      (2) Spinovestibular tract
      (3) Cerebellovestibular tracts
      (4) Reticulovestibular tracts
   b. **Efferent connections of the vestibular nuclei** (see Fig. 8-36)
      (1) Medial longitudinal fasciculus
         (a) The vestibular nuclei send axons into the medial longitudinal fasciculus, which connects the nuclei of CN III, CN IV, and CN VI.
         (b) Descending axons in the fasciculus also run into the cervical spinal cord and coordinate eye movements and head posture.
      (2) Vestibulospinal tracts
         (a) Direct tracts descend to the spinal cord from the vestibular nuclei.
         (b) The tracts facilitate the contraction of the extensor muscles, which support the body against collapse by the pull of gravity. (See the syndrome of **decerebrate rigidity** in section XIV E 1.)
      (3) Vestibulocerebellar pathways. These afferent and efferent pathways reflect the original derivation of the cerebellum as a vestibular system component (see Fig. 9-11). They are believed to coordinate the axial muscles to maintain the upright posture.
      (4) Vestibuloreticular pathways. Afferent and efferent connections of the vestibular nuclei with the reticular formation mediate the nausea, vomiting, pallor, and hypotension that accompany vestibular system disorders (motion sickness).
      (5) Vestibulothalamocortical pathway. The effects of vestibular stimulation reach conscious appreciation in the form of nausea and vertigo and contribute to a sense of balance. Some pathway presumably exists to the thalamus and cerebral cortex, in keeping with other conscious sensations; however, the exact course of this pathway is unclear.

7. **Three major functions of the vestibular system**
   a. The vestibular system **provides information about movement of the head** (linear or angular acceleration or deceleration) and **changes in head position** in relation to the pull of gravity. This aids in:
      (1) Coordinating the position of the eyes, head, and neck
      (2) Providing a sense of balance
   b. The vestibular system **increases the tone in the antigravity muscles**, which support the body against the pull of gravity.
   c. The vestibular system **tends to hold the eyes on a target when the head moves**, which is to say vestibular impulses counter-roll the eyes against the direction of head movement to keep them on their original fixation point.

8. **Clinical effects of vestibular nerve lesions.** An acute lesion of the vestibular nerve causes:
   a. Severe vertigo, with falling and past-pointing to the side of the lesion
   b. Nystagmus (oscillating eye movements) and oscillopsia (a sense of oscillation of objects viewed)
   c. Autonomic effects include:
      (1) Nausea and vomiting
      (2) Pallor
      (3) Sweating
      (4) Hypotension

E. **CN VIII, cochlear component** (Fig. 8-37)

1. **Cochlear receptor.** The **organ of Corti**, within the cochlea of the inner ear, is tonotopically organized to detect sounds of low to high frequencies. The tonotopic organization extends through the auditory pathway up to and including the auditory receptive cortex.

2. The **cochlear (spiral) ganglion.** The spiral ganglion, in the modiolus or core of the cochlea, contains the primary bipolar auditory neurons.

3. **Extra-axial course of the cochlear nerve**
   a. The central processes of the bipolar neurons unite into the cochlear (auditory) nerve in the

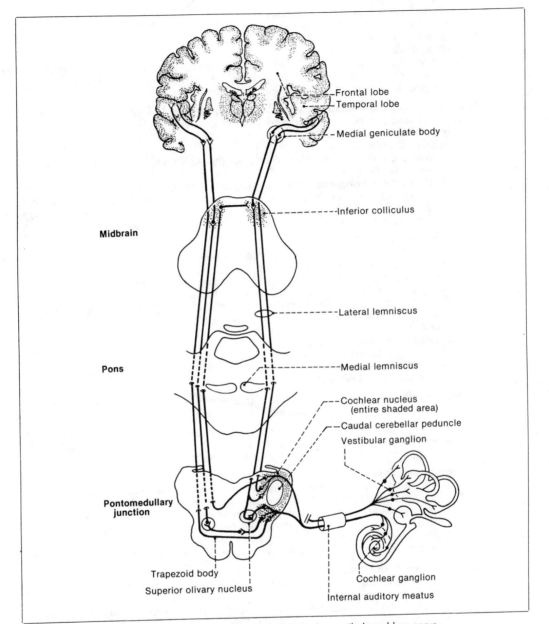

Figure 8-37. Cochlear pathways of CN VIII, the vestibulocochlear nerve.

distal end of the internal auditory canal. The cochlear nerve runs centrally through the auditory meatus in company with the vestibular nerve and CN VII.
  b. After crossing the subarachnoid space, the cochlear nerve enters the brainstem at the lateral recess of the fourth ventricle.

4. Intra-axial course of cochlear afferents
  a. The nerve divides into two divisions, one for the dorsal cochlear nucleus and the other for the ventral (see Fig. 8-37).
  b. The cochlear nuclei, which contain the secondary neuron of the auditory pathway, drape saddlebag fashion around the caudal cerebellar peduncle (see Fig. 8-37).

5. Efferent (secondary) pathways from the cochlear nuclei
  a. Most cochlear efferents synapse in:
    (1) Supplementary nuclei of the auditory pathway, including the:
      (a) Superior olivary complex

(b) Nuclei of the trapezoid body

(c) Nuclei of the lateral lemniscus

(2) Inferior colliculus

(3) Reticular formation

b. The secondary cochlear axons and the tertiary and quaternary axons from supplementary auditory nuclei form a trapezoidal configuration in the caudal pontine tegmentum, which is called the **trapezoid body** (see Figs. 8-31 and 8-37).

6. Efferent tertiary and quaternary pathways from the supplementary auditory nuclei

    a. From the superior olivary nuclei and nuclei of the trapezoid body, the main efferent pathway is the lateral lemniscus.

    b. Additional pathways lead:

        (1) Into the reticular formation to mediate the startle response to sound and to control the stapedius muscles

        (2) Back into the organ of Corti. An olivocochlear efferent tract crosses the pons, enters the contralateral cochlear nerve, and runs to the organ of Corti. This pathway may influence the reception of sound at the organ of Corti. Not ending on muscle or gland effectors, it is not generally included in the theory of nerve components.

7. Lateral lemniscus

    a. The lateral lemniscus forms at the level of the trapezoid body and ascends in the dorsolateral pontine and midbrain tegmentum.

    b. Since the lateral lemniscus contains decussated and nondecussated axons, interruption of one lateral lemniscus does not lead to unilateral deafness.

    c. The lateral lemniscus comes into contact with the medial lemniscus at midbrain levels, making a **lemniscal crescent** in the midbrain tegmentum consisting of the lateral, spinal, trigeminal, and medial lemnisci (see Fig. 8-32).

    d. Axons of the lateral lemniscus end in the:

        (1) Nuclei scattered along its course

        (2) Inferior colliculus of the quadrigeminal plate

        (3) Medial geniculate body of the thalamus

8. Inferior colliculus of the quadrigeminal plate. Neurons of the inferior colliculus relay to the medial geniculate body via the brachium of the inferior colliculus (see Figs. 8-23A and 8-34).

9. Medial geniculate body and thalamocortical radiation. The medial geniculate body is the specific thalamic sensory relay nucleus for hearing. It projects through the deep hemispheric white matter to the auditory receptive cortex of the temporal lobe.

10. Auditory receptive cortex

    a. The auditory cortex occupies the transverse gyri of Heschl in the temporal lobe.

    b. The transverse gyri are in the floor of the lateral (sylvian) fissure (see Fig. 13-7).

        (1) Low tones are represented in the anterolateral part of the transverse gyri.

        (2) High tones are represented in the posteromedial portion of the transverse gyri.

    c. The transverse gyri and surrounding cortex are usually larger in the left cerebral hemisphere, a fact that may relate to the normal dominance of the left hemisphere for language.

11. Clinical effects of lesions of the auditory nerve and central pathways

    a. Interruption of the organ of Corti or the cochlear nerve causes diminished hearing or complete deafness ipsilaterally. Irritation may cause tinnitus.

    b. The bilaterality of representation in the lateral lemnisci means that unilateral lesions of the auditory pathway, from lemniscal origin to and including the receptive cortex, do not cause unilateral deafness.

    c. Abnormalities in the conduction of auditory impulses through CN VIII and its central pathways can be detected by surface electrodes on the head, the **B**rainstem **A**uditory **E**voked **R**esponses (BAER) test.

F. CN V, the trigeminal nerve (Fig. 8-38)

    1. CN V has a motor root and a sensory root.

    2. Motor root

        a. The motor nucleus (SVE) of CN V is in the rostral pontine tegmentum. The motor axons exit laterally under the cover of the sensory root (see Fig. 8-1).

        b. The motor root crosses the subarachnoid space to exit from the skull through the foramen ovale with the mandibular division of CN V (see Fig. 8-17).

        c. It innervates the chewing muscles (the temporalis, the pterygoids, and the masseter) and the tensor tympani and tensor veli palatini.

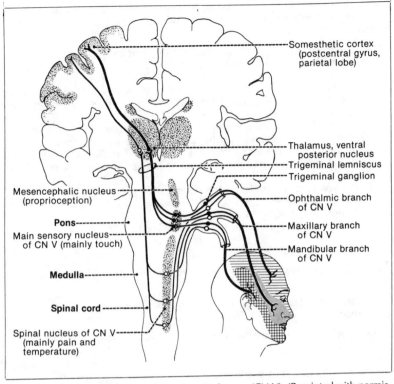

Figure 8-38. Sensory pathways of the trigeminal nerve (CN V). (Reprinted with permission from DeMyer W: *Technique of the Neurologic Examination: A Programmed Text,* 3rd ed. New York, McGraw-Hill, 1980, p 292.)

3. **Trigeminal (syn: semilunar or gasserian) ganglion (GSA)**
   a. The trigeminal ganglion contains the primary unipolar neurons for CN V. It is the largest sensory ganglion of the peripheral nervous system (PNS).
   b. The peripheral divisions consist of:
   - **(1)** V1, ophthalmic division
   - **(2)** V2, maxillary division
   - **(3)** V3, mandibular division
   c. The three divisions gather into one huge sensory root proximal to the ganglion to enter the dorsolateral aspect of the basis pontis (see Figs. 8-1 and 8-2).

4. **Three trigeminal nuclei: mesencephalic, main sensory, and spinal**
   a. The **mesencephalic nucleus** is anomalous because it is the only example of dorsal root–type neurons within the central nervous system (CNS).
   - **(1)** Peripheral axons of the mesencephalic nucleus follow the sensory root into the three major peripheral sensory divisions and also enter the motor root.
   - **(2)** The axons are thought to serve as proprioceptive afferents from the ocular, facial, masticatory, and pharyngeal muscles.
   b. The main **sensory nucleus** receives afferents from the trigeminal ganglion and subserves touch from the face, eyeball, and mucous membranes of the head.
   c. The **spinal nucleus** of CN V subserves pain and temperature sensation for the facial skin; eyeball; mucous membranes of the sinuses, nose, and mouth; the teeth; and the meninges.

5. **Intra-axial course of primary trigeminal afferent axons**
   a. Upon entering the pons, the afferent trigeminal axons, like the spinal afferents, typically branch to end at various levels of the trigeminal nuclei and reticular formation.
   b. The descending or spinal root of CN V conveys C fibers for pain and temperature sensation. It corresponds to and is continuous with the dorsolateral fasciculus of Lissauer.
   c. The spinal nucleus of CN V consists of substantia gelatinosa. It extends from the medulla into, and is continuous with, the substantia gelatinosa of the cervical level of the spinal

cord. Thus, the substantia gelatinosa is one continuous topographic nuclear column, extending the length of the spinal cord and mediating pain and temperature for the entire body.

6. **Efferent pathways from the trigeminal sensory nuclei**
   a. The **trigeminal lemniscus** arises from the trigeminal sensory nuclei. It has two components.
      (1) The first component, from the spinal nucleus of CN V, decussates at the medullary level and joins the medial lemniscus at pontine levels to ascend to the thalamus (see Fig. 8-38).
      (2) A second, uncrossed component arises from more rostral portions of CN V nuclei and ascends to the thalamus as the ipsilateral trigeminal lemniscus.
   b. Other connections of the trigeminal sensory nuclei mediate clinically important reflexes by running directly to cranial nerve nuclei or to them through the reticular formation. These include:
      (1) The jaw jerk, a muscle stretch reflex (MSR) [CN V–CN V reflex]
      (2) The corneal reflex (CN V–CN VII reflex)
      (3) Tearing (CN V–CN VII reflex)
      (4) Sneezing (CN V–reticular formation reflex)

G. **Decussations of the pons**

1. The **auditory pathways** partially decussate through the trapezoid body and superior olivary nuclei.

2. The **pontocerebellar pathways** from the nuclei of the basis pontis decussate to form the middle cerebellar peduncle (see Fig. 8-30).

3. The **cerebellovestibular pathway** partially decussates across the roof of the fourth ventricle (see Fig. 9-11).

H. **Anatomical features of the pontomidbrain junction**

1. The bulging belly of the pons abruptly replaces the midbrain, which forms a narrow **isthmus** between it and the cerebral hemispheres (see Fig. 8-6).

2. The cerebral peduncle with its pyramidal tract disappears abruptly into the pontine belly.

3. The aqueduct becomes continuous with the rostral tip of the fourth ventricle.

4. The anterior medullary velum joins the inferior colliculus of the quadrigeminal plate, and CN IV emerges at this point.

5. The rostral tip of the cerebellum ends at the pontomidbrain plane (see Fig. 8-6).

6. Ventrally, the basilar artery branches into the posterior cerebral arteries (see Fig. 15-9).

XI. MIDBRAIN

A. **Gross external anatomy** (see Fig. 8-23A)

B. The **tegmental gray matter of the midbrain** consists of:

1. **Two cranial nerve nuclei** (see Fig. 8-11)
   a. Oculomotor nucleus of CN III with a GSE and a GVE component (Edinger-Westphal nucleus)
   b. Trochlear nucleus of CN IV

2. **Two supplementary motor nuclei**
   a. **Red nucleus**, which receives the cerebellorubrothalamic tract after it decussates
   b. **Substantia nigra**, which projects to the basal nuclei of the forebrain

3. **Reticular formation**

C. **Quadrigeminal plate**

1. The quadrigeminal plate consists of superior and inferior colliculi and closely related brachia (see Fig. 8-23A). It is the tectum of the midbrain.
   a. The **superior colliculus** consists of layers of fibers and neurons connected to the reticular formation and adjacent accessory nuclei of the optic system. It receives axons from the retina via the superior brachium.

b. The **inferior colliculus** receives the medial lemniscus and relays to the medial geniculate body by the inferior brachium.

2. Both colliculi send a number of decussating and nondecussating pathways (tectospinal tracts) to the reticular formation, adjacent midbrain nuclei, and the spinal cord.

3. While the colliculi are integrating centers for optic and auditory reflexes, we know of no specific syndromes of quadrigeminal plate lesions in man.

D. Composition of the midbrain basis. The midbrain basis contains the following tracts, shown topographically in Fig. 8-35:

1. Corticopontine tract, two components
   a. Frontopontine tracts
   b. Temporopontine tracts

2. Pyramidal tract, two components
   a. Corticobulbar tract
   b. Corticospinal tract

E. Decussations of the midbrain

1. The **dentatorubral** and **dentatothalamic tracts** of the rostral cerebellar peduncle (the brachium conjunctivum) decussate in the caudal part of the pontine tegmentum (see Fig. 8-32).

2. The corticobulbar pathway for volitional horizontal eye movements decussates in the tegmentum caudally.

3. Other decussations include efferent pathways between the colliculi, decussations of their tectospinal tracts, and decussation of the rubrospinal tracts, but the functions of these connections in humans are unknown.

XII. CORTICOBULBAR TRACTS

A. Definition. Corticobulbar tracts are the efferent fibers that arise in the frontoparietal sensorimotor (paracentral) cortex and end on neurons of the brainstem tegmentum. This definition excludes the corticopontine tracts.

B. Function. The corticobulbar tracts, via reticular formation pathways, control voluntary movements of the cranial nerve muscles, and by reaching sensory nuclei, modulate sensory transmission.

C. Course

1. From the paracentral cortex, the corticobulbar fibers descend through the white matter and internal capsule to enter the midbrain basis. In the midbrain basis, the corticobulbar fibers occupy a medial position near the frontopontine fibers (see Fig. 8-33).

2. As they descend in the brainstem basis, groups of corticobulbar fibers veer dorsally into the tegmentum at various levels. Some fibers veer directly into the tegmentum, some descend various distances in the medial lemniscus before ending, and some may veer dorsally initially and then recurve rostrally.

3. In principle, the corticobulbar fibers decussate, but a larger number remain ipsilateral than in the corticospinal system.

D. Termination of corticobulbar tracts

1. Corticobulbar tracts end in:
   a. Reticular formation and satellite nuclei scattered along the brainstem
   b. Cranial nerve and sensory nuclei

2. The vast majority of the corticobulbar motor pathways are routed through reticular formation and satellite nuclei. Only a tiny minority of corticobulbar axons end directly on cranial nerve motor nuclei.

E. Corticobulbar pathways to cranial nerve motor nuclei

1. Optomotor nuclei: CN III, CN IV, and CN VI. The pathways for horizontal and vertical eye movements take different courses.
   a. For **horizontal eye movements**, the corticobulbar fibers decussate in the caudal midbrain/

rostral pontine tegmentum and synapse in reticular formation on or near the CN VI nuclei. Then the pathway ascends through the medial longitudinal fasciculus to the CN III nucleus.

    b. For **vertical eye movements**, the corticobulbar pathway enters the pretectal region (a diencephalic region of satellite nuclei just rostral to the superior colliculus); the pathway then relays directly to the CN III and CN IV nuclei.

2. Motor nuclei: CN V, CN VII, CN IX, CN X, CN XI, and CN XII

    a. Except for CN VII, the motor nuclei of this group are regarded as receiving about an equal number of decussated and nondecussated fibers. After unilateral corticobulbar tract interruption, the muscles have some weakness, which is usually bilateral and mild, not strongly lateralized and severe.

    b. CN VII nucleus. Lower motoneurons (LMNs) of CN VII have a topographic organization for the facial muscles.

        (1) The LMNs for the frontalis (forehead) muscles and, to a lesser extent, the orbicularis oculi, receive bilateral corticobulbar fibers.

        (2) LMNs for the lower facial muscles receive almost exclusively contralateral (decussated) corticobulbar fibers.

        (3) An upper motoneuron (UMN) lesion of the corticobulbar fibers paralyzes only the lower facial muscles. The patient has a flat nasolabial fold and cannot retract the corner of the mouth. The weakness is contralateral if the lesion affects the tract prior to its decussation.

        (4) Destruction of the nucleus of CN VII or of the trunk of the nerve paralyzes all ipsilateral facial muscles.

F. Corticobulbar pathways to cranial nerve sensory nuclei

    1. Corticobulbar fibers end in the sensory nuclei of the brainstem, including the:

        a. Nuclei gracilis and cuneatus

        b. Nucleus of the tractus solitarius

        c. All components of the trigeminal nerve nucleus

    2. These corticobulbar fibers are thought to inhibit or enhance sensory transmission through the various sensory nuclei. This allows selective attention or selective inattention to various stimuli.

XIII. RETICULAR FORMATION

    A. Definition. Reticular formation consists of widely spaced neuronal perikarya loosely arranged into nuclear groups (see Fig. 3-9B). The perikarya are separated by huge dendritic trees and connected by immense numbers of highly collateralized afferent and efferent axons. As a type of neuronal organization, reticular formation is highly characteristic of the brainstem tegmentum.

    B. Morphology of reticular formation neurons

        1. Although reticular formation neurons differ in size and shape, the large neurons characteristic of reticular formation have:

            a. A large nucleus

            b. Long, smooth-surface dendrites that extend 0.5 mm or more from the perikaryon

            c. Bundles of dendrites that form dendrodendritic contacts and that are arranged at right angles to the brainstem

            d. Long, highly branched axons (Golgi type I neurons) that collateralize locally and that bifurcate into long ascending and descending branches. Branches of a given axon may reach both the spinal cord and cerebrum (Fig. 8-39).

        2. The reticular formation contains few if any Golgi type II neurons.

    C. Extent of the reticular formation

        1. The reticular formation extends throughout the length of the brainstem tegmentum. It fills space that is not occupied by cranial nerve nuclei, supplementary sensory and motor nuclei, or named long and short tracts.

        2. The **caudal limit** is generally regarded as the medullocervical junction, but the reticular nuclei of the spinal cord and lamina VII may forecast the reticular formation proper of the brainstem level.

        3. The **rostral limit** is less easily stated. Technically, the reticular formation ends at the mid-

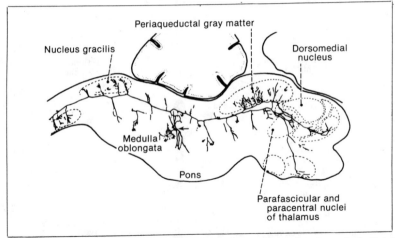

Figure 8-39. Sagittal section of the brainstem of a 2-day-old rat, showing a single Golgi silver-impregnated gigantocellular neuron of the reticular formation. The *arrow* indicates the perikaryon. The axon branches profusely to all parts of the diencephalon, brainstem, and spinal cord. (Adapted with permission from Scheibel ME, Scheibel AB: Structural substrates for integrative patterns in the brainstem reticular core. In *Reticular Formation of the Brain*. Edited by Jasper HH, et al, Boston, Little, Brown, 1958, p 46.)

brain–diencephalic junction, but morphologically and functionally, it may extend into the diencephalon.

D. What are the nuclei of the reticular formation?

1. In contrast to the densely packed perikarya of the regular nuclei, the reticular formation perikarya tend to form much looser nuclear groups, often with vague boundaries. Neuroanatomists, therefore, differ as to their identification.

2. The classification of many satellite nuclei clustered around the cranial nerve nuclei and scattered along tracts and that of catecholaminergic nuclei is controversial.

3. Finally, the recognized nuclear groupings of the reticular formation may not match some centers demonstrated by physiologic evidence.

E. Classification of reticular formation nuclei into four nuclear regions (Fig. 8-40)

1. **Raphe nuclei** extend the entire length of the median/paramedian plane of the brainstem. The midline decussation of brainstem tracts forms the raphe itself.

2. **Medial (central) gigantocellular nuclei** extend through the pontomedullary tegmentum, lateral to the raphe nuclei. They contain the conspicuous gigantocellular neurons seen in Figure 8-39.

3. **Lateral parvicellular (small-celled) nuclei** extend from the medullocervical region into the midbrain. They are just lateral to the magnocellular group (see Fig. 8-40) in the medulla and pons. The midbrain also contains the interpeduncular nucleus (not shown in Fig. 8-40).

4. **Cerebellar reticular formation nuclei** mainly are connected with the cerebellum. Some authorities do not include these three nuclei in the reticular formation because of their strong cerebellar connections.

F. Afferents to the reticular formation

1. **Overview of afferent connections**
   a. The **lateral parvicellular nuclei** receive the majority of afferents to the reticular formation. The lateral nuclei relay to the **medial gigantocellular nuclei**, which originate the majority of efferents.
   b. The reticular formation receives collaterals from most of the ascending and descending pathways that traverse the brainstem, whatever the origin of the pathway in spinal cord or

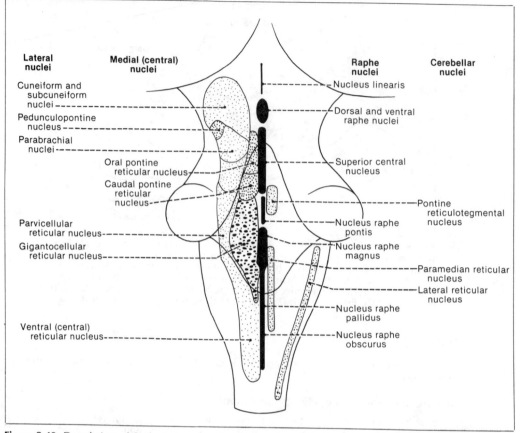

Figure 8-40. Dorsal view of the brainstem showing the location of the four groups of reticular formation nuclei.

brain and whatever its function: visceral or somatic, motor or sensory, or purely internuncial. Thus, the reticular formation receives the most varied, heterogeneous input of any neuronal grouping in the nervous system.

c. In principle, the afferents from sensory pathways reach the reticular formation from collaterals of axons from secondary neurons, not by direct, primary afferents.

d. The afferent fibers bypassing the reticular formation are the discriminative or one-to-one systems designed to preserve the order of the information transmitted. They include the:
   (1) Dorsal column pathway through the medial lemniscus
   (2) Retinogeniculocalcarine tract
   (3) Tonotopic fibers of the auditory system

e. The auditory and optic systems do reach the reticular formation, as can be inferred by the prompt startle response to loud sound or a sudden bright light, but the one-to-one component of these systems probably bypasses the reticular formation.

2. **Spinal afferents** include:
   a. Spinoreticular tracts
   b. Collaterals from spinothalamic tracts

3. **Brainstem afferents** include:
   a. Sensory collaterals of secondary/tertiary tracts from the sensory nuclei of cranial nerves:
      (1) Trigeminal
      (2) Cochlear
      (3) Vestibular
      (4) Nucleus solitarius
   b. **Tectoreticular tracts** from the superior and inferior colliculi (the midbrain tectum)
   c. **Reticuloreticular pathways.** Reticular formation neurons interconnect by means of innumerable axodendritic and dendrodendritic connections.

4. **Cerebellar afferents** come particularly from the nucleus fastigius of the deep cerebellar

nuclei. The cerebellar nuclei of the reticular formation in turn project to the deep nuclei and cerebellar cortex.

   5. Limbic system afferents come from the:
   a. Basal forebrain and hypothalamus via the medial forebrain bundle
   b. Mamillary bodies of the hypothalamus via the mamillotegmental tract
   c. Periaqueductal gray matter via diffuse axonal projections
   d. Habenular nuclei of the diencephalon via the habenulointerpeduncular tract

   6. Basal ganglia afferents. The globus pallidus sends fibers to the pedunculopontine nucleus of the midbrain reticular formation.

   7. Cerebral cortex afferents. Direct corticobulbar pathways and collaterals reach most of the reticular formation but end predominantly in the:
   a. Gigantocellular nuclei of the pons and medulla, which originate the reticulospinal tracts
   b. Cerebellar nuclei of the reticular formation

G. Efferents from the reticular formation. The reticular formation integrates the great variety of afferent information it receives, runs it through multisynaptic circuits of appropriate complexity, and disperses the efferent axons widely. Reticular efferents influence almost all parts of the CNS, from the spinal cord to the cerebral cortex.

   1. Reticular formation efferents run in the afferent pathways listed in section XIII F, making these two-way pathways.

   2. Efferent reticular formation pathways also include:
   a. Reticulobulbar tracts to all cranial nerve nuclei
   b. Reticulospinal tracts, which run in the ventrolateral columns of the spinal cord
   c. Reticulothalamic tracts
   d. Specific neurotransmitter pathways

H. Overview of reticular formation functions

   1. Methods of determining reticular formation functions
   a. Transecting or destroying tegmental regions (the reticular formation has a safety factor: bilateral destruction generally is required at a given level to abolish the function)
   b. Stimulating various regions to determine the physiologic effects, which are usually the opposite of the effect of destructive lesions.
   c. Recording, by means of implanted electrodes, the electrical activities of the reticular formation neurons during specific activities such as waking, sleeping, or breathing

   2. Range of reticular formation functions
   a. Mental activity. The reticular formation mediates consciousness, attention span, alerting responses, and the sleep–wake cycle.
   b. Homeostasis and neurovegetative reflexes. The reticular formation mediates reflexes that control the activity of viscera and glands in the interest of homeostasis.
      (1) In concert with the forebrain, reticular formation centers control breathing, pulse, blood pressure, gastrointestinal and genitourinary system motility, electrolyte balance, pupillary size, and ocular movements.
      (2) Reticular formation circuitry mediates the reflexes of the upper gastrointestinal and respiratory tracts: coughing, sneezing, swallowing, vomiting, hiccuping, gagging, chewing, sucking, and feeding.
   c. Somatomotor and sensorimotor reflexes
      (1) The reticular formation mediates postural reflexes, extensor and flexor muscle tone, and vestibular reflexes affecting the eyes and somatic muscles.
      (2) Stimulation of the gigantocellular effector zone in the medullary reticular formation tends to inhibit somatomotor activity by reducing MSRs, flexion reflexes, extensor tone, and cortically induced movements.
      (3) Stimulation of the gigantocellular effector zone in the pontine reticular formation and in the mesencephalic reticular nuclei tends to facilitate somatomotor activity, including cortically induced movements.
      (4) Destructive lesions tend to cause the opposite effect.
      (5) Although these effects occur in animal experiments, clinical use of this information is difficult because natural lesions rarely affect discrete nuclear regions of the reticular formation.
   d. Effects of stimulation of the raphe nuclei and the periaqueductal gray matter
      (1) In animal experiments, stimulation of the nucleus raphe magnus of the medulla or of the periaqueductal gray matter abolishes the response to pain.

(2) Reticulospinal pathways are presumed to reduce the transmission of pain impulses by inhibitory effects on the neurons of the substantia gelatinosa.

(3) The raphe nuclei of the medulla may also belong to a sleep-inducing system of the brainstem.

I. Rostral–caudal dichotomy of reticular formation function. Transection of the tegmentum at the midpontine level divides the reticular formation into rostral and caudal halves.

1. The **rostral half** of the reticular formation is essential for arousal, consciousness, and the waking state.

2. The **caudal half** of the reticular formation is essential for automatic breathing; for vestibular reflexes; for cardiovascular, pulmonary, and gastrointestinal reflexes mediated through CN VII, CN IX, and CN X; and for genitourinary and defecation reflexes.

J. Function of the rostral half of the reticular formation: the ascending reticular activating system

1. Destruction of the rostral pontine reticular formation causes transitory loss of consciousness, while destruction of the midbrain reticular formation permanently abolishes consciousness. The unconscious individual maintains breathing and blood pressure and other reflexes mediated through the caudal half of the reticular formation.

2. Stimulation of the rostral reticular formation causes the converse of destruction; that is, stimulation of an electrode implanted in the rostral reticular formation will arouse a sleeping animal.

3. The rostral half of the reticular formation projects to the forebrain by an **ascending reticular activating system**, which mediates alerting responses and consciousness and maintains the cerebrum in a waking state.

    a. The ascending reticular activating system activates the cerebral cortex directly and, via thalamic connections, indirectly. Thus, the maintenance of the conscious waking state requires three neuronal pools and their interconnections, the:

        (1) Rostral reticular formation (midbrain tegmentum)

        (2) Thalamus

        (3) Cerebral cortex

    b. Bilateral destruction of any of these three neuronal groups results in unconsciousness, as does interruption of their connecting fiber pathways that run through diencephalic and cerebral white matter.

K. Functions of the caudal half of the reticular formation. Lesions of the caudal half of the pontine or the medullary tegmentum result in:

1. Respiratory dysrhythmia or apnea and elimination of respiratory-related reflexes

2. Abolition of reflexes mediated through CN VII, CN IX, and CN X

3. Hypotension and Horner syndrome because of loss of sympathetic pathways that descend from the hypothalamus through the reticular formation and its reticulospinal connections

L. Central pathways for the control of breathing

1. Breathing serves three different functions: speech, automatic emotional expression, and homeostasis.

    a. Speech is controlled by pyramidal pathways.

    b. Automatic emotional expression (laughing, crying, sighing, and the utterance of expletives) is controlled by limbic–extrapyramidal pathways.

    c. Homeostasis (oxygen and carbon dioxide levels and acid–base balance) is controlled by the reticular formation and its reticulospinal pathways.

    d. All pathways ultimately act through the same LMNs of the cranial, phrenic, and intercostal nerves, and all centers are ultimately interconnected. (At this point you may want to review the effects of spinal cord lesions on breathing; see Chapter 7, section VIII B.)

2. Pyramidal pathways for the volitional control of breathing by the waking brain.

    a. A center in the parasylvian area of the left cerebral hemisphere controls speech. The speech center and all centers for the volitional control of breathing act through pyramidal pathways.

    b. The forebrain, in the waking state, also provides a general drive to breathe, mediated in part through pyramidal pathways.

    c. Sleep, coma, diffuse cerebral disease, and pyramidal tract interruption reduce the drive to breathe provided by the forebrain but do not cause respiratory failure because the reticular formation centers maintain breathing automatically.

3. Limbic–extrapyramidal respiratory pathways for control of emotional expression

  a. The neural drive for automatic crying, laughing, sighing, and expletive speech presumably arises in limbic circuits of the forebrain.

  b. After loss of voluntary speech because of a left parasylvian lesion or after bilateral corticobulbar tract lesions, the patient may still cry, laugh, sigh, or utter expletives. Bilateral corticobulbar tract lesions may even exaggerate the patient's crying or laughing (see section XIV C 3).

  c. Emotional states in general may increase or decrease breathing.

    (1) Patients with anxiety commonly hyperventilate, which may cause syncope or epileptic seizures.

    (2) Young children may react to anger or frustration by breath-holding spells that terminate in loss of consciousness.

M. Reticular formation lesions and respiratory dysrhythmias

  1. Lesions at various levels of the reticular formation alter the rate and depth of breathing in characteristic ways (Fig. 8-41).

  2. The more caudal the lesion in the reticular formation, the more disastrous the effects on breathing. Lesions of the caudal-most medullary reticular formation or of the medullocervical junction cause complete respiratory arrest (apnea).

N. Medullary respiratory centers for homeostatic (automatic) breathing

1. Function

  a. Centers in the pontomedullary reticular formation collaborate to produce an automatic, rhythmic drive to breathe, which maintains oxygen and carbon dioxide levels in the blood.

  b. They automatically maintain a level of breathing adequate to support life even after hemispheric destruction or rostral brainstem transection, although such lesions alter the respiratory rhythm (see Fig. 8-41).

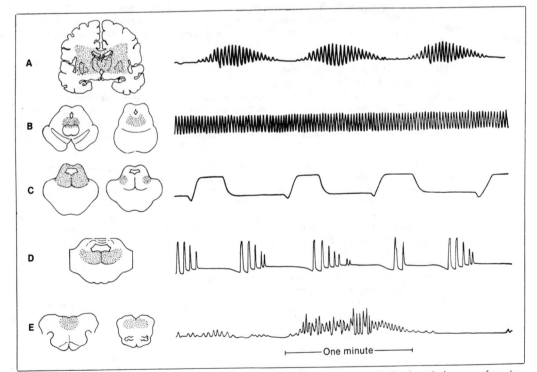

Figure 8-41. Correlation of intra-axial brainstem lesions (*shaded areas*) at successive levels with the type of respiratory dysrhythmia produced. (*A*) Cheyne-Stokes respiration. (*B*) Central neurogenic hyperventilation. (*C*) Apneustic breathing. (*D*) Cluster breathing. (*E*) Ataxic breathing. (Adapted with permission from Plum D, Posner J: *The Diagnosis of Stupor and Coma.* Philadelphia, Davis, 1966, p 16.)

2. Afferent pathways to the medullary respiratory centers come from the:
  a. Remainder of the reticular formation
  b. Descending motor pathways, including:
   (1) Collaterals from corticobulbar and corticospinal pathways
   (2) Limbic pathways, as yet undetermined, but inferred from functional considerations
  c. Ascending sensory pathways
   (1) Afferent stimulation in general increases reticular formation activity and increases breathing.
   (2) Stimulation of skin afferents increases breathing, while section of thoracic dorsal roots decreases breathing. These two facts suggest an ascending spinal pathway, as yet unknown, or collaterals from the long ascending tracts.
   (3) Pain has a variable effect on breathing. Severe pain may increase or decrease breathing, depending in part on its emotional impact. Pleuritic or chest wall pain, a "stitch in the side," always inhibits breathing.
   (4) Afferents from the throat and lungs via CN IX and CN X mediate inhibitory or excitatory respiratory reflexes.

3. Anatomical location of medullary respiratory centers. Current evidence suggests **two groups of respiratory neurons.**
  a. Group I, a **dorsal respiratory group** of neurons, is located in the ventrolateral part of the nucleus solitarius. It consists primarily of inspiratory neurons (Fig. 8-42).
  b. Group II, a **ventral respiratory group** of neurons, is located in the ventrolateral part of the medulla, in association with the nuclei ambiguus and retroambigualis.
   (1) Group II consists both of inspiratory and expiratory neurons.
   (2) This assembly of neurons extends into the medullocervical junction, nearly to the level of C1.

4. Medullary chemoreceptors. The ventrolateral part of the medulla contains receptors, perhaps neurons themselves, sensitive to the carbon dioxide concentration, bicarbonate ion, and acid–base balance. These receptors, acting through the neurons of the dorsal or ventral respiratory group, increase or decrease breathing to alter carbon dioxide levels as needed for acid–base balance.

5. Reticulospinal efferent tracts from the medullary respiratory centers
  a. The reticulospinal pathways from the medullary respiratory centers decussate ventral to the obex (the caudal tip of the fourth ventricle) to descend to the LMNs for the diaphragm (C3–C5) and intercostal muscles (T2–T12) [see Fig. 8-42].
  b. The reticulospinal tracts can be interrupted by either a **transverse** or a **sagittal cut.**
   (1) A **sagittal cut** a few millimeters long through the obex and subjacent neural tissue divides the tracts as they decussate.
   (2) A **transverse cut** through the ventrolateral quadrants of the spinal cord at C1 or C2 interrupts the reticulospinal tracts as they descend to the LMNs after decussating.
   (3) As is customarily required to abolish reticular formation functions completely, the transverse cut has to be bilateral because of some nondecussating or double-decussating fibers.

6. Ondine's curse and the dichotomy between volitional and automatic breathing
  a. Pyramidal tract section abolishes voluntary breathing and the normal drive to breathe that arises in the waking forebrain. The patient survives because the pontomedullary respiratory centers function automatically.
  b. After destruction of the medullary respiratory centers or section of the reticulospinal pathways, the patient maintains breathing through the forebrain and pyramidal tracts but cannot breathe automatically. If the patient sleeps, which removes the forebrain drive to breathe, respiration stops (sleep apnea) and the patient may die. Ondine's curse condemns the patient to remain awake forever in order to breathe, never to enjoy Keats' "sleep full of sweet dreams and quiet breathing."
  c. Sudden infant death syndrome (SIDS or crib death). Infants with SIDS fail to maintain automatic respiration when they go to sleep; they are found dead the next morning. The defect may be in the respiratory centers of the medulla or in its afferent or efferent pathways. However, the exact defect in SIDS is not known.

XIV. CLINICAL SYNDROMES OF BRAINSTEM AND INTRA-AXIAL CRANIAL NERVE LESIONS

A. The symptoms and signs of a brainstem lesion depend on the **longitudinal site** along the

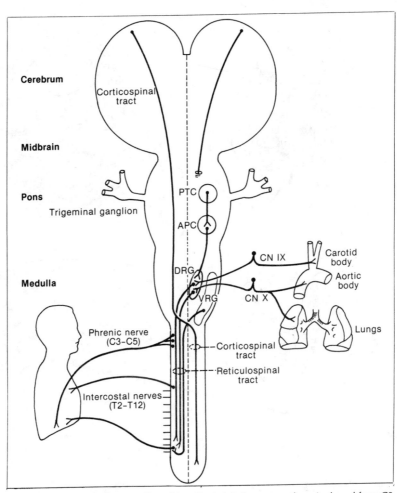

Figure 8-42. Neuroanatomy of breathing. By their influence on the spinal cord from C3 to T12, the corticospinal tracts control volitional breathing and the reticulospinal tracts control automatic breathing. *PTC* = pneumotaxic center; *APC* = apneustic center; *DRG* = dorsal respiratory group of neurons, mainly inspiratory, associated with the dorsal motor nucleus of the vagus nerve; *VRG* = ventral respiratory group of mixed inspiratory–expiratory neurons associated with the nuclei ambiguus and retroambigualis.

brainstem, in the midbrain, pons, or medulla, and on the **cross-sectional site**, in the basis or tegmentum.

B. Classic brainstem syndromes characteristic of the lesion site

  1. Alternating right- and left-sided signs of unilateral brainstem lesions
    a. Interruption of a cranial nerve in the brainstem causes ipsilateral LMN paralysis.
    b. Interruption of the pyramidal tract, which will decussate, or of a long sensory tract, which has decussated, causes contralateral signs.
    c. The term alternating refers to the fact that the signs of interruption of the long tract alternate with (i.e., are on the opposite side of) the cranial nerve signs.

  2. Alternating hemiplegia, hemianesthesia, and hemihyperkinesia
    a. Alternating cranial nerve signs and hemiplegia. A frequent syndrome involves a somite cranial nerve palsy such as CN III, CN VI, or CN XII palsy, and contralateral hemiplegia. The combination occurs because the somite nerves exit ventrally in the paramedian plane and run near the pyramidal tract where a single lesion may affect a nerve and the tract (Fig. 8-43).
    b. Alternating hemianesthesia. Interruption of the medial lemniscus along with cranial nerve palsy, with or without pyramidal tract involvement, causes contralateral hemianesthesia.
    c. Alternating hemihyperkinesia (see section XIV E 3)

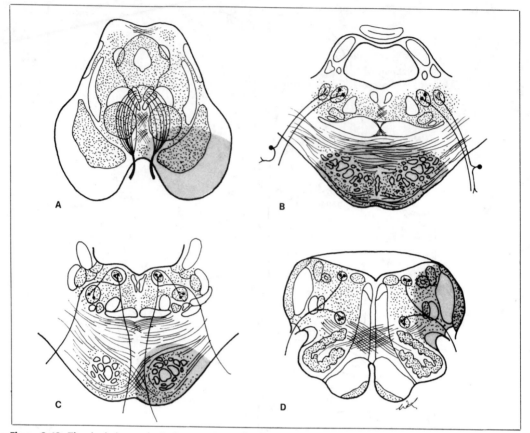

Figure 8-43. The *shaded areas* depict lesions of various brainstem levels. (A) Midbrain, CN III level. (B) Rostral pons, CN V level. (C) Caudal pons, CN VI and CN VII levels. (D) Medulla, CN IX level.

C. Specific medullary syndromes

1. Lateral medullary (Wallenberg) syndrome

a. A lesion of the lateral part of the medulla produces a classic syndrome with alternating signs. This part of the medulla receives its blood from the posterior inferior cerebellar artery and frequently undergoes infarction in patients with cerebrovascular disease.

b. Like the Brown-Séquard syndrome of spinal cord hemisection, the lateral medullary syndrome critically tests your knowledge of neuroanatomy (Table 8-5; see Fig. 8-43D).

2. Bulbar palsy. The medulla, a bulb-like expansion of the spinal cord, innervates the muscles of the tongue, palate, pharynx, and larynx through CN IX, CN X, and CN XII. LMN paralysis of these muscles, resulting in dysphagia and dysarthria, is called "true" bulbar palsy.

3. Pseudobulbar palsy

a. Definition. Pseudobulbar palsy is a syndrome of dysphagia, dysarthria, and emotional lability, characterized by exaggerated laughing or crying. It is caused by weakness of bulbar muscles due to bilateral but partial interruption of the corticobulbar tracts. Bilateral, complete destruction of the corticobulbar and corticospinal (pyramidal) tracts results in the **locked-in syndrome** (see section XIV D 1).

b. Patients with pseudobulbar palsy laugh or cry involuntarily in response to slight provocation, and they switch rapidly from one to the other if the examiner suggests a humorous or sad situation.

c. Since the lesion is in the motor cortex or somewhere along the corticobulbar tracts, not in the bulbar nerves, the syndrome is referred to as "pseudobulbar palsy," in contrast to "true" LMN bulbar palsy.

d. The neurophysiologic drive for the emotional expression released by the corticobulbar lesion is unclear, but it is presumed to arise in limbic or extrapyramidal centers.

Table 8-5. Lateral Medullary Syndrome of Wallenberg

Signs and Symptoms	Structure Involved
Ipsilateral	
Facial pain; dysesthesia or anesthesia	Descending root of CN V
Dysphagia and dysarthria	CN IX or the nucleus ambiguus
Paralysis of palatal elevation, pharyngeal constric- tors, and vocal cord	CN X
Ataxia, dysmetria, and intention tremor	Spinocerebellar tract or cerebellar hemisphere
Horner syndrome of miosis, ptosis, and anhidrosis of the face	Descending autonomic tract in the lateral re- ticular formation
Contralateral	
Loss of pain and temperature in the body and ex- tremities	Lateral spinothalamic tract
General	
Nausea, vomiting, vertigo, and hiccuping	Reticular formation and vestibular connec- tions

D. Specific pontine syndromes

1. **Locked-in syndrome of the pontine basis**
   a. **Definition.** The locked-in syndrome consists of complete quadriplegia and bulbar and facial palsy due to complete interruption of both pyramidal tracts. The lesion is usually in the basis pontis and is due to an infarct, a neoplasm, trauma, or demyelination (see Fig. 8-43B).
   b. The patient is conscious but can make only vertical eye movements. All other voluntary movements, including horizontal eye movements, are completely paralyzed.
      (1) The patient retains vertical eye movements because the corticobulbar pathway for ver- tical movements runs directly from the cerebrum into the pretectal region and mid- brain.
      (2) In contrast, the corticobulbar pathway for horizontal eye movements loops caudally into the pons, where the lesion interrupts it (see Chapter 10, section VII E, F).
   c. Since the lesion of the basis spares the midbrain tegmentum, the patient retains con- sciousness and can see, hear, and communicate by moving the eyes up and down for yes and no. Thus, the patient, although conscious and mentally intact, is "locked-in" to himself by the paralysis.

2. **Caudal pontine respiratory syndrome.** Caudal pontine tegmental lesions may cause apneus- tic breathing (see Fig. 8-41C) along with interruption of CN VI or CN VII.

E. Specific midbrain syndromes

1. **Decerebrate rigidity**
   a. **Definition.** Decerebrate rigidity is a characteristic driven posture that follows anatomic or physiologic transection of the midbrain. The patient is comatose and assumes a position dictated by the pull of the antigravity muscles (Fig. 8-44).
   b. Experimentally, the syndrome is produced by a surgical transection of the midbrain at the midcollicular level. This lesion effectively disconnects the cerebrum or decerebrates the individual.
   c. Any driven posture or similar release phenomenon requires two conditions:
      (1) A lesion that "releases" a subordinate mechanism to display an action
      (2) Integrity of a subordinate mechanism to produce the drive that is released and that causes the posture
   d. Midbrain transection incites or releases decerebrate rigidity.
   e. The vestibular system drives the decerebrate rigidity. The decerebrate rigidity disappears after:
      (1) Destruction of the vestibular nerves, vestibular nuclei, or transection of the vestibulo- spinal tracts
      (2) Division of the dorsal roots
      (3) Division of the ventral roots (which, of course, eliminates all neurally driven muscular activity)

2. **Parkinson's disease** (paralysis agitans)
   a. **Definition.** Parkinson's disease is a syndrome of tremor at rest and rigidity of the muscles,

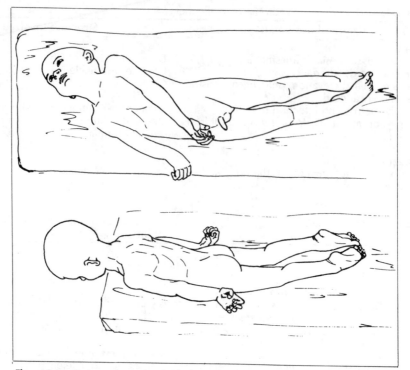

Figure 8-44. Posture of a patient with decerebrate rigidity. The patient is arched back (opisthotonos), holds the arms and legs rigidly extended, and shows flexion and pronation of the hands and plantar flexion of the feet. (Adapted with permission from Penfield W, Jasper H: *Epilepsy and the Functional Anatomy of the Human Brain*. Boston, Little, Brown, 1954, p 380.)

caused by a lesion, usually degeneration, of the pigmented neurons of the substantia nigra, which deprives the striatum of dopaminergic fibers.

    b. If the lesion is unilateral, the patient shows only contralateral parkinsonism.

3. Miscellaneous hyperkinesias. Rostral midbrain lesions, interrupting connections with the diencephalon and basal motor nuclei and red nuclei, result in a variety of contralateral involuntary movements varying from tremor to hemichorea and hemiballismus. The lesion also frequently interrupts CN III.

4. Coma plus oculomotor paralysis and pupillodilatation. Lesions of the midbrain tegmentum cause coma. Frequently the CN III nucleus or its fibers are also interrupted, causing in addition:

    a. Paralysis of ocular rotatory muscles

    b. Enlarged pupils due to interruption of parasympathetic fibers to the iris

F. Figure 8-45 is a **localizing diagnosticon for brainstem lesions.**

XV. CLINICAL SYNDROMES OF EXTRA-AXIAL CRANIAL NERVE LESIONS

A. Anatomical proximity of cranial nerves. Lesions at the conjunction of the cranial nerves, where they attach to the brainstem, travel through the subarachnoid space, and converge to exit from the skull, lead to characteristic syndromes because the lesion affects more than one nerve.

B. Characteristic sites of conjunction of cranial nerves include the:

    1. Parasellar region, cavernous sinus, and superior orbital fissure, where the optic chiasm and CN III, CN IV, CN V, and CN VI come into conjunction

    2. Cerebellopontine angle, where CN VI, CN VII, and CN VIII run in conjunction and CN V, CN IX, and CN X are nearby

    3. Jugular foramen, where CN IX, CN X, and CN XI exit (see Fig. 8-22)

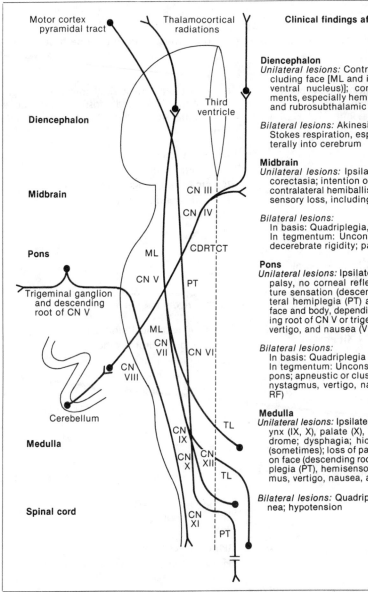

Clinical findings after destructive lesions

Diencephalon
Unilateral lesions: Contralateral hemisensory loss, including face [ML and its terminal nucleus (posterior ventral nucleus)]; contralateral involuntary movements, especially hemiballism (subthalamic nucleus and rubrosubthalamic connections)

Bilateral lesions: Akinesia, unconsciousness; Cheyne-Stokes respiration, especially if lesion extends bilaterally into cerebrum

Midbrain
Unilateral lesions: Ipsilateral cranial nerve (III) palsy, corectasia; intention or postural tremor (CDRTCT) or contralateral hemiballism, hemiplegia (PT), and hemisensory loss, including face (ML)

Bilateral lesions:
In basis: Quadriplegia, pseudobulbar palsy
In tegmentum: Unconsciousness, hyperventilation, decerebrate rigidity; parkinsonism (SN)

Pons
Unilateral lesions: Ipsilateral cranial nerve (V, VI, or VII) palsy, no corneal reflex; loss of pain and temperature sensation (descending root of CN V); contralateral hemiplegia (PT) and hemisensory loss (ML) in face and body, depending on involvement of descending root of CN V or trigeminal lemniscus; nystagmus, vertigo, and nausea (VP and RF)

Bilateral lesions:
In basis: Quadriplegia (locked-in syndrome)
In tegmentum: Unconsciousness if in rostral half of pons; apneustic or cluster breathing if in caudal half; nystagmus, vertigo, nausea, and vomiting (VP and RF)

Medulla
Unilateral lesions: Ipsilateral cranial nerve palsy: of pharynx (IX, X), palate (X), or tongue (XII); Horner's syndrome; dysphagia; hiccups; loss of corneal reflex (sometimes); loss of pain and temperature sensation on face (descending root of CN V); contralateral hemiplegia (PT), hemisensory loss on body (ML); nystagmus, vertigo, nausea, and vomiting (VP and RF)

Bilateral lesions: Quadriplegia; ataxic breathing or apnea; hypotension

Figure 8-45. Localizing diagnosticon for brainstem lesions (exclusive of central ocular pathways). *CDRTCT* = cerebello-dentato-rubro-thalamo-cortical tract; *ML* = medial lemniscus; *PT* = pyramidal tract; *TL* = trigeminal lemniscus; *Roman numerals* = cranial nerve nuclei; *SN* = substantia nigra; *VP* = vestibular pathways; *RF* = reticular formation.

STUDY QUESTIONS

Directions: Each question below contains five suggested answers. Choose the **one best** response to each question.

1. Testing the sense of taste would be most important in a patient presenting with

(A) loss of hearing
(B) diplopia
(C) dystaxia
(D) dysphagia
(E) hemifacial paralysis

2. The gag reflex involves which of the following cranial nerve pathways?

(A) CN VII afferent and CN VII efferent
(B) CN VIII afferent and CN IX efferent
(C) CN IX or CN X afferent and CN IX or CN X efferent
(D) CN X afferent and CN XI efferent
(E) CN IX afferent and CN XII efferent

3. A basic function of the vestibular system is to

(A) move the eyes against the direction of head movement
(B) detect sounds of low frequency
(C) agitate the eyeballs to prevent visual fatigue of the retinal image
(D) elevate the eyes against the pull of gravity
(E) none of the above

4. Assuming support of breathing and blood pressure, if required by the site of the lesion, which surgical lesion would abolish consciousness?

(A) Transection of the rostral part of the cervical cord
(B) Transection of the pontine basis
(C) Hemispherectomy
(D) Transection of the midbrain tegmentum
(E) Removal of the cerebellum

5. Decerebrate rigidity can be abolished by transection of the

(A) diencephalon
(B) cerebellum
(C) corticospinal tracts
(D) vestibulospinal tracts
(E) spinocerebellar tracts

6. A patient with a skull fracture through the floor of the right middle fossa has no tear secretion on that side. The most likely cause is damage to the

(A) ciliary ganglion
(B) chorda tympani
(C) greater superficial petrosal nerve
(D) pericarotid sympathetic plexus
(E) superior cervical ganglion

7. The posterior plane of cutaneous innervation by the trigeminal nerve is at the

(A) occipitocervical junction
(B) lambdoid suture plane
(C) interaural plane
(D) coronal suture plane
(E) intercanthal line

8. The descending root of CN V ends at the

(A) pontomedullary junction
(B) mid-medullary level
(C) obex
(D) upper cervical level
(E) upper thoracic level

9. On the right side a patient shows paralysis of palatal elevation, of the vocal cord, and of the trapezius and sternocleidomastoid muscles. The gag reflex is absent on the right, and the patient has moderate difficulty swallowing. A site for a lesion that would explain all of these findings is

(A) left cerebellopontine angle
(B) right cavernous sinus
(C) left pontine tegmentum
(D) right jugular foramen
(E) right cerebral peduncle and interpeduncular fossa

10. The maxillary division of the trigeminal nerve supplies the

(A) helix of the ear
(B) skin of the upper lip
(C) skin over the angle of the mandible
(D) forehead
(E) none of the above

11. CN VII innervates the

(A) stapedius muscle
(B) levator palatini
(C) omohyoid muscle
(D) lateral pterygoid muscles
(E) geniohyoid muscle

12. The site at which the smallest lesion produces complete loss of consciousness with minimal effects on other functions is the

(A) medullary tegmentum
(B) caudal pontine tegmentum
(C) rostral midbrain tegmentum
(D) dorsolateral diencephalon
(E) medial hemispheric wall in the cingulate gyri

13. In the locked-in syndrome, the lesion usually involves the

(A) midbrain tectum
(B) midbrain tegmentum
(C) midbrain or pontine basis
(D) pontine tegmentum
(E) medullary pyramids

14. If the palate fails to elevate on the right side when a patient says "Ah," one would suspect a lesion of the

(A) right vagus nerve
(B) right glossopharyngeal nerve
(C) right spinal accessory nerve
(D) recurrent branch of the ansa hypoglossi on the left
(E) trigeminal nerve on the right

15. An operation that would abolish automatic breathing is

(A) transection of the basis of the midbrain
(B) transection of the pons at a rostral level
(C) transection of the pyramids
(D) a sagittal cut limited to the dorsal part of the cervicomedullary junction
(E) a sagittal cut limited to the pyramidal decussation at the cervicomedullary junction

16. The decerebrate posture generally indicates a lesion of the

(A) pons
(B) medulla
(C) midbrain
(D) cerebellum
(E) diencephalon

17. The corneal reflex involves an afferent and efferent arc, which is mediated by

(A) CN V only
(B) CN III only
(C) CN III and CN VII
(D) CN III and CN VIII
(E) CN V and CN VII

Directions: Each question below contains four suggested answers of which **one or more** is correct. Choose the answer

A   if **1, 2, and 3** are correct
B   if **1 and 3** are correct
C   if **2 and 4** are correct
D   if **4** is correct
E   if **1, 2, 3, and 4** are correct

18. The pyramidal tract appears on the surface of the brain at which of the following locations?

(1) Internal capsule
(2) Basis pedunculi
(3) Basis pontis
(4) Medullary pyramids

19. Well-demonstrated sites of termination of the primary vestibular afferent fibers include the

(1) inferior olivary nucleus
(2) cochlear nuclei
(3) nucleus of CN III
(4) flocculonodular lobe of the cerebellum

SUMMARY OF DIRECTIONS

A	B	C	D	E
1, 2, 3 only	1, 3 only	2, 4 only	4 only	All are correct

---

20. Accurate descriptions of the lateral lemniscus include which of the following?

(1) It consists nearly exclusively of crossed axons
(2) It ascends in the dorsolateral part of the tegmentum
(3) It contains a considerable number of primary auditory afferent axons
(4) It terminates in a specific thalamic relay nucleus

21. Classic clinical signs of a unilateral brainstem lesion include which of the following?

(1) Ipsilateral lower motoneuron (LMN) cranial nerve palsy
(2) Prolonged coma
(3) Contralateral hemiplegia
(4) Ipsilateral loss of superficial sensation

22. The dorsal group of respiratory neurons have which of the following characteristics?

(1) They are directly sensitive to changes in carbon dioxide levels
(2) They send mainly uncrossed reticulospinal pathways into the cord
(3) They function mainly as expiratory neurons
(4) They are associated with the nucleus solitarius

23. Characteristics of CN III include which of the following?

(1) It is the rostral-most motor cranial nerve
(2) It is the first somite cranial nerve
(3) It is the first cranial nerve with autonomic axons
(4) It exits dorsally from the brainstem

24. Statements that describe the brainstem tegmentum include which of the following?

(1) It conveys the long sensory tracts
(2) It contains the reticular formation
(3) Its rostral portion contains large pigmented nuclei
(4) It contains all of the somite cranial nerve nuclei

25. Anatomical features of the pontomedullary junction include which of the following?

(1) It is the site of attachment of CN V, CN VI, and CN VII
(2) It is the narrowest part of the fourth ventricle
(3) The nucleus ambiguus crosses into the pons at the plane of the junction
(4) The dorsal spinocerebellar tracts turn dorsally just rostral to the plane

26. Signs that could result from a C1 spinal cord lesion and that could also result from a posterior fossa lesion include

(1) ptosis and pupilloconstriction (Horner's syndrome)
(2) laryngeal paralysis
(3) paralysis of the trapezius muscle
(4) paralysis of the tongue

Directions: The groups of questions below consist of lettered choices followed by several numbered items. For each numbered item select the **one** lettered choice with which it is **most** closely associated. Each lettered choice may be used once, more than once, or not at all.

Questions 27–31

Match the anatomical features listed below with the appropriate brainstem level.

(A) Midbrain
(B) Pons, rostral level
(C) Pons, middle level
(D) Pons, caudal level
(E) Medulla, caudal level

27. Largest diameter of the brainstem
28. Smallest diameter of the brainstem
29. Thinnest roof plate
30. Narrowest site of communication between the ventricles
31. Largest indentation in the basis

Questions 32–36

Match each spinal cord structure listed below with its closest homologous or analogous structure in the brainstem.

(A) Hypoglossal nucleus
(B) Medial longitudinal fasciculus
(C) Edinger-Westphal nucleus
(D) Vestibular nerve
(E) Motor nucleus of CN VII

32. Nucleus of the spinal accessory nerve
33. Ground bundles
34. Sacral parasympathetic nuclei
35. Ventral somatomotor neurons
36. Dorsal roots

Questions 37–40

Match each ganglion with the cranial nerve to which it contributes sensory axons.

(A) CN I
(B) CN VII
(C) CN V
(D) CN VIII
(E) CN III

37. Gasserian ganglion
38. Olfactory ganglion
39. Sphenopalatine ganglion
40. Vestibular ganglion

ANSWERS AND EXPLANATIONS

1. The answer is E. (*VI C 2 f*) Testing the sense of taste would be most important in a patient who had hemifacial paralysis, which would indicate a lesion of CN VII. The taste fibers and the motor fibers of the cranial nerve run together through the middle ear. The taste fibers then depart through the chorda tympani nerve, and the motor fibers continue through the facial canal to exit at the stylomastoid foramen. If the lesion is in the facial nerve proximal to the origin of the chorda tympani nerve, loss of taste indicates the location of the lesion. Sparing the sense of taste suggests that the lesion is distal to the takeoff of the taste fibers.

2. The answer is C. [*VI C 3 f (3) (b)*] The gag reflex involves an afferent arc over CN IX or CN X and an efferent arc to the levator palatini muscle, which is supplied by CN X or, in some instances, predominantly by CN IX.

3. The answer is A. [*X D 2 a, 6 b (1) (b), 7 c*] A basic function of the vestibular system is to counter-roll the eyes against the direction of head movement. This reflex, in alliance with the fixation reflexes, permits the eyes to remain on target even though the head and body are moving. Otherwise, movement of the body might interfere with the continued alignment of the eyes on the visual target.

4. The answer is D. (*XIV D 1 c; Figure 8-45*) Large parts of the nervous system can be removed or transected without abolishing consciousness. A cerebral hemisphere or the entire cerebellum can be removed. The spinal cord or the brainstem, from the caudal pontine levels on down, can be transected without abolishing consciousness if blood pressure and breathing are supported. Midbrain transection permanently abolishes consciousness.

5. The answer is D. (*XIV E 1 d, e*) Decerebrate rigidity is a postural syndrome that occurs after midbrain transection. It is driven by the vestibulospinal system. Therefore, after the syndrome has been produced, section of the vestibulospinal tracts will abolish it.

6. The answer is C. [*VI C 2 f (3); Table 8-3; Figure 8-18*] The greater superficial petrosal nerve leaves CN VII at the geniculate ganglion and crosses the floor of the middle fossa to reach the sphenopalatine ganglion, where the axons synapse. The ganglionic neurons then innervate the lacrimal glands.

7. The answer is C. [*VI C 1 a (2); Figures 8-17 and 8-38*] The junction between the innervation of the cranial nerves and the spinal nerves occurs at or near the interaural plane. This is a line roughly connecting the external auditory canals over the vertex of the head. This line does not correspond to any particular underlying bony line marks, such as the coronal or lambdoidal sutures.

8. The answer is D. (*X F 4 b, c*) The descending root of CN V ends in the upper cervical region, where an expansion of the substantia gelatinosa receives the pain and temperature fibers from the face. The substantia gelatinosa is one continuous nuclear mass representing the entire body from the tip of the coccyx in the caudal region of the cord on up to the lips in the rostral region of the cervical cord.

9. The answer is D. (*XV B 3; Figure 8-13*) CN IX, CN X, and CN XI exit from the skull through the jugular foramen. A lesion at that foramen would interrupt all three nerves and paralyze the ipsilateral palatal, pharyngeal, sternocleidomastoid, and trapezius muscles. This is one example of several syndromes that occur when a single, often small, lesion affects a conjunction of cranial nerves at the base of the skull.

10. The answer is B. (*X B 4 c; Figure 8-38*) The trigeminal nerve receives its name from its three large sensory divisions. The ophthalmic division innervates the forehead; the maxillary innervates the skin over the upper lip, maxilla, and nares; and the mandibular innervates the skin over the mandible, except for the skin over the angle, which is innervated by cervical nerves.

11. The answer is A. [*VI C 2 e (1) (a); Figure 8-19*] CN VII innervates the stapedius muscle. The function of this muscle is to dampen the oscillations of the ossicles of the inner ear. This action appears to protect the ear against excessively loud sounds. Stapedius muscle paralysis causes the patient to experience normal sounds as uncomfortably loud, a symptom called hyperacusis.

12. The answer is C. (*XIII I, J 1, 3*) In general, brain lesions that impair consciousness are found somewhere between the rostral pontine tegmentum and the medial hemispheric wall extending through the midbrain and diencephalon. The lesion site that causes the most severe, enduring loss of consciousness with the least destruction of tissue is in the midbrain tegmentum. The ascending reticular activating system funnels through this region into the diencephalon and the hemispheres. This narrow portion of the brain is appropriately called the cerebral isthmus.

13. The answer is C. (*XIV D 1*) The locked-in syndrome is complete paralysis of all voluntary movements except for vertical eye movements, although the patient retains consciousness and normal mental functions. Such a state occurs after bilateral interruption of the pyramidal tracts, usually in the basis pontis but sometimes in the midbrain. If the lesion were at the medullary level, the patient would retain some chewing and other facial movements.

14. The answer is A. (*VI C 4 e; Figure 8-21*) Several cranial nerves innervate the tongue, palate, and pharynx. Of these cranial nerves, the most important one for palatal elevation is generally the vagus nerve (CN X). Interruption of the right vagus nerve would cause paralysis of elevation of the palate on the right side.

15. The answer is D. [*XIII N 3 b, 5 b (1), 6 b; Figure 8-42*] To abolish automatic breathing, the experimenter could destroy the caudal medullary tegmentum, which contains the critical respiratory neurons necessary to drive respiration. Section of the reticulospinal tracts that decussate ventral to the obex at the cervicomedullary junction to enter the cord, or of the reticulospinal tracts in the cord, would accomplish the same end.

16. The answer is C. (*XIV E 1 a; Figure 8-44*) Lesions at various levels of the brainstem may cause characteristic changes in the patient's breathing or posture. Midbrain transection results in a characteristic driven posture called decerebrate rigidity. The patient has opisthotonos, extension and pronation of the arms, extension of the lower extremities, and plantar flexion of the feet.

17. The answer is E. (*X F 5 b*) Many of the brainstem reflexes involve an afferent arc over one of the cranial nerves and an efferent arc over another cranial nerve. The corneal reflex with its afferent arc mediated through CN V and its efferent arc through CN VII exemplifies this fact.

18. The answer is C (2, 4). (*II D 1 a, 2; XII*) The pyramidal tracts begin in the cerebral motor cortex and pass down through the internal capsule, which is still within the deep white matter of the brain. They appear on the surface of the brain at the basis pedunculi, disappear again into the nuclei of the basis pontis, and emerge again on the surface of the brain as the medullary pyramids.

19. The answer is D (4). (*X D 5 b*) Primary vestibular fibers end in the vestibular nuclei, the reticular formation, the interstitial nucleus of the vestibular nerve, and some pass directly to the flocculonodular lobe of the cerebellum. The latter are unique direct connections not found in the other sensory pathways to the cerebellum, all of which first synapse at spinal cord or brainstem levels.

20. The answer is C (2, 4). (*X E 7*) The lateral lemniscus consists of about equal numbers of crossed and uncrossed auditory axons. These are secondary, rather than primary, auditory afferent fibers, many of which originate in the superior olivary nucleus. The lateral lemniscus terminates in a specific thalamic relay nucleus, the medial geniculate body.

21. The answer is B (1, 3). (*XIV B 1 a, 2 a*) One classic type of brainstem syndrome consists of an ipsilateral lower motoneuron (LMN) cranial nerve palsy and contralateral hemiplegia. A lesion of one side of the basis of either the midbrain or the pons would cause a CN III palsy and contralateral hemiplegia in the midbrain and a CN VI palsy and contralateral hemiplegia in the pontine basis. In both of these sites, the exiting cranial nerve runs through or in close proximity to the pyramidal tract fibers prior to their decussation at the cervicomedullary junction.

22. The answer is D (4). (*XIII L 1, N 3 a*) The dorsal group of respiratory neurons are mainly inspiratory and send crossed reticulospinal pathways into the spinal cord. They are anatomically associated with the nucleus solitarius. They are not directly sensitive to changes in carbon dioxide or oxygen levels.

23. The answer is A (1, 2, 3). [*III D 1 a; IV C 2 d (2); V C 1 a*] CN III has a number of unique characteristics. It is the rostral-most motor cranial nerve, the first somite cranial nerve, and the first cranial nerve to have autonomic axons. It exits ventrally from the brainstem as do the other somite nerves except for CN IV, which exits dorsally.

24. The answer is E (all). (*II E 2 a, b; XIV E 2*) The brainstem tegmentum conveys all of the long sensory tracts and contains the somite and cranial nerve motor nuclei except for those of CN XI. Its reticular formation occupies the area not devoted to nuclei and tracts. Large pigmented neurons occupy the substantia nigra and interpeduncular nucleus in the ventral part of the midbrain tegmentum. Destruction of the substantia nigra results in parkinsonism.

25. The answer is D (4). (*X C 1, 7, 9*) The pontomedullary sulcus is the line of attachment of CN VI, CN VII, and CN VIII. It corresponds to the plane of the widest part of the fourth ventricle and of the tallest part, the fastigium. None of the cranial nerve motor nuclei of the pons or medulla cross the plane. The vestibular nuclei cross the plane, and CN VI and CN VII nuclei are in the pons just rostral to the plane.

26. The answer is B (1, 3). [*VI C 5 d (2), XIII K 3*] A lesion of C1 may cause signs that can also be caused by lesions in the posterior fossa. Ptosis and pupilloconstriction may result from a lesion of the descending autonomic pathways through the medulla and spinal cord, down to the level of T1. The spinal accessory nerve, which innervates the trapezius muscles, arises in the rostral part of the cervical cord and enters the posterior fossa through the foramen magnum. The accessory fibers of the vagus nerve, which travel with the spinal accessory nerve, arise from the medulla, not the spinal part of the spinal accessory nerve, and hence would not be affected by a C1 lesion.

27–31. The answers are 27-C, 28-E, 29-E, 30-A, 31-A. (*II A–D; Figures 8-1, 8-2, and 8-3*) The widest part of the brainstem is the midpontine level. The size of the brainstem diminishes, going caudally from the midpontine level into the medulla or rostrally from the midpontine level into the midbrain. The smallest cross-sectional diameter is located at the caudal medullary level. On the dorsal surface of the brainstem, the caudal medullary level has the thinnest roof plate. The roof plate of the entire medulla consists of the posterior medullary velum, which is purely membranous and posteriorly has an aperture by which ventricular fluid can escape into the subarachnoid space around the brainstem. The roof plate of the pons consists of the anterior medullary velum, which is a thin sheet containing some nerve fibers. On the contrary, the tectum, or roof plate, of the midbrain consists of a thick lamina of nerve cells and fibers known as the quadrigeminal plate.

Internally, the narrowest site of communication between the ventricles is the aqueduct of the midbrain. In the pons, the aqueduct expands to form the fourth ventricle, which has its widest lateral diameter at the plane of the pontomedullary sulcus. From that point, the fourth ventricle narrows to an apex at the obex, which is at the junction of the medulla and spinal cord. The fourth ventricle then continues into the central canal of the spinal cord.

32–36. The answers are 32-E, 33-B, 34-C, 35-A, 36-D. (*Table 8-4*) The brainstem as a whole and the medulla in particular can be interpreted as merely expanded and somewhat elaborated spinal cord. Both the brainstem and spinal cord have a similar embryogenesis, with alar and basal plates, and both have a basically segmental plan, with somites extending from the spinal cord to the midbrain level. Both have a central cavity, the central canal in the spinal cord and the aqueduct and fourth ventricle in the brainstem. The major differences are the fact that the brainstem has a well-developed reticular formation and has branchial arch nuclei. The best possible spinal cord homologue of the branchial arch nuclei is the spinal accessory nucleus in the rostral part of the cervical cord. Several brainstem structures have direct homologues in the spinal cord. The hypoglossal nucleus consists of ventral somatomotor neurons just like the ventral somatomotor neurons of the spinal cord gray matter. The medial longitudinal fasciculus is a brainstem ground bundle, which interconnects the somitic CN III, CN IV, and CN VI in the same way that the ground bundles of the spinal cord convey the short intra- and intersegmental pathways for the cord. The Edinger-Westphal nucleus consists of the preganglionic parasympathetic neurons of CN III in the same way that the sacral parasympathetic nuclei are preganglionic neurons for the pelvic splanchnic nerve. The dorsal roots of the spinal nerves correspond to the ganglia on CN IX and CN X, the gasserian ganglion, and also the special sensory ganglia of CN VIII, with its cochlear and vestibular divisions. The numerous similarities of structure between brainstem and spinal cord stop at the rostral end of the brainstem. Rostral to that level, in the diencephalon and cerebrum, the anatomical arrangements differ drastically. The spinal cord has no direct homologue for the cerebral cortex.

37–40. The answers are: 37-C, 38-A, 39-C, 40-D. (*VI A*) Various cranial nerves have one or more ganglia along their course. CN VIII has two ganglia, the spiral ganglion, which serves the auditory part of the nerve, and the vestibular ganglion, which serves the vestibular component of the nerve. CN V receives its sensory axons from the gasserian ganglion, which is outside the CNS, but it also has a unique ganglion in the CNS called the mesencephalic nucleus of CN V, which also provides sensory axons. No other nerves have a similar arrangement. CN I has the two olfactory ganglia, one on each side of the nasal septum. They produce the shortest cranial nerve of all. Its axons run only from the ganglion beneath the cribriform plate, through the cribriform plate, to synapse on the olfactory bulb. Some cranial nerves that are essentially motor in function do not have their own ganglion and probably receive their sensory fibers from the gasserian ganglion. Examples include CN III, CN IV, and CN VI, which innervate the ocular rotatory muscles. The sphenopalatine ganglion of CN VII contributes postganglionic axons that enter a peripheral branch of CN V to reach the lacrimal gland. The geniculate ganglion contributes taste fibers to CN VII, which ultimately run through the lingual branch of CN V.

9

Cerebellum

I. GROSS ANATOMY OF THE CEREBELLUM

A. Definition. The cerebellum is a fist-sized, transversely fissured mass of central nervous system (CNS) tissue attached to the dorsum of the pons by peduncles (Fig. 9-1; see Fig. 1-3).

B. Composition. The cerebellum basically consists of the following parts (see Fig. 1-8*B*):

1. A cortex sulcated into numerous folia

2. Deep white matter

3. Paired deep nuclei

4. Paired peduncles, which convey afferent and efferent nerve fibers (see Fig. 9-10)

C. Location and anatomical relationships of the cerebellum

1. The cerebellum occupies the posterior fossa, along with the medulla, the pons, and most of the midbrain.

2. The **cerebellar tentorium** roofs the posterior fossa, separating the cerebellum from the overlying temporo-occipital lobes of the cerebrum.

3. Supported by its peduncles, the cerebellum overhangs the anterior and posterior medullary vela (the tectum, or roof, of the fourth ventricle) [see Fig. 9-3].

4. When the peduncles are sliced across, the cerebellum falls free from the pons and thus from the neuraxis.

5. Removal of the cerebellum fully exposes the rhomboid fossa, the floor of the fourth ventricle.

D. Transverse subdivision of the cerebellum into three lobes

1. Transverse clefts or fissures, which are much deeper than the folia, separate the groups of folia into **lobes** and **lobules** (Figs. 9-2 and 9-3; see Fig. 9-1). The three cerebellar lobes are:
   a. Anterior lobe
   b. Posterior lobe
   c. Flocculonodular lobe

2. Figure 9-2 depicts the cerebellar lobes as if they were flattened out. In reality, the flocculonodular lobe is rolled underneath. (Compare Figures 9-1, 9-2, and 9-3.)

E. Three sagittal subdivisions of the cerebellum

1. Two parasagittal cuts slice out a midline **vermis** from the two cerebellar hemispheres (see Fig. 9-2).

2. Any sagittal or parasagittal cut reveals the characteristic foliar pattern of the cerebellum and the deeper fissures that demarcate the three major lobes and the minor lobules (see Fig. 9-3).

F. Cerebellar tonsils

1. A cerebellar tonsil forms the medioventral border of each cerebellar hemisphere (see Fig. 9-1*B*).

2. Between the two tonsils is a space, the **cerebellar vallecula**. In the depths of the vallecula, one can see the median **foramen of Magendie**, a perforation in the posterior medullary

A

Primary fissure   Anterior lobe   Vermis

Hemisphere

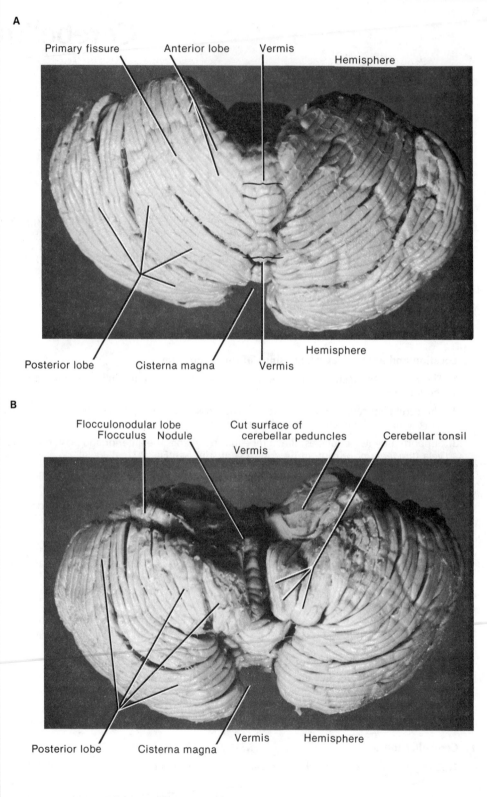

Posterior lobe   Cisterna magna   Vermis

Hemisphere

B

Flocculonodular lobe   Cut surface of
Flocculus   Nodule   cerebellar peduncles   Cerebellar tonsil
Vermis

Posterior lobe   Cisterna magna   Vermis   Hemisphere

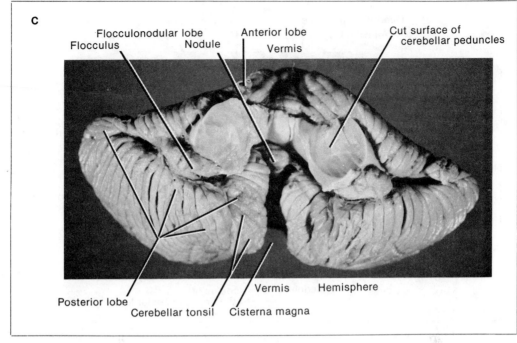

Figure 9-1. Gross photographs of the cerebellum. (A) Superior surface. (B) Inferior surface. (C) Anterior view, showing the transversely sectioned cerebellar peduncles.

velum by which cerebrospinal fluid (CSF) enters the subarachnoid space from the fourth ventricle.

3. Dissecting the tonsils off discloses the entire posterior medullary velum.

4. Whenever the intracranial pressure increases, the tonsils tend to herniate downward, out of the posterior fossa and through the foramen magnum (see Fig. 2-15). By compressing the medullocervical junction, tonsilar herniation causes quadriplegia and respiratory arrest.

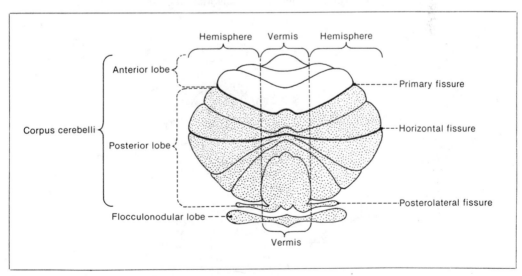

Figure 9-2. Diagrammatic dorsal view of the cerebellum showing three sagittal subdivisions (hemisphere, vermis, and hemisphere) and three transverse subdivisions (anterior lobe, posterior lobe, and flocculonodular lobe) [Larsell's nomenclature].

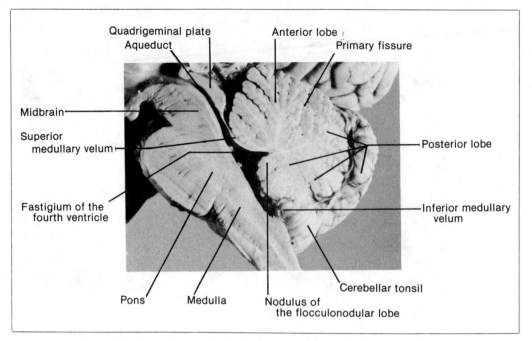

Figure 9-3. Gross photograph of sagittal section of the cerebellar vermis and brainstem.

G. Deep nuclei of the cerebellum

1. Three paired nuclear masses, buried in the cerebellar white matter, overlie the fourth ventricle (Fig. 9-4).

2. In medial-to-lateral order, the nuclei are:
   a. **Fastigial nucleus** (nucleus fastigii), whose name comes from its location near the fastigium of the fourth ventricle
   b. **Interpositus nucleus**
      (1) The interpositus nucleus is so named because of its interposition between the dentate and fastigial nuclei.
      (2) It consists of two nuclei: nucleus emboliformis and nucleus globosus.

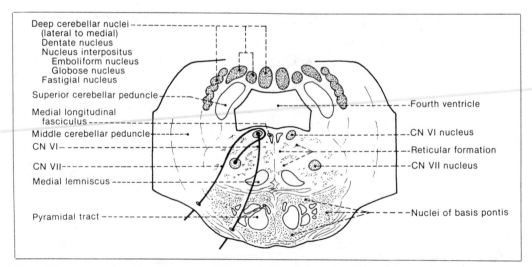

Figure 9-4. Transverse section of the pons, middle cerebellar peduncle, fourth ventricle, and overlying deep cerebellar nuclei.

c. **Dentate nucleus** (nucleus dentatus), which is the largest and most lateral of the cerebellar nuclei, receiving its name from its corrugated or tooth-like outline, which closely resembles the inferior olivary nucleus

II. ONTOGENY, PHYLOGENY, AND FUNCTION OF THE CEREBELLUM

A. Ontogeny

1. The cerebellum develops as two hillocks, one in each of the paired rhombic lips of the pons (Fig. 9-5).

2. The hillocks unite in the midline at the roof plate to form the solid cerebellar mass.

3. Since the cerebellum is a thickening in the dorsal wall of the neural tube, not an evagination, it has no ventricular cavity, even though it overlies the fourth ventricle.

B. Phylogeny and function

1. In vertebrates, the first part of the cerebellum to appear was the flocculonodular lobe.

2. Originally the flocculonodular lobe developed out of the vestibular nuclei. It retains, even in primates, direct afferent and efferent vestibular connections reflecting its phylogenetic origin.

3. The flocculonodular–vestibular system coordinated reflex contractions of the axial muscles to relate the position and movement of the head, eyes, and trunk to each other and to the planes of space and the pull of gravity.

4. As the cerebrum came to produce willed movements of the trunk and elaborating limbs, the cerebellum was then adapted to coordinate the contractions of axial and appendicular muscles during willed postures and willed movements. The cerebropontocerebellar pathway enlarged in parallel with the enlargement of:
   a. Cerebral motor cortex and pyramidal tracts
   b. Basis pontis
   c. Inferior olivary complex
   d. Cerebellar hemispheres and dentate nucleus

5. The essential clinical sign of cerebellar lesions is **dystaxia**; that is, incoordination of muscular contractions during willed movement or willfully sustained postures.

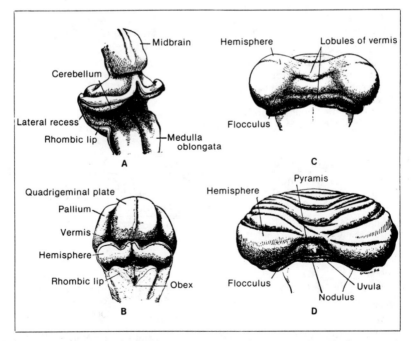

Figure 9-5. Ontogeny of the cerebellum. (*A*) Six weeks (6 ×). (*B*) Two months (4 ×). (*C*) Four months (3 ×). (*D*) Five months (2.8 ×). (Reprinted with permission from Arey LB: *Developmental Anatomy*. Philadelphia, WB Saunders, 1946, p 441.)

C. Phylogenetic/functional nomenclature of the cerebellar lobes

1. The cerebellum consists of three units having different phylogenetic ages, connections, and functions: the archicerebellum, the paleocerebellum, and the neocerebellum. These terms correspond to Larsell's lobar subdivisions of the cerebellum (Table 9-1).

a. The **archicerebellum** (the flocculonodular lobe, or vestibulocerebellum) is the original part of the cerebellum, elaborated in relation to the vestibular nuclei.

b. The **paleocerebellum** (the anterior lobe, or spinocerebellum) receives the proprioceptive trunk and limb afferents from the spinal cord.

c. The **neocerebellum** (the posterior lobe, or cerebrocerebellum) receives the corticoponto-cerebellar pathway and the pathway from the inferior olivary nucleus.

2. In turn, each of these three phylogenetic/anatomical/functional subdivisions projects to its own midline nucleus (see Table 9-1).

III. CEREBELLAR CORTEX

A. Neuronal layers and neuronal types

1. The cerebellar cortex has three layers of neuronal perikarya: **molecular, Purkinje cell,** and **granular** (Fig. 9-6).

2. The three cortical layers contain five types of neurons in all (Table 9-2 and Fig. 9-7).

3. Although each type of neuronal perikaryon occupies only one of the cortical layers, either the dendrites or axons or both extend into or through the other layers.

B. Orientation of cerebellar neurons

1. Many cortical neurons and their processes have a definite spatial orientation to the plane of the folia. Figure 9-7 shows a folium cut across at right angles to its long axis, like slicing a loaf of bread.

2. Orientation of Purkinje dendrites

a. Figure 9-7 shows that the dendrites of the Purkinje neurons and Golgi type II neurons poke up into the molecular layer.

b. The Purkinje neuron dendrites are flattened to occupy only one plane, a plane across the long axis of the folium.

c. To remember the orientation of the Purkinje cell dendrites, place your hands flat on the sides of your head with your palms on your ears. The plane of your fingers is now **across** (transverse to) the long axis of the folia and, therefore, represents the actual flat plane of the dendrites of your own Purkinje neurons (and the Golgi type II neurons and stellate neurons, as well).

3. Orientation of granule neuron axons (see Fig. 9-7)

a. The axons of the granule neurons ascend into the molecular layer where they bifurcate.

b. After they bifurcate, these axons run parallel to the long axis of the folia and parallel to each other, hence the name parallel fibers.

c. Visualize the parallel axons as electrical wires running across the dendritic trees of several Purkinje, Golgi type II, and stellate neurons, upon which they synapse.

Table 9-1. Organization of the Cerebellum into Triads

Larsell's Lobar Subdivisions	Phylogenetic/ Functional Subdivisions	Afferent Peduncle	Efferent Peduncle	Deep (Midline) Nucleus	Olivary Nucleus (Medulla)
Flocculonodular lobe	Archicerebellum (vestibulocerebel-lum)	Caudal	Caudal	Fastigial	Medial accessory
Corpus cerebelli Anterior lobe	Paleocerebellum (spinocerebellum)	Rostral and caudal	Rostral	Interpositus (emboliform and globose)	Dorsal accessory
Posterior lobe	Neocerebellum (cerebrocerebellum)	Middle	Rostral	Dentate	Inferior

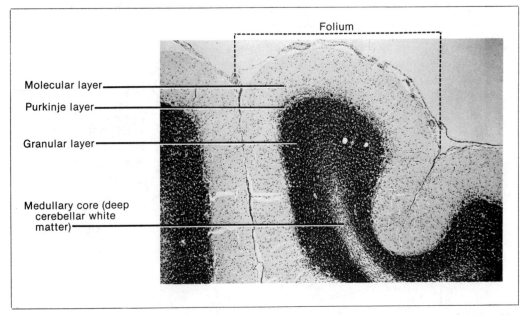

Folium

Molecular layer

Purkinje layer

Granular layer

Medullary core (deep
   cerebellar white
   matter)

Figure 9-6. Photomicrograph of a Nissl-stained transverse section of cerebellar folia, showing the three layers of the cerebellar cortex (40 ×).

4. Orientation of stellate neuron dendrites and axons (see Fig. 9-7)
   a. The inner stellate neurons of the molecular layer have their dendrites in the transverse plane of the folia, like Purkinje and Golgi type II neurons.
   b. Their axons also run in the transverse plane. Thus they run at right angles to the parallel fibers or tangential to the contour of the folia. Hence, they are called tangential fibers. Their terminal axons form baskets around Purkinje neurons (see Fig. 9-7).

5. Intrafolial and interfolial connections
   a. The parallel fibers connect the Purkinje, inner stellate, and Golgi type II neuron dendrites laterally, forming extended intrafolial connections.
   b. The tangential fibers connect the Purkinje neurons in the anterior–posterior plane, forming intrafolial and transfolial or interfolial connections.

C. Termination of afferent fibers in the cerebellar cortex

   1. The majority of afferents to the cerebellar cortex end as climbing fibers or mossy fibers.

   2. Climbing fibers originate from the inferior olivary nuclei.
      a. After collateralizing to the deep cerebellar nuclei, they ascend to the cortex and climb directly up onto the Purkinje neuron dendrites, hence their name.
      b. The relationship of the climbing fibers to Purkinje cells is nearly one to one.

   3. Mossy fibers originate in the remaining cerebellar motor and sensory afferent systems. After

Table 9-2. Five Types of Neurons in the Cerebellar Cortex and the Layers That Contain Their Perikarya

Neuron	Layer
Outer stellate Inner stellate (basket)	Molecular
Purkinje	Purkinje
Golgi type II Granule	Granular

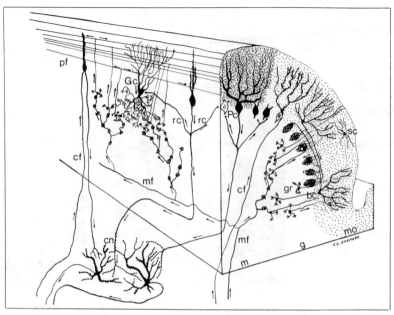

Figure 9-7. Stereogram of a transversely cut cerebellar folium, as the neurons and inter-neuronal connections would appear in Golgi silver impregnations. *bc* = basket cells; *cf* = climbing fiber; *cn* = deep cerebellar nuclei; *g* = granular layer; *Gc* = Golgi cell; *gr* = granule cell; *m* = medullary layer; *mf* = mossy fiber; *mo* = molecular layer; *Pc* = Purkinje cell; *pf* = parallel fiber; *rc* = recurrent collateral; *sc* = stellate cell. (Reprinted with permission from Crosby EC, Humphrey T, Lauer EW: *Correlative Anatomy of the Nervous System*. New York, Macmillan, 1962, p 196.)

collateralizing to the deep cerebellar nuclei, the mossy fibers end in the glomeruli of the granular layer of the cerebellar cortex, where they may affect thousands of granular neurons.

D. Cerebellar glomeruli

    1. The mossy fibers end in rosette-like terminals, which enter into a synaptic arrangement called a **glomerulus** (Fig. 9-8).

        a. The perikarya of the granule neurons cluster around the glomeruli, which are free of nuclei.

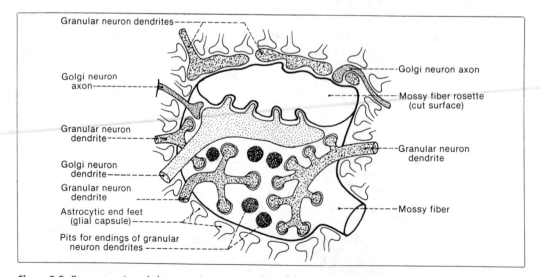

Figure 9-8. Reconstruction of electron microscope studies of the synaptic connections in a cerebellar glomerulus.

    b. A glomerulus consists of:
      (1) Rosette-like endings of mossy fibers
      (2) Claw-like dendritic terminals of the granule neurons
      (3) Axons of Golgi type II neurons (these axon terminals encounter the axon terminals of the mossy fibers, thus constituting an axo-axonic synapse)
      (4) Some dendritic branches from Golgi type II neurons; thus, mossy fiber endings come in contact with both axons and dendrites of Golgi type II neurons
      (5) A glial capsule, which surrounds each glomerulus
  2. The parallel fibers of the granule neurons convey the output from the cerebellar glomeruli into the molecular layer.

E. Synaptic connections of the neurons of the cerebellar cortex
  1. The Purkinje cell is the focal neuron of the cerebellar cortex because of the following.
    a. All afferent pathways ultimately converge on the Purkinje cell.
    b. Purkinje axons are the only way out of the cerebellar cortex, its "final common pathway."
      (1) A small minority of Purkinje axons leave the cerebellum. They synapse directly on vestibular nuclei.
      (2) The vast majority of Purkinje axons remain within the cerebellum, where they synapse on the deep cerebellar nuclei. The deep nuclei originate most of the efferent fibers that leave the cerebellum.
    c. Purkinje axons, in a curious arrangement, send a recurrent collateral back to adjacent Purkinje cells and to Golgi type II neurons (see Fig. 9-7).
  2. Table 9-3 summarizes the synaptic connections of cerebellar cortical neurons.
  3. Summary of excitatory and inhibitory synapses of the cerebellar cortex
    a. All incoming climbing and mossy fibers produce **excitatory** synapses.
    b. Four of the five types of intrinsic neurons of the cerebellar cortex produce **inhibitory** synapses.
    c. Only the granule neuron axons (parallel fibers) produce excitation (Table 9-4).

Table 9-3. Five Neuron Types of the Cerebellar Cortex* and Their Synaptic Connections

Neuron Type	Afferent Connections	Axonal Distribution
Outer stellate	Receive parallel fibers from granule neurons	Axons synapse on outer part of Purkinje neuron dendrites
Inner stellate	Receive parallel fibers from granule neurons	Axons form tangential fibers that synapse on Purkinje dendrites via basket collaterals
Purkinje	• Climbing fibers from extracerebellar sources • Parallel fibers from axons of the granule neurons of the cerebellar cortex • Basket fibers from the inner stellate neurons • Axons from the outer stellate neurons • Noradrenergic afferents from nucleus locus ceruleus	Most Purkinje axons run to deep nuclei. A few Purkinje axons, originating in the flocculonodular lobe, bypass the deep nuclei to reach the vestibular nuclei. Purkinje axons also send recurrent collaterals back to themselves and to Golgi type II neurons
Golgi type II	Receive mossy fiber and climbing fiber synapses on dendrites in granular layer and receive parallel axons on dendrites that extend into the molecular layer	Send axons to cerebellar glomeruli to synapse on mossy fiber rosettes
Granule	Receive rosette endings from mossy fibers in cerebellar glomeruli	Send parallel fibers to the Purkinje neuron dendrites and inner and outer stellate neurons of the molecular layer and those parts of Golgi type II neuron dendrites that penetrate the molecular layer

*The neurons are listed in order from superficial to deep as they appear in the cerebellar cortex (see Fig. 9-7).

Table 9-4. Inhibitory and Excitatory Synaptic Relationships of the Cerebellar Cortex and Deep Nuclei

---

Inhibitory intrinsic neurons of the cerebellar cortex
 Golgi type II neurons of the granular layer
 Purkinje neurons
 Inner and outer stellate neurons

Excitatory intrinsic neurons of the cerebellar cortex
 Granule neurons

Excitatory extrinsic and intrinsic fibers
 Climbing fibers and mossy fibers, both the direct fibers to the cerebellar cortex and their collaterals to the midline nuclei
 Parallel fibers from granule neurons

Inhibitory intrinsic fibers*
 Basket fibers
 Purkinje fibers

Cerebellar nuclei
 Inhibited by Purkinje fibers
 Excited by collaterals from climbing and mossy fibers and may have own intrinsic excitatory pacemaker

---

*There are no inhibitory extrinsic fibers, at least from somatic afferent systems.

IV. CEREBELLAR CIRCUITS

A. General plan

1. Like all integrating centers, the cerebellum has well-defined afferent and efferent pathways and internal circuitry.
   a. Its **afferent pathways** arise in sensory systems, motor cortex, and reticular formation.
   b. Its **internal circuitry** converges on the Purkinje cells, most of which relay through the cerebellar nuclei.
   c. Its **efferent pathways** arise from the cerebellar nuclei, which influence other parts of the CNS acting on the lower motoneurons (LMNs).
2. All afferents enter the cerebellum through one of the three cerebellar peduncles, and all efferents leave through one.
3. Since the peduncles attach the cerebellum to the pons and only the pons, all afferent and efferent pathways of the cerebellum run through the pons during at least a part of their course.

B. Afferent cerebellar pathways

1. The motor and sensory afferents entering the cerebellum run dorsally in one of the peduncles, send a collateral to a deep cerebellar nucleus, and proceed through the medullary cores of the folia to reach the cerebellar cortex.

2. **Sensory system afferents**
   a. Sensory system afferents come from proprioceptors:
      (1) Muscle spindles
      (2) Vestibular end organs
      (3) Joint receptors
   b. Other somatic sensory systems project to the vermis, but their function and clinical significance are unknown.

3. **Motor system afferents** come from:
   a. Corticopontocerebellar system
   b. Olivocerebellar system

4. **Reticular formation afferents** come from:
   a. "Cerebellar nuclei" of reticular formation (see Chapter 8, section XIII F 4)
   b. Nucleus locus ceruleus (see Chapter 14, section II C 2 a)

5. **Topographic distribution of afferents in the cerebellar cortex**

a. **Vestibular afferents** end mainly in the flocculonodular lobe, caudal vermis, and lingula.
b. **Spinocerebellar** and **trigeminocerebellar afferents** end in the cortex of the vermis, predominantly of the anterior lobe. These cerebellar afferents end somatotopically with the lower extremity represented most rostrally (Fig. 9-9).
c. **Pontine basis afferents** of the corticopontocerebellar relay system decussate in the basis and end mainly in the cortex of the contralateral cerebellar hemisphere with no overlap in the vermis.
d. **Olivary afferents** end in a topographical medial-to-lateral manner.
    (1) The smaller nuclei of the inferior olivary complex project to the vermian cortex.
    (2) The main inferior olivary nucleus projects to the cortex of the contralateral cerebellar hemisphere.
e. **Nucleus locus ceruleus** afferents project to the cerebellar cortex diffusely.

C. Cerebellar peduncles

  1. Location. On each side of the pons, three peduncles—the **rostral (superior)**, **middle**, and **caudal (inferior)**—unite into one stalk of fibers that attaches the cerebellum to the pons (Fig. 9-10).

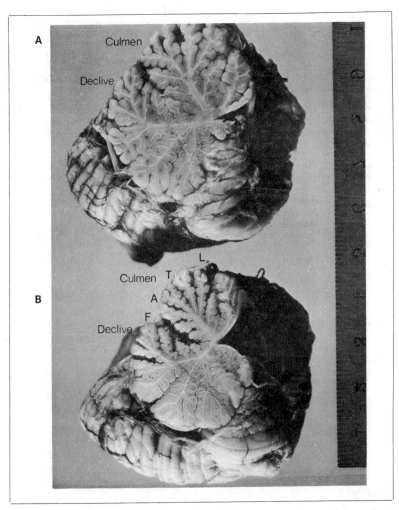

Figure 9-9. Sagittal sections through the cerebellar vermis. (*A*) Normal control. (*B*) Cerebellum of alcoholic patient who had dystaxia of the legs and trunk (rostral vermis syndrome). The cerebellar vermis receives the spinocerebellar and trigeminocerebellar tracts in topographic order. The cerebellum in *B* shows atrophy of the culmen, which receives the leg and trunk fibers. *L* = leg area; *T* = trunk; *A* = arm; *F* = face. (Courtesy of Dr. Jans Muller, Indiana University School of Medicine, Indianapolis, IN.)

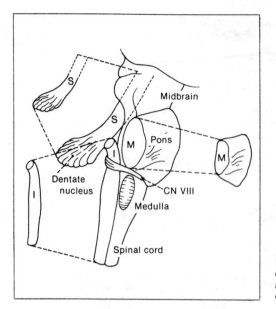

Figure 9-10. Exploded lateral view of the cerebellar peduncles. *S* = superior or rostral cerebellar peduncle; *M* = middle cerebellar peduncle; *I* = inferior or caudal cerebellar peduncle.

2. The caudal and rostral peduncles contain afferent and efferent tracts; the middle peduncle is purely afferent (Table 9-5).

3. The **caudal** peduncle is largely afferent but conveys some cerebellovestibular efferents.
   a. It has two components: the **restiform body** and the **juxtarestiform body** (see Table 9-5).
   b. The juxtarestiform body conveys the vestibulocerebellar and cerebellovestibular pathways (Fig. 9-11).

4. The **middle** peduncle is solely afferent. It conveys the pontocerebellar pathway.
   a. It is the largest and most lateral of the cerebellar peduncles.
   b. It mainly consists of decussated fibers from the nuclei of the contralateral half of the basis pontis.

5. Rostral peduncle
   a. It conveys two major efferent pathways from the dentate nucleus: the dentatothalamic and the dentatorubral tracts.
   b. The ventral spinocerebellar tract, an afferent pathway, curves dorsally to enter through this peduncle.

Table 9-5. Major Tracts in the Cerebellar Peduncles

Peduncle	Tracts	Afferent/Efferent
Caudal (inferior)	Restiform body	
	Dorsal spinocerebellar tract	A
	Olivocerebellar tract	A
	Arcuatocerebellar tract	A
	Reticulocerebellar tract	A
	Juxtarestiform body	
	Direct and secondary vestibulo-cerebellar tracts	A
	Cerebellovestibular tracts	E
Middle	Pontocerebellar tracts	A
Rostral (superior)	Ventral spinocerebellar tract	A
	Trigeminocerebellar tract	A
	Tectocerebellar tract	A
	Brachium conjunctivum (dentatorubrothalamic tract)	E

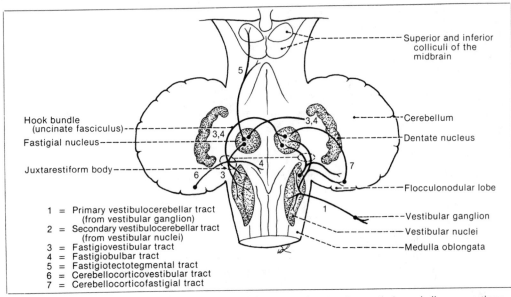

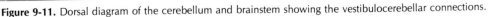

Figure 9-11. Dorsal diagram of the cerebellum and brainstem showing the vestibulocerebellar connections.

V. CEREBROCEREBELLOPYRAMIDAL PATHWAY

A. Clinical importance

1. The single most important cerebellar circuit connects the cerebellum with the cerebral motor cortex and, through the pyramidal tract of the latter, to the LMNs. In its entirety, it consists of a **cerebrocortico-ponto-cerebellocortico-dentato-thalamo-cortico-pyramido-LMN** circuit (Fig. 9-12).

2. Interruption of the coordinating influence of the cerebellum on the motor cortex causes the clinical signs of cerebellar dysfunction.

B. Decussations and laterality of cerebellar signs

1. Notice in Figure 9-12 the two decussations of the cerebrocerebellar circuit.
   a. One is in the pontocerebellar pathway through the basis pontis and the middle cerebellar peduncle.
   b. The other is in the pathway through the rostral cerebellar peduncle as it passes through the midbrain to the thalamus.

2. Notice that the circuit brings the coordinating influence of one cerebellar cortex to bear upon the **contralateral** motor cortex. The pyramidal tract from that motor cortex will then decussate before reaching the LMNs. Thus, the entire circuit has three clinically significant decussations, which you should know.

3. Because of the three decussations, a lesion in one cerebellar hemisphere will impair coordination in the **ipsilateral** extremities.

4. Thus, the clinical aphorism is that cerebral hemisphere lesions cause **contralateral** motor signs (the pyramidal syndrome; see Table 7-3) and cerebellar hemisphere lesions cause **ipsilateral** motor signs (the cerebellar syndrome; see section VI B).

5. Interruption of the dentatothalamic pathway **before** it decussates causes **ipsilateral** signs; interruption **after** it decussates causes **contralateral** signs. Think through the circuit in Figure 9-12 to understand this statement.

VI. CLINICAL EFFECTS OF CEREBELLAR LESIONS

A. Conditions under which cerebellar signs occur

1. The cerebellum functions to coordinate the sequence and strength of muscular contractions during:
   a. Willed postures, such as the vertical posture or holding the hands out

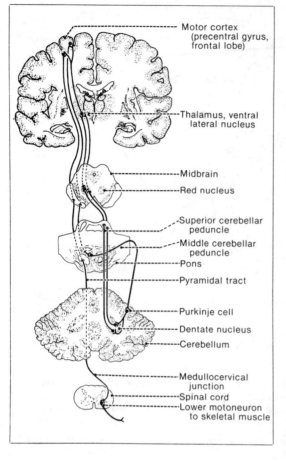

Motor cortex
(precentral gyrus,
frontal lobe)

Thalamus, ventral
lateral nucleus

Midbrain

Red nucleus

Superior cerebellar
peduncle

Middle cerebellar
peduncle

Pons

Pyramidal tract

Purkinje cell

Dentate nucleus

Cerebellum

Medullocervical
junction

Spinal cord

Lower motoneuron
to skeletal muscle

Figure 9-12. Diagram of the cerebrocerebellocerebral circuit. Commence at the cerebral motor cortex and trace through the circuit, noting the sites of the decussations.

  b. Willed movements of the trunk, limbs, and bulbar muscles

2. Unless the patient can make a voluntary muscular contraction (i.e., one mediated through the motor cortex and the pyramidal pathways), the cerebellum and its pathways cannot be tested. Therefore, the cerebellum and its pathways cannot be tested during:
  a. Sleep
  b. Coma
  c. Paralysis due to interruption of the pyramidal tract

3. Cerebellar lesions have no clinically apparent effect on mentation, consciousness, memory, sensory perception, or autonomic functions.

B. Signs and syndromes of cerebellar lesions

1. Clinical signs of a cerebellar lesion include:
  a. Dystaxia and **dysmetria** [due to incoordination of axial and appendicular muscles; dystaxia of axial (truncal) and leg muscles leading to a broad-based, unsteady gait]
  b. Dysarthria (due to incoordination of speech muscles)
  c. Nystagmus (due to incoordination of eye muscles)
  d. Hypotonia (the physiologic basis of hypotonia that follows cerebellar lesions is unclear)

2. Four cerebellar syndromes can be recognized, based on the location of the lesion (Fig. 9-13).
  a. The **cerebellar hemisphere syndrome** consists of dystaxia and hypotonia of the ipsilateral extremities. The most common causes are neoplasms and infarction.
  b. The **rostral vermis syndrome** consists of dystaxia of the legs and trunk during walking; there is little or no involvement of the upper extremities or of the speech or eye muscles. This syndrome occurs most frequently in chronic alcoholic patients. Alcoholism causes selective degeneration of the "leg region" of the anterior vermis. (Review Figure 9-9.)
  c. The **caudal vermis syndrome** (flocculonodular lobe syndrome) consists of the inability to maintain upright posture due to truncal dystaxia. Nystagmus may also be present. This syn-

Distribution of deficits	Dysarthria	Arm overshoot	Hypotonia	Dystaxia of Arms	Dystaxia of Gait and trunk	Dystaxia of Legs	Nystagmus	Clinical syndrome	Lobe or lobes affected
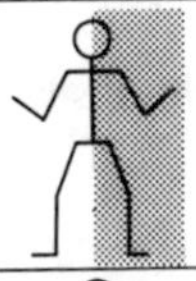 (figure)	+	+	+	+	+	+	Bidirectional, coarser to side of lesion. Fast component to sides of gaze	Cerebellar hemisphere syndrome	Mainly posterior lobe, variably anterior lobe
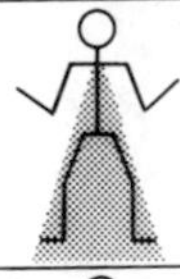 (figure)	0	±	+	±	+	+	0	Rostral vermis syndrome	Anterior lobe
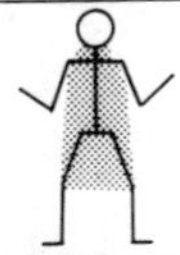 (figure)	0	0	±	0	+	±	Variable	Caudal vermis syndrome	Flocculonodular and posterior lobes
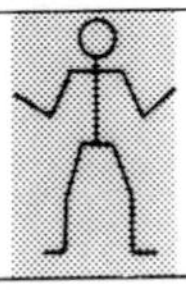 (figure)	+	+	+	+	+	+	Variable	Pancerebellar syndrome	All lobes

Figure 9-13. Summary of the four cerebellar syndromes.

drome occurs most commonly with tumors of the vermis (e.g., ependymoma of the fourth ventricle, cerebellar astrocytoma, or medulloblastoma).

    d. The **pancerebellar syndrome** consists of the full picture of bilateral dystaxia, dysarthria, nystagmus, and hypotonia of all voluntary muscles. The most common causes are degenerative diseases, multiple sclerosis, and intoxications. Acute alcoholic intoxication, for example, causes the complete pancerebellar syndrome.

  3. Since the causes of the various syndromes differ, identifying the syndrome correctly is nearly tantamount to recognizing the cause.

  4. Signs of interruption of cerebellar pathways
    a. Interruption of dentatothalamic/dentatorubral pathways may cause a **terminal tremor** (i.e., a tremor of an extremity, which increases as the part nears its endpoint). For example, such a tremor may occur when the fingertip is brought in to touch the nose.
    b. Interruption, even surgical transection, of either spinocerebellar or cerebropontocerebellar pathways causes little or only transient cerebellar dysfunction.

VII. SUMMARY OF THE CEREBELLAR TRIADS. As a mnemonic exercise, review the cerebellar triads, as listed here and in Table 9-1.

  A. Three sagittal divisions: vermis and two hemispheres

  B. Three transverse divisions into lobes: anterior, posterior, and flocculonodular

  C. Three phylogenetic/functional subdivisions, which correspond to the lobes: archicerebellum (vestibulocerebellum, the flocculonodular lobe), paleocerebellum (spinocerebellum, the anterior lobe), and neocerebellum (cerebrocerebellum, the posterior lobe)

  D. Three layers of cortex: molecular, Purkinje cell, and granular, from superficial to deep

  E. Three pairs of midline nuclei: the fastigial nucleus, the nucleus interpositus (composed of the emboliform and globose nuclei), and the dentate nucleus, in medial to lateral order

  F. Three endings of the Purkinje axons: recurrent collateral to the axon itself, to a midline nucleus, or to a vestibular nucleus

G. **Three neuronal sources of synapses in the cerebellar glomeruli:** mossy fiber endings, dendrites of granule cells, and dendrites and axons of Golgi type II neurons

H. **Three peduncles on each side:** the caudal (inferior), middle, and rostral (superior)

I. **Three olivary nuclei:** medial accessory, dorsal accessory, and inferior olivary

J. **Three major decussations**, which bring the cerebellar influence back to the ipsilateral LMNs (see Fig. 9-13).

STUDY QUESTIONS

Directions: Each question below contains five suggested answers. Choose the **one best** response to each question.

1. Most efferent axons in the superior cerebellar peduncles arise in

(A) deep nuclei of the cerebellum
(B) stellate neurons of the cerebellar cortex
(C) Purkinje cells
(D) Golgi type II neurons of the cerebellar cortex
(E) none of the above

2. A middle-aged patient of questionable sobriety shows dystaxia of the lower extremities; he has little or no arm dystaxia, dysarthria, or nystagmus. He most likely has a lesion of

(A) the spinocerebellar tracts in the cord
(B) the vermis of the anterior lobe of the cerebellum
(C) the central tegmental tract
(D) the tuber and pyramis
(E) the dentatorubrothalamic tract at the midbrain level

3. Dystaxia resulting from lesions of the cerebellar hemisphere reflects dysmodulation of impulses relayed through which pathway?

(A) Dentatovestibulospinal
(B) Olivocerebellar
(C) Dentatorubral
(D) Dentatothalamocerebrocortical
(E) Spinocerebellar

4. The part of the cerebellum that may undergo transforaminal herniation and strangle the medullocervical junction is the

(A) rostral vermis
(B) flocculonodular lobe
(C) caudal (inferior) peduncle
(D) tonsil
(E) anterior medullary velum

Directions: Each question below contains four suggested answers of which **one or more** is correct. Choose the answer

    A   if **1, 2, and 3** are correct
    B   if **1 and 3** are correct
    C   if **2 and 4** are correct
    D   if **4** is correct
    E   if **1, 2, 3, and 4** are correct

5. Which of the following lesions would reduce the afferent fibers to the deep cerebellar nuclei?

(1) Transection of the inferior cerebellar peduncle
(2) Section of the auditory nerve
(3) Destruction of Purkinje neurons
(4) Destruction of cerebellar granule cells and Golgi type II neurons

6. A cerebellar glomerulus consists of which of the following?

(1) Mossy fiber rosettes
(2) Contacts from axons and dendrites of Golgi type II neurons
(3) Dendrites of granule neurons
(4) Glial capsule

7. Excitatory neurons of the cerebellar cortex include which of the following?

(1) Purkinje neurons
(2) Inner stellate (basket) neurons
(3) Golgi type II neurons
(4) Granule neurons

8. Correct statements concerning the cerebellar peduncles include which of the following?

(1) The middle peduncle conveys mostly crossed pontocerebellar axons
(2) All cerebellar peduncles attach the cerebellum to the pons
(3) The inferior (caudal) peduncle conveys spinocerebellar axons
(4) The inferior peduncle conveys mostly afferent fibers

9. The molecular layer of the cerebellar cortex contains which of the following neural elements?

(1) Dendrites of Purkinje neurons
(2) Stellate neurons
(3) Parallel and climbing fibers
(4) Cerebellar glomeruli

10. An ependymoma expanding in the fourth ventricle would most likely encroach upon which of the following structures early in its course?

(1) The nodule of the flocculonodular lobe
(2) Cochlear nuclei
(3) The juxtarestiform body
(4) The middle cerebellar peduncle

11. Correct statements about the parallel fibers include which of the following?

(1) They make a T-like bifurcation, with the axons running transverse to the axis of the folia
(2) They arise in the neurons of the granular layer
(3) They make the majority of their synapses in the granular layer
(4) They synapse on dendrites of Purkinje, stellate, and Golgi type II neurons

12. Correct statements about the Purkinje neurons include which of the following?

(1) They are located in the second layer of the cerebellar cortex
(2) They extend their dendrites into the molecular layer and their axons through the granular layer
(3) They have dendritic trees that are at right angles to the long axis of the folia
(4) They send numerous axons to the olivary nuclei and basis pontis

13. The examiner can best detect cerebellar dysfunction of the arms and legs if the patient

(A) is asleep
(B) is quadriplegic
(C) is comatose
(D) has a locked-in syndrome
(E) is awake and not paralyzed

Directions: The group of questions below consists of lettered choices followed by several numbered items. For each numbered item select the **one** lettered choice with which it is **most** closely associated. Each lettered choice may be used once, more than once, or not at all.

Questions 14–18

Match the source of the afferent fibers listed below with the part of the cerebellar cortex to which each fiber most strongly projects.

(A) Cerebellar hemisphere
(B) Anterior lobe of the vermis
(C) Tonsil
(D) Flocculonodular lobe
(E) All parts of the cerebellum equally

14. Spinocerebellar tracts
15. Trigeminocerebellar tract
16. Principal inferior olivary nuclei, lateral part
17. Vestibular nerve and nuclei
18. Nucleus locus ceruleus

ANSWERS AND EXPLANATIONS

1. The answer is A. (*IV A 1 c*) The superior cerebellar peduncle conveys afferent and efferent cerebellar fibers. The majority of efferent fibers that leave the cerebellum arise in the deep nuclei, mainly the dentate nuclei, and exit through the superior peduncle. The largest group of afferents in the peduncle consists of the ventral spinocerebellar tract.

2. The answer is B. (*VI B 2 b*) The vermis of the anterior lobe of the cerebellum represents the body parts in an inverted manner, with the feet and legs being most rostral and superior and the upper parts of the body being more caudal and inferior. This region of the vermis undergoes degeneration in alcoholic patients. Dystaxia predominantly affects the lower extremities and gait; there is relatively little dystaxia of the arms and little or no dysarthria.

3. The answer is D. (*V A 1; Figure 9-12*) The dystaxia after cerebellar lesions reflects dysmodulation of impulses relayed through the dentatothalamocerebrocortical pathway. This pathway brings the coordinating influence of the cerebellum to bear upon the motor cortex, which in turn projects its influence through the pyramidal tract to the contralateral muscles.

4. The answer is D. (*I F 4*) In response to increased intracranial pressure, as may result from edema or various space-occupying lesions, the cerebellar tonsils, which are dorsolateral to the fourth ventricle, herniate through the foramen magnum and compress the medullocervical junction. The patient suffers quadriplegia due to compression of the pyramidal tracts and arrest of respiration due to compression of the reticulospinal tracts.

5. The answer is B (1, 3). [*III E 1 b (2); IV B 1*] The deep cerebellar nuclei receive collaterals from the afferent fibers that run through the deep cerebellar white matter to the cortex. These include the afferents from inferior olivary nuclei and the proprioceptive sensory systems. Some direct primary vestibular afferent fibers reach the deep nuclei. The Purkinje neurons, the only efferent neurons of the cerebellar cortex, mostly synapse on the deep nuclei.

6. The answer is E (all). (*III D 1 b*) The cerebellar glomeruli are peculiar synaptic arrangements consisting of mossy fiber rosettes, axons and dendrites from Golgi type II neurons of the granular layer, and the dendrites of granule neurons themselves. A glial capsule surrounds the whole conglomeration. The axons of the granule neurons, which enter the molecular layer, provide the output from the glomerulus.

7. The answer is D (4). (*III E 3 c; Table 9-4*) All of the neurons of the cerebellar cortex apparently are inhibitory except for the granule neurons. These, however, are the most numerous neuron type in the cerebellar cortex.

8. The answer is E (all). (*IV C 1–3*) The various peduncles have different fiber components. The simplest is the middle peduncle, which conveys mostly crossed pontocerebellar axons. The superior peduncle contains both efferents and afferents. The inferior, or caudal, peduncle is mainly afferent like the middle peduncle; the majority of its fibers are olivocerebellar.

9. The answer is A (1, 2, 3). (*III B 2 a, 3 c, C 2 a; Table 9-2*) The neural elements in the molecular layer of the cerebellar cortex consist of the inner and outer stellate neurons, the dendrites of Pukinje and Golgi type II neurons, and the climbing fibers that accompany the Purkinje dendrites. In addition, the molecular layer contains the parallel fibers from the granular layer. The cerebellar glomeruli are confined to the granular layer.

10. The answer is B (1, 3). (*Figures 9-1C, 9-3, 9-11*) A tumor of the fourth ventricle will encroach on the nodule of the flocculonodular lobe. Expanding laterally, the tumor would encroach on the juxtarestiform body, which forms the immediate lateral boundary of the ventricle, before it would encroach on the restiform body or the middle cerebellar peduncle. An intraventricular tumor would not affect the cochlear nuclei, which drape laterally around the caudal peduncle and are thus outside of the fourth ventricle.

11. The answer is C (2, 4). (*III B 3*) The parallel fibers are axons that arise by T-like bifurcations of axons of the granular layer of the cerebellar cortex. These axons enter the molecular layer and run parallel to the axis of the folia. They synapse on neurons that extend their dendrites into the molecular layer, namely the Purkinje neurons, inner and outer stellate neurons, and Golgi type II neurons of the granular layer.

12. The answer is A (1, 2, 3). (*III A 1, B 2 a; Figure 9-7*) The Purkinje neurons are the only type of neuron in the second layer of the cerebellar cortex. Their dendrites extend into the granular layer and are flattened at right angles to the long axis of the folia. Purkinje axons run through the molecular layer and medullary cores of the folia to the deep nuclei of the cerebellum. Some Purkinje axons bypass the deep nuclei to end in the vestibular nuclei. The proximal portion of the Purkinje axon sends collaterals back to their own perikarya or to neighboring Purkinje perikarya.

13. The answer is E. (*VI A 2*) Lesions of the cerebellum cause dystaxia (incoordination) of muscular contractions when the patient voluntarily employs the muscles, either to sustain a posture, such as the vertical posture, or to move a part of the body. Such actions are only possible in responsive patients with intact pyramidal pathways. A comatose or sleeping patient or one with interrupted pyramidal tracts, as in the locked-in syndrome or quadriplegia, would not make willful muscular contractions of the arms, legs, or trunk and would not show cerebellar signs.

14–18. The answers are: 14-B, 15-B, 16-A, 17-D, 18-E. [*IV B 5 a, b, d (2) e*] The afferent tracts to the cerebellum generally terminate in specific regions. The vermis receives the bulk of the spinocerebellar tracts and the trigeminocerebellar tract.

The hemispheres receive projections from the principal olivary nuclei and from the basis pontis.

The flocculonodular lobe is the oldest part of the cerebellum phylogenetically and the part from which the whole cerebellum takes its origin. It originally received the vestibular connections, both through direct connections to the vestibular nerve and through the vestibular nuclei, and it retains these connections even though the phylogenetically newer parts of the cerebellum are much larger in higher animals. From its original role as an integrating center for the vestibular system in controlling the axial muscles, the cerebellum has now accepted the role of coordinating the appendicular or limb muscles. The parts of the cerebellum that perform this function have increased in size in accordance with the size of the cerebral motor cortex and the cortical efferent system through the pyramidal and corticopontocerebellar tracts.

The rostral vermis also receives projections from the visual and auditory systems, although the functional role of these projections is not well understood. Many of the afferent pathways to the cerebellum also send collaterals to the deep cerebellar nuclei as they pass through the deep cerebellar white matter on their way to the cerebellar cortex. The nucleus locus ceruleus projects diffusely to the cerebellum just as it projects diffusely to most other parts of the CNS.

I. MOTOR AND SENSORY COMPONENTS OF THE OPTIC SYSTEM

A. The **sensory component** of the optic system produces the special sense of vision. It acts through CN II (the optic nerve) and its special central pathways.

B. The **motor component** fixates the eyeballs on targets, moves them conjugately to locate or pursue targets, controls the size of the pupil and the focusing of light rays on the retina, and elevates the eyelids. The motor system acts through its own central pathways and CN III (oculomotor), CN IV (trochlear), and CN VI (abducens).

C. **Clinical testing of the sensory and motor functions of the optic system.** The neuroanatomy of the optic system becomes meaningful only if the methods of clinical testing are known (see Table 10-6).

II. ANATOMY OF THE EYEBALL

A. **Frontal aspect of the eye.** Ocular structures seen from the front consist of the cornea, iris, and conjunctiva.

1. The **cornea**, a transparent disk, covers the iris.

2. The **iris** is an opaque pigmented diaphragm with a central opening, the **pupil** (Fig. 10-1), which varies in size.

3. The **conjunctiva**, a mucous membrane, covers the exposed surface of the eyeball peripheral to the cornea.

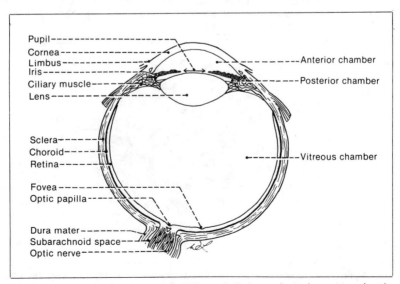

Figure 10-1. Horizontal section of the right eyeball as seen from above. Note that the optic papilla and optic nerve are medial to the fovea.

B. A **transverse section of the eyeball** discloses three main layers: the sclera, choroid, and retina (see Fig. 10-1).

1. The **sclera**, the outer tunic, consists of tough, fibrous connective tissue. Seen through the conjunctiva, it is the "white of the eyes." The sclera continues intracranially through the optic foramen as the **dura mater**.

2. The **choroid**, a vascular coat, contains capillaries and venules. It extends forward as the **ciliary body** and **iris**.

3. The **retina** is the neuronal layer of the eyeball.

C. Ophthalmoscopic anatomy of the optic fundus

1. With an ophthalmoscope, the physician can look through the patient's pupil to examine the living retinal tissue and blood vessels in the back or **fundus** of the eye (Fig. 10-2).
   a. Notice the **optic disk** (optic papilla) and the **macula lutea** with its **fovea centralis**.
   b. Arteries emerge from the optic disk, and veins converge upon it. The vessels travel across the retinal surface between it and the entering light rays. The arteries ramify toward, but do not encroach on, the macula, leaving it an avascular area.
   c. The fundus appears reddish because the neuronal layers of the retina are completely transparent and the light reflects off the pigment cell layer and the rich vascular plexus of the choroid.

2. A **transverse section of the fundus** shows a slight elevation of the margin of the optic disk where optic axons from the retinal neurons converge upon it. These axons form the **optic nerve** after piercing the **lamina cribrosa** of the sclera (Fig. 10-3).
   a. The optic disk and macula each show a depression, the **physiologic cup** and the **fovea centralis**, respectively.
   b. The optic disk appears pink where the optic nerve axons run across its outer part because capillaries accompany the otherwise transparent axons.
   c. The physiologic cup, in the center of the disk where the large vessels perforate, has no nerve fibers and thus no capillaries. The scleral white of the lamina cribrosa shines through.

3. **Ophthalmoscopic anatomy of optic atrophy and papilledema**
   a. Optic atrophy refers to degeneration of optic nerve fibers. The optic nerve may undergo **anterograde degeneration** after retinal lesions. Because they lack collaterals, the fibers may undergo **retrograde degeneration** back into the retina after optic nerve interruption. Subsequently, the capillaries, which give the nerve fiber layer of the disk its normal color, atrophy. The optic disk then appears white because the entire white lamina cribrosa, denuded of capillaries and axons, shines through.
   b. Papilledema refers to swelling of the nerve fiber layer of the optic papilla (disk).
      (1) The subarachnoid space extends out along the optic nerve to the eyeball (see Figs. 10-1 and 10-3). The ophthalmic artery and ophthalmic vein also run with the optic nerve.

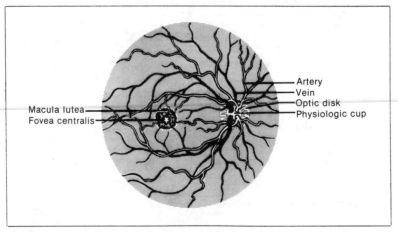

Macula lutea
Fovea centralis

Artery
Vein
Optic disk
Physiologic cup

Figure 10-2. Anatomy of the optic fundus as seen by ophthalmoscopy. The macula is the visual center of the retina. The area surrounding the macula is referred to as the periphery of the retina.

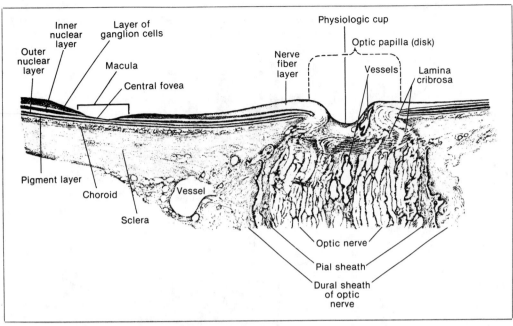

Inner
nuclear
layer

Outer
nuclear
layer

Layer of
ganglion cells

Macula

Central fovea

Pigment layer

Choroid

Vessel

Sclera

Physiologic cup

Optic papilla (disk)

Nerve
fiber
layer

Vessels

Lamina
cribrosa

Optic nerve

Pial sheath

Dural sheath
of optic
nerve

Figure 10-3. Section of the retina through the fovea centralis and the optic papilla. The drawing does not show the blood vessels on the retinal surface and traversing the physiologic cup. (Reprinted with permission from Bloom W, Fawcett D: *A Textbook of Histology.* Philadelphia, WB Saunders, 1970, p 795.)

　　(2) Increased intracranial pressure will reflect out into the subarachnoid space and collapse the ophthalmic vein. Fluid leaks into the optic papilla and surrounding retina from the dammed-up blood vessels. Ophthalmoscopy shows an elevated, swollen optic papilla, engorged veins, and obliteration of the physiologic cup.

　4. Myelinated nerve fibers may occur around the optic disk because the retina and optic nerve arise by evagination of the diencephalon.
　　a. Optic nerve myelin comes from oligodendroglia, which normally extend only to the lamina cribrosa.
　　b. Sometimes oligodendroglia extend beyond the lamina. Ophthalmoscopy discloses them as a whitish patch on the disk margin.

D. Neurons and layers of the retina

　1. The retina essentially contains six types of neurons distributed in three layers (Fig. 10-4; Table 10-1).
　2. Rod and cone (receptor) layer of the retina
　　a. The rods and cones are the receptors for light.
　　b. They are on the scleral side of the retina. Therefore, light must penetrate the overlying retinal layers to reach the rods and cones.
　　c. Cones are concentrated at the macula and fovea centralis, where they are not covered by overlying retinal elements or blood vessels (see Fig. 10-3). The eyeballs align so that the cones receive the central ray of light from the object viewed (see Fig. 10-6).
　　d. The retinal receptors peripheral to the macula are mainly **rods**.
　3. Rods and cones make the retina a dual organ.
　　a. The retina mediates two types of vision, central and peripheral, based on the location of the rods and cones.
　　b. Central vision is mediated by the cones, since they are concentrated in the macula. The cones mediate two functions: acuity and color vision.
　　　(1) Acuity, the ability to discriminate lines or points at a distance, is tested by having the patient read letters from a chart.
　　　(2) Color vision is tested by color recognition.
　　c. Peripheral vision is mediated by the rods, since they occupy the peripheral retina around the macula. The peripheral retina has three functions:
　　　(1) Awareness of the periphery of the visual field

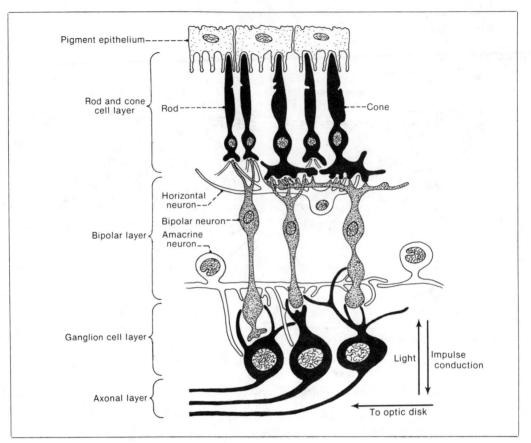

Figure 10-4. Retinal neurons as diagrammed from electron microscopy.

        (2) Night vision
        (3) Motion detection
  4. Bipolar (internuncial) layer of the retina
      a. The middle retinal layer contains three types of neurons: bipolar, horizontal, and amacrine (see Fig. 10-4).
          (1) Bipolar neurons predominate. They connect the rods and cones with the ganglion cell layer.
          (2) Horizontal neurons have their perikarya in the outer part (scleral side) of the bipolar layer.
          (3) Amacrine neurons have their perikarya in the inner part (corneal side) of the bipolar layer.

Table 10-1. Three Layers and Six Neuronal Types of the Retina

Layers and Neurons	Function

Outer layer (scleral side of the retina)
  Rod neurons
  Cone neurons
	Receptor layer for light rays

Middle layer
  Bipolar neurons
  Horizontal neurons
  Amacrine neurons
	Layer of retinal interneurons

Inner layer (corneal side of the retina) Ganglionic neurons	Efferent layer, originating axons of the optic nerve

    b. Horizontal and amacrine cell processes defy classification as dendrites or axons.
      (1) Horizontal cell processes come in contact with the axodendritic synapses between the rod and cone cells and the bipolar cells (see Fig. 10-4).
      (2) Amacrine cell processes come in contact with the synapses between the bipolar neurons and the dendrites of the ganglion layer neurons (see Fig. 10-4).
    c. Since the connections of the bipolar, horizontal, and amacrine neurons all remain within the retina, they constitute its internuncial layer.

5. Ganglionic (efferent) layer of the retina
    a. The efferent layer of the retina consists of multipolar neurons exhibiting dendritic/axonal polarization.
    b. The ganglionic layer, on the corneal surface of the retina, originates the optic nerve axons. They travel across the corneal surface of the retina to converge on the optic papilla (Fig. 10-5).

6. Course of ganglionic axons across the retina
    a. The axons from the macula converge directly on the optic papilla, forming a **maculopapillary bundle**.
    b. The axons of the ganglion cells surrounding the macula take an increasingly curved course to the optic papilla.

III. VISUAL PATHWAY: RETINO-GENICULO-CALCARINE PATHWAY

A. Physical optics of image formation on the retina

    1. The physical optics of the eye invert the retinal image (Fig. 10-6).

    2. The actual retinal image is a real image based on physical optics. Neural actions then translate this physical image into a physiologic event that we can call a **visual image**. The mind learns to project the visual image back to the original site of the visual stimulus.
      a. If a light ray strikes the **nasal** half of the retina, the mind projects, perceives, or interprets the object correctly as located in the **temporal** half of space (see Fig. 10-6).
      b. If a light ray strikes the **superior** half of the retina, the mind projects the visual image to the **inferior** half of space.

    3. Figure 10-6 depicts image formation as if it were simply a pinhole camera effect. In reality, the cornea and lens refract the light rays and focus them on the retina. Only the central ray, which strikes the macula, does not undergo refraction, making the macula the site where vision is most acute.

B. Representation of the visual fields. To understand best the arrangement of axons in the visual pathways, consider the phylogeny of vision.

    1. Lower animals view an arrow by **panoramic vision**, integrating it as one continuous visual field because of the total decussation of the optic nerve fibers (Figs. 10-7 and 10-8).

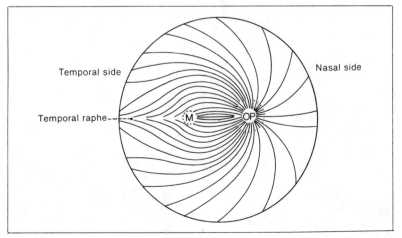

Figure 10-5. Fundus of the right eye. The fibers from the macula (*M*) run straight to the optic papilla (*OP*), forming a maculopapillary bundle. The fibers peripheral to the macula take an increasingly curved course.

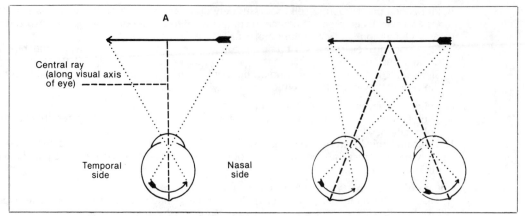

Figure 10-6. Retinal image formed by monocular (*A*) and binocular (*B*) fixation.

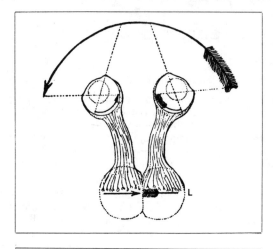

Figure 10-7. Discontinuous representation of the visual image if the optic nerve does not decussate. *L* = visual center. (Reprinted with permission from Ramón y Cajal S: *Recollections of My Life, Memoirs of the American Philosophical Society*, vol 8. Cambridge, MA, MIT Press, 1937, p 472.)

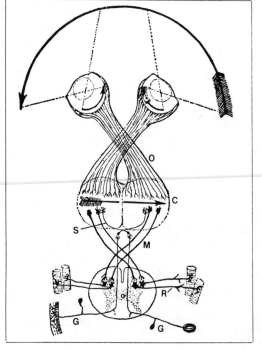

Figure 10-8. Continuous representation of the visual image resulting from decussation of the optic nerve in a lower animal with panoramic vision. Compare with Figure 10-9, which represents binocular stereoscopic vision. *C* = visual center; *G* = ganglion; *M* = crossing motor fibers; *O* = decussated optic nerve; *R* = motor root of spinal nerve; *S* = decussated central sensory pathway. (Reprinted with permission from Ramón y Cajal S: *Recollections of My Life, Memoirs of the American Philosophical Society*, vol 8. Cambridge, MA, MIT Press, 1937, p 473.)

2. Primates view an arrow by **stereoscopic binocular vision**, integrating two visual fields. This arrangement requires a shift from total decussation of the optic nerve at the optic chiasm (the primitive arrangement) to partial decussation (the advanced arrangement) [Fig. 10-9].

3. In submammalia, the midbrain tectum, corresponding to the superior colliculus, receives the retinal fibers and mediates vision. These animals have no cortex as such and no primary visual receptive cortex.

4. In higher animals, a **retinogeniculate tract** synapses in the lateral geniculate body of the thalamus. A **geniculocalcarine tract** relays visual impulses to the calcarine region of the occipital lobe (see Fig. 10-9). In higher animals, the cerebral cortex, not the midbrain tectum, mediates vision.

5. The retinogeniculate pathway proximal to the retina consists of the optic nerve, optic chiasm, and optic tract. Study in Figure 10-9 the different visual field defects caused by lesions at these three sites.

C. Optic nerve and chiasm

1. The optic nerve begins behind the lamina cribrosa. It enters the skull through the optic foramen, in company with the ophthalmic artery and vein. From the optic nerve, the optic axons enter the optic chiasm.

2. The optic axons undergo a partial decussation at the chiasm (see Fig. 10-9). Figure 10-10 presents the actual pattern of the chiasmatic decussation.
   a. Fibers from the **temporal** half of the macula and peripheral retina run in the ipsilateral optic tract. Recall that the temporal half of the retina mediates the visual field in the nasal half of space (see Fig. 10-6).
   b. Fibers from the **nasal** half of each retina cross in the chiasm to reach the contralateral optic tract.

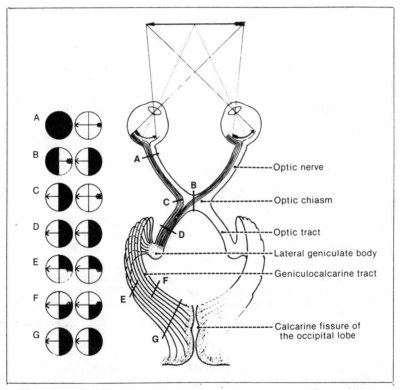

Figure 10-9. Visual pathway from the retina to the calcarine cortex, showing the visual field defects resulting from lesions at sites *A–G*. The optic axons synapse in the lateral geniculate body, a feature not shown because of the scale of the drawing. *A* = complete blindness, left eye; *B* = complete bitemporal hemianopia; *C* = complete left nasal hemianopia; *D* = complete right homonymous hemianopia; *E* = complete right superior homonymous quadrantanopia; *F* = complete right inferior homonymous quadrantanopia; *G* = complete right homonymous hemianopia.

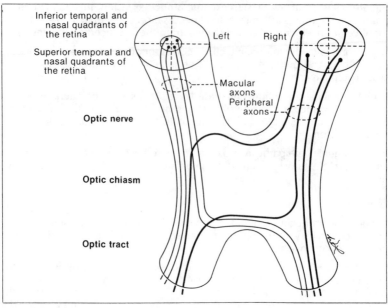

Figure 10-10. Actual pattern of decussation of the optic axons in the optic chiasm as viewed from above. Macular projection shown on *left*; peripheral macular projection on *right*.

  c. The decussating axons form two knees.
    (1) The knee of axons from the **inferior** nasal retinal quadrant serves the **superior** temporal fields.
    (2) The knee of axons from the **superior** nasal retinal quadrant serves the **inferior** temporal fields.
  d. The macular fibers (maculopapillary bundle) decussate posteriorly, forming a ''chiasm within a chiasm.''
  e. Lesions that encroach on the chiasm may selectively affect these bundles, producing various field defects. For example, a lesion at the junction of the optic nerve and chiasm would produce complete blindness of the ipsilateral eye (due to interruption of the optic nerve) and a contralateral superior temporal quadrantanopia (due to interruption of the inferior nasal retinal fibers) [see Fig. 10-10].

D. Neighborhood anatomy of the optic chiasm

  1. The optic chiasm sits just **below** the third ventricle and floor of the diencephalon, to which it attaches, and **above** the pituitary gland.

  2. Obstruction of the flow of cerebrospinal fluid (CSF) through the cerebral aqueduct or the foramina of Luschka and Magendie causes the ventricular system to enlarge. The floor of the diencephalon balloons down onto the chiasm, producing visual impairment, including visual field defects.

  3. The optic chiasm sits just above the sella turcica, which houses the pituitary body. Pituitary tumors encroach on the bottom of the chiasm, producing a superior bitemporal quadrantanopia by interrupting first the decussating axons of the inferior nasal quadrants.

  4. Laterally, aneurysms of the carotid artery and circle of Willis may encroach on the chiasm.

E. Optic tract

  1. The optic tract runs from the optic chiasm to the lateral geniculate body by encircling the midbrain–diencephalic junction (see Figs. 8-1 and 8-2).

  2. The axons of the optic tract separate into two streams: a retinogeniculate tract and a retinopretectal tract.
    a. The **retinogeniculate tract** enters the lateral geniculate body. These axons mediate vision.
    b. The **retinopretectal tract** continues past the geniculate body to enter the pretectal region, a region of the diencephalon just rostral to the midbrain tectum. These axons mediate the pupillary light reflexes (see section VI B 6).

F. Lateral geniculate body and geniculocalcarine tract

1. The lateral geniculate body, a thalamic sensory relay nucleus, retains the topographic representation of the retinal axons. Its axons form the **geniculocalcarine tract** (optic radiation), which skirts the venticular wall in the **external sagittal stratum** (Fig. 10-11).

2. The geniculocalcarine tract preserves the retinal topography in its course and in the pattern of axonal termination in the calcarine cortex.

 a. Interruption of the **superior** fibers of the geniculocalcarine tract or **superior** bank of the

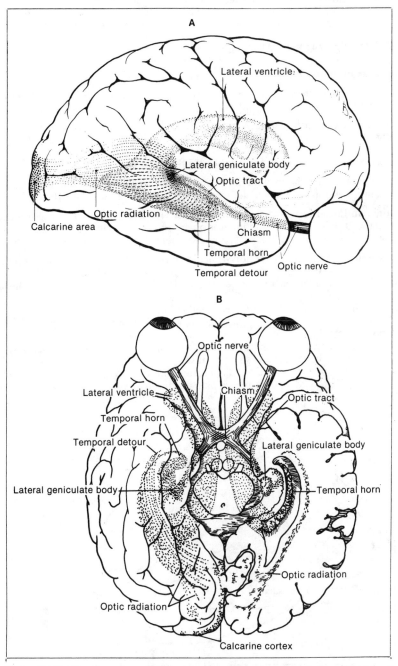

Figure 10-11. Phantom view of the cerebrum to show the anatomical relationship of the optic pathways to the cerebral wall. (*A*) Lateral view of the cerebrum. (*B*) Ventral view of the cerebrum. On the left, the temporal lobe is sectioned. (Reprinted with permission from Cushing H: *Trans Arn Neurol Assoc* 47:374–423, 1921.)

calcarine fissure causes contralateral **inferior** homonymous quadrantanopia (see Fig. 10-9).

b. Interruption of the **inferior** fibers of the tract or **inferior** bank of the calcarine cortex will cause contralateral **superior** homonymous quadrantanopia.

c. Complete interruption of the geniculocalcarine tract or calcarine cortex causes contralateral homonymous hemianopia (see Fig. 10-9).

d. To remember the topography of the retina in the geniculocalcarine tract and calcarine cortex, merely set the eyeball back along the tract (Fig. 10-12); then recall the inversion of the visual field in relation to the retinal image (see Fig. 10-6).

e. With the eyeball superimposed on the occipital pole, the macula is represented **posteriorly** and the periphery of the retina more **anteriorly** (see Fig. 10-12).

IV. ACTIONS OF EXTRAOCULAR MUSCLES

A. Types of ocular muscles

1. Each eye has 11 muscles, classified as smooth or striated and as intraocular or extraocular (Fig. 10-13).

2. The **orbicularis oculi**, a striated muscle sphincter, closes the eyelids. It is classified as a facial rather than an ocular muscle because of its branchial origin and innervation by CN VII.

B. Extraocular striated muscles for rotation of the eyeball

1. One of the seven striated extraocular muscles, the levator palpebrae, elevates the eyelid. The remaining six rotate the eyeball around one of its three axes (Fig. 10-14).

2. Origin and insertion of the rotator muscles. Five of the six ocular rotator muscles originate from the annulus of Zinn. The inferior oblique muscle originates from the anterior rim of the orbit. All six rotator muscles insert on the sclera (Fig. 10-15). Table 10-2 lists their actions.

3. Law of tonic oppositional action of ocular muscles. The muscles of one eyeball act in agonist–antagonist pairs or sets. The muscle or muscles that rotate the eyeball in one direction are opposed by a muscle or muscles that rotate it in the opposite direction. The law holds true for voluntary movements as well as when the eyes are at rest.

a. With the eyes still, either looking straight ahead or deviated, the agonist–antagonist sets of muscles receive equal tonic innervation, which cancels out their opposing actions. Thus, a positive mechanism maintains the position of the eyes.

b. Two lines of evidence demonstrate the tonic innervation: electromyography and deviation of the eye following paralysis of a muscle.

(1) An electromyographic needle inserted into any ocular rotator muscle with the eye not moving records a continuous play of muscular contraction (tonic innervation). Other

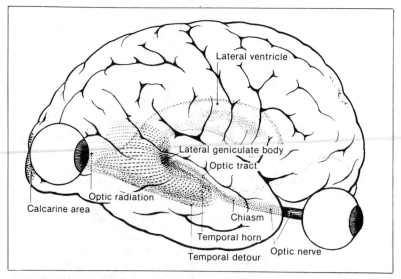

Figure 10-12. Superimposition of the eyeball on the occipital lobe provides a mnemonic for remembering the topographic representation of the retina and visual fields. (Reprinted with permission from Cushing H: *Trans Am Neurol Assoc* 47:374–423, 1921.)

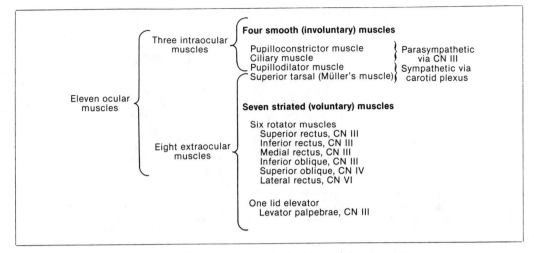

Figure 10-13. The eleven ocular muscles and their innervation.

skeletal muscles receive no nerve impulses and are electrically silent when the part they act on is at rest.

(2) Following ocular muscle paralysis, the tonic innervation of the intact antagonistic muscle will rotate the eyeball toward its direction (e.g., in lateral rectus palsy, the medial rectus muscle pulls the eye into adduction).

(3) Ocular muscle paralysis and the resultant ocular malalignment causes the retinal image to miss the macula of the affected eye. The image from the unaffected eye remains on the macular target. The mind then "sees" two visual images, a condition called **double vision** or **diplopia**.

C. Actions of the medial and lateral recti

1. The lateral rectus muscle **abducts** the eye, rotating the cornea **laterally**. Its paired antagonist, the medial rectus muscle, **adducts** the eye, rotating the cornea **medially**.

2. The medial and lateral recti have only one action because they pull "on center." They adduct or abduct the eye around its vertical axis.

D. Because they may pull "off center," the remaining ocular muscles produce secondary and tertiary rotations, which vary with the position of the eyeball (see Table 10-2).

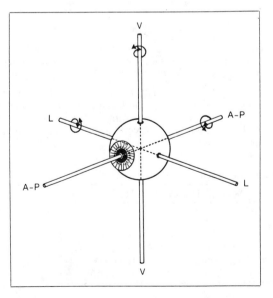

Figure 10-14. The three rotational axes of the eye. *V* = vertical; *L* = lateral; *A–P* = anteroposterior.

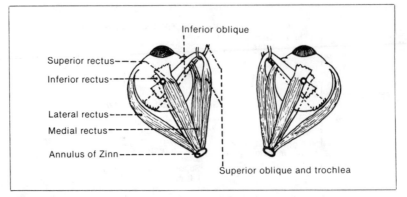

Figure 10-15. The eyeballs as seen from above, showing the origin and insertion of the ocular rotator muscles. All ocular rotator muscles originate from the annulus of Zinn except for the inferior oblique muscle, which originates from the anterior rim of the orbit.

E. Actions of the superior and inferior recti

1. The primary action of the superior and inferior recti is to **elevate** or **depress** the eyeball by rotating it around its lateral (**transverse**) axis.

2. With the eye abducted, the superior rectus acts only as an elevator and the inferior rectus acts only as a depressor.

3. With the eye adducted, the elevator action of the superior rectus converts to adduction and intorsion and the depressor action of the inferior rectus converts to adduction and extorsion. (Torsions rotate the eye around its **anterior–posterior** axis.)

F. Actions of the superior and inferior oblique muscles

1. The primary action of the superior and inferior oblique muscles is to **depress** or **elevate** the eye when it is adducted.

2. With the eye abducted by the lateral rectus muscle, the depressor action of the superior oblique muscle converts to intorsion and abduction.

3. With the eye abducted, elevation by the inferior oblique muscle converts to abduction and extorsion.

4. Thus, when the eye is adducted, elevation or depression by the superior or inferior recti decreases. In compensation, the power of the oblique muscles to elevate or depress the eye increases.

G. Two muscles elevate the eyelid: the levator palpebrae and superior tarsal muscles.

1. The **levator palpebrae muscle**, a striated muscle innervated by CN III, originates from the optic foramen. It inserts into the tarsal plate of the upper eyelid. It holds up the eyelid tonically and further elevates it phasically when the person voluntarily looks up.

2. The **superior tarsal muscle**, a smooth muscle innervated by the carotid sympathetic nerve, originates from connective tissue of the orbit and inserts into the tarsal plate. It acts tonically and involuntarily to set the height of the palpebral fissure. For example, if a person is frightened, the muscle further elevates the eyelid, giving a "bright-eyed" appearance; however, it does not elevate the lid during voluntary gaze upward.

Table 10-2. Movements of Individual Ocular Muscles

Muscle	Primary Action	Secondary Action	Tertiary Action
Medial rectus	Adduction		
Lateral rectus	Abduction		
Superior rectus	Elevation	Adduction	Intorsion
Inferior rectus	Depression	Adduction	Extorsion
Superior oblique	Depression	Abduction	Intorsion
Inferior oblique	Elevation	Abduction	Extorsion

V. PERIPHERAL INNERVATION OF THE EYES

A. Six nerves innervate the eyes (Table 10-3).

B. CN III (oculomotor nerve; see Fig. 8-15)

1. **Functional components**
   a. The **general somatic efferent (GSE) axons** that innervate the ocular rotator muscles and the levator palpebrae originate in the oculomotor nucleus of the rostral midbrain tegmentum, just ventral to the periaqueductal gray matter. Longitudinally, the nucleus coincides with the superior colliculus.
   b. The **general visceral efferent (GVE) parasympathetic axons** that innervate the pupilloconstrictor and ciliary muscles arise in the Edinger-Westphal nucleus, which forms a rostrodorsal cap over the oculomotor nucleus proper.

2. **Intra-axially**, CN III runs ventrally to exit into the subarachnoid space of the interpeduncular fossa (see Fig. 8-34).

3. **Extra-axially**, CN III encounters the posterior cerebral artery in the interpeduncular fossa.
   a. At the site of exit, the parasympathetic axons of CN III cluster in the dorsomedial sector of the nerve (Fig. 10-16).
   b. The posterior cerebral artery may impinge on the pupilloconstrictor fibers if it is enlarged by an aneurysm or displaced by herniation of a cerebral hemisphere (see Fig. 2-15). Then, pupillodilation will precede paralysis of the ocular rotator muscles.
   c. After clearing the posterior cerebral artery, CN III enters the lateral dural leaf of the cavernous sinus (Fig. 10-17).
   d. Clearing the the cavernous sinus, CN III enters the superior orbital fissure (see Fig. 8-13).
      (1) The **GSE axons** innervate the four rectus muscles and the inferior oblique muscle (see Fig. 8-15).
      (2) The **parasympathetic** axons follow the inferior oblique branch of CN III to the ciliary ganglion.

4. The **ciliary ganglion** contains the parasympathetic postganglionic neurons innervating the

Table 10-3. Innervation of the Eye by Its Six Nerves

Number and Name of Nerve	Innervation	Clinical Effects of Interruption of Nerve
Efferent		
CN III (oculomotor nerve)	Striated muscle: superior, medial, and inferior recti; inferior oblique	Diplopia, eye abducted and turned down
	Levator palpebrae	Ptosis (paralysis of volitional lid elevation)
	Smooth muscle: pupilloconstrictor	Pupil dilated and fixed to light
	Ciliary muscle	Loss of lens thickening
CN IV (trochlear nerve)	Striated muscle: superior oblique	Diplopia, most severe on looking down and in; eye extorted; head tilted to side opposite paralyzed eye
CN VI (abducens nerve)	Striated muscle: lateral rectus	Diplopia, most severe on looking to side of paralysis; eye turned in (adducted)
Carotid sympathetic nerve	Smooth muscle: superior tarsal and and pupillodilator	Horner's syndrome (ptosis, miosis, hemifacial anhidrosis, vasodilation)
Afferent		
CN II (optic nerve)	From retina	Blindness
CN V (trigeminal nerve)	Proprioceptive afferent	No known clinical effect
	Corneal/conjunctival afferents	Anesthesia of cornea with loss of corneal reflex

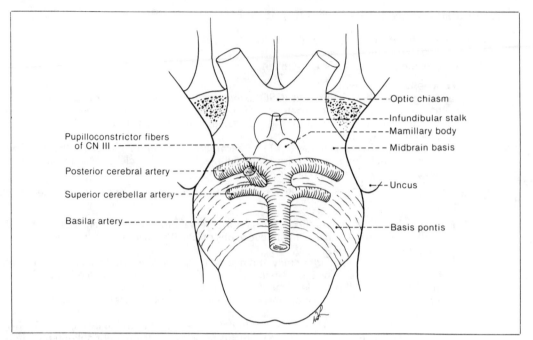

Pupilloconstrictor fibers of CN III

Posterior cerebral artery

Superior cerebellar artery

Basilar artery

Optic chiasm
Infundibular stalk
Mamillary body
Midbrain basis
Uncus
Basis pontis

Figure 10-16. The pupilloconstrictor parasympathetic axons occupy the dorsomedial sector of CN III after it exits into the interpeduncular fossa and encounters the posterior cerebral artery.

pupilloconstrictor and ciliary muscles (see section VI D 1 c). The postganglionic axons from the ciliary ganglion reach the eyeball in the **short ciliary** nerves (Fig. 10-18).

5. Short ciliary nerves
   a. These nerves convey three types of axons:
     (1) Postganglionic parasympathetic axons to the pupilloconstrictor and ciliary muscles
     (2) Postganglionic sympathetic vasomotor axons to smooth muscle of the intraocular blood vessels
     (3) Afferent fibers from the nasociliary branch of CN V from the interior of the eyeball
   b. Although all three types of axons run through the ciliary ganglion and the short ciliary nerves, only the parasympathetic axons actually synapse in the ganglion.

6. Long ciliary nerves (see Fig. 10-18) convey two types of fibers:
   a. Afferents, mainly pain afferents, from the cornea and iris through the nasociliary branch of CN V
   b. Sympathetic efferents to the pupillodilator muscle

7. Signs of CN III interruption
   a. Lateral and downward rotation of the eye occurs because actions of the lateral rectus and superior oblique muscles are unopposed. The patient experiences diplopia. The patient's attempts to adduct and depress the eye result in intorsion (due to the unopposed action of the superior oblique muscle); the eye will not adduct.
   b. The **pupil is dilated and fails to constrict** in response to light or in accommodation for near vision.
   c. Ptosis is present. After paralysis of the levator palpebrae muscle, the ptosis is severe, and the lid does not elevate when the patient looks upward. After paralysis of the superior tarsal muscle, the ptosis is mild, and the lid does elevate when the patient looks up, if the levator palpebrae muscle is intact.
   d. The **lens fails to adjust in accommodation for near and far vision**, due to ciliary muscle paralysis.

C. CN IV (trochlear nerve)

   1. CN IV contains GSE axons for the superior oblique muscle and GSA axons from it for proprioception.

   2. Intra-axially, the axons originate in the trochlear nucleus, which is embedded in the medial longitudinal fasciculus ventral to the inferior colliculus and aqueduct. The axons undergo a

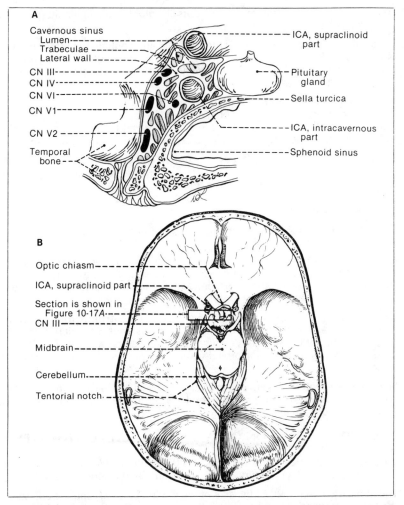

Figure 10-17. (A) Transverse (coronal) section through the cavernous sinus and sella turcica. CN III, CN IV, and CN VI and the two sensory branches of CN V run through the lateral wall of the cavernous sinus; CN VI runs through the lumen. *ICA* = internal carotid artery; *V1* = ophthalmic division of CN V; *V2* = maxillary division of CN V. (B) Interior view of the base of the skull. The rectangle is the section shown in Figure 10-17A.

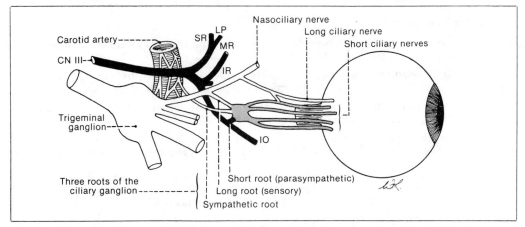

Figure 10-18. Lateral aspect of the right eye showing its innervation. Muscular branches of CN III: *IO* = inferior oblique; *IR* = inferior rectus; *LP* = levator palpebrae; *MR* = medial rectus; *SR* = superior rectus.

complete internal decussation and exit dorsally into the subarachnoid space caudal to the inferior colliculus.

3. Extra-axially, CN IV wraps around the midbrain and continues ventrally between the posterior cerebral and superior cerebellar arteries (see Fig. 15-9). After entering the lateral wall of the cavernous sinus (see Fig. 10-17), it emerges into the superior orbital fissure to end on the superior oblique muscle, its only muscle.

4. Unique anatomical features of CN IV
   a. It undergoes complete internal decussation.
   b. It exits from the dorsal aspect of the brainstem and travels around the midbrain.
   c. It has the smallest diameter of the 12 pairs of cranial nerves and is the least myelinated.

5. Signs of CN IV interruption. The eye is extorted and elevated because the action of the intact inferior oblique muscle is unopposed. The patient has diplopia, which worsens during attempts to look down when the eye is adducted.

D. CN VI (abducens nerve)

1. CN VI contains GSE axons for the lateral rectus muscles and GSA axons from it for proprioception.

2. Intra-axially, CN VI commences in the abducens nucleus beneath the floor of the fourth ventricle near the pontomedullary junction. Running ventrally, the axons enter the subarachnoid space at the pontomedullary sulcus, between the internal auditory artery and the anterior inferior cerebellar artery (see Fig. 15-9).

3. Extra-axially, CN VI takes a long intracranial course. It turns rostrally, running along the length of the belly of the pons to enter the cavernous sinus where it runs in the lumen, in contrast to CN III, CN IV, and CN V, which run in the lateral wall (see Fig. 10-17). CN VI enters the orbit through the superior orbital fissure to innervate the lateral rectus muscle, its only muscle.

4. Signs of CN VI interruption. The eye remains adducted because tonus of the medial rectus muscle is unopposed. The patient complains of diplopia, which is most severe during attempts to abduct the eye.

VI. ACTIONS AND INNERVATION OF SMOOTH MUSCLES OF THE EYES

A. The four **smooth muscles** of the eye consist of three intraocular muscles (the pupilloconstrictor, pupillodilator, and ciliary) and one extraocular muscle (the superior tarsal).

1. The pupillary muscles adjust the size of the pupil. The ciliary muscle adjusts the thickness of the lens. The superior tarsal muscle adjusts the height of the palpebral fissure.

2. Parasympathetic axons via CN III and the ciliary ganglion innervate the pupilloconstrictor and ciliary muscles.

3. Sympathetic axons via the carotid sympathetic nerve innervate the pupillodilator and superior tarsal muscles.

B. Pupillary muscles

1. The iris, a diaphragm between the cornea and lens, contains a central aperture of variable diameter, the pupil (see Fig. 10-1).

2. Pupillodilator muscle fibers originate in the outer part of the iris and run radially to insert into the pupillary margin. Their contraction **enlarges** the diameter of the pupil.

3. Pupilloconstrictor muscle fibers encircle the pupillary border of the iris, forming a sphincter. Their contraction **reduces** the diameter of the pupil.

4. Control of pupillary size
   a. The pupils are almost exactly round, equal in size, and centered in the iris. They continuously change size.
      (1) Light, accommodation for near vision, and drowsiness or sleep **reduce** pupillary size.
      (2) Alertness, fright, pain, and strong emotion **increase** pupillary size. In fact, almost any pathway through the limbic system/hypothalamus or reticular formation may influence pupillary size.
   b. The pupil may constrict because of **increased** stimulation of the pupilloconstrictor muscle or **decreased** stimulation of the pupillodilator muscle. The reverse holds true regarding dilation.

c. Paralysis of one of the two muscles will allow its antagonist to act unopposed, and the pupil will assume the size dictated by the pull of the intact muscle.

5. Direct and consensual pupillary light reflexes

a. Each pupil constricts directly upon illumination of its eye, the **direct** pupillary light reflex. Each pupil also constricts upon illumination of the opposite eye, the **consensual** pupillary light reflex.

b. Normally, both pupils constrict equally when either the direct or the consensual reflex is elicited. Thus, illumination of one eye causes equal constriction of both pupils.

6. Arc of the pupillary light reflex

a. The **afferent arc** is CN II; the **efferent arc** is CN III (Fig. 10-19).

b. The afferents of the pupillary light reflex presumably are collaterals of the axons that synapse in the lateral geniculate body. They depart from the optic tract as the **retinopretectal tract**.

c. These fibers or their pretectal connections disperse bilaterally from the pretectal region to the Edinger-Westphal nucleus. The bilateral dispersion of the pathway accounts for the normal equality of the direct and consensual pupillary light reflexes.

7. Effects of CN II and CN III lesions on pupillary light reflexes

a. Interruption of one optic nerve will abolish the direct pupillary light reflex of the affected eye **and** the consensual reflex of the opposite eye.

  (1) The consensual reflex of the affected eye upon illumination of the other eye will remain intact.

  (2) Both pupils remain equal and will still constrict equally when the intact eye is illuminated.

b. Interruption of CN III (parasympathetic component) abolishes both the direct and consensual pupillary reflex of the affected eye.

  (1) The direct pupillary light reflex of the opposite eye and its consensual reflex to illumination of the affected eye remain intact.

  (2) The pupil of the affected eye is larger than that of the unaffected eye because the action of the pupillodilator muscle is unopposed.

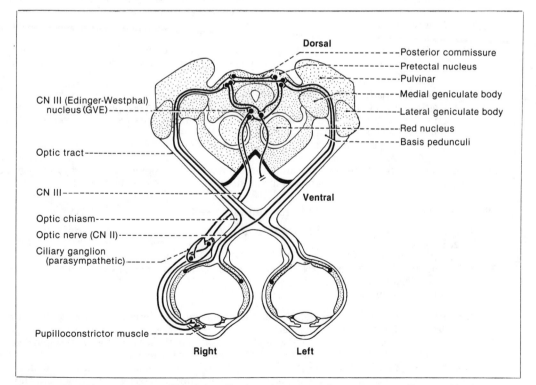

Figure 10-19. Pathway for the pupillary light reflex from the retina to the pretectum–midbrain and back to the pupilloconstrictor muscle. *GVE* = general visceral efferent. (Redrawn with permission from Crosby E, Humphrey T, Lauer E: *Correlative Anatomy of the Nervous System*, New York, Macmillan, 1962, p 236.)

C. Brainstem pathways for pupillary control

1. Hypothalamic centers and their descending pathways

a. Stimulation of the hypothalamus demonstrates overlapping areas that cause pupillodilation by sympathetic stimulation or by parasympathetic inhibition.

b. The **parasympathetic inhibitory pathway** runs directly from the hypothalamus through the periventricular/periaqueducal gray matter to the Edinger-Westphal nucleus.

c. The **sympathetic excitatory pathway** takes a lateral course.

(1) It enters the midbrain by running through the substantia nigra.

(2) Then it shifts to descend through the brainstem in proximity to the lateral spinothalamic tract. Its interruption in the medullary tegmentum accounts for the Horner syndrome component of the lateral medullary wedge syndrome (see Table 8-5).

(3) In the cervical cord, the descending sympathetic pathway shifts to the lateral white column, near the plane of the denticulate ligaments. The axons end in the ciliospinal center of Budge, which contains the preganglionic neurons for the cervical sympathetic chain (see Fig. 6-4).

2. Ascending brainstem pathways for pupillodilation. Two ascending pathways cause pupillodilation by inhibition of the Edinger-Westpthal nucleus.

a. One ascends in the paramedian reticular formation, near the medial longitudinal fasciculus.

b. The other runs in or is identical to the lateral spinothalamic tract. It is in close proximity to the descending excitatory sympathetic pupillodilator pathway. This pathway, at least in part, mediates the ciliospinal pupillodilation reflex (see section VI E 6).

D. Ciliary muscle and the accommodation reflex for near vision

1. Accommodation for near vision requires the integration of three actions: convergence of the eyes, pupilloconstriction, and lens thickening.

a. **Convergence** requires contraction of the medial recti, an act that occurs reflexly when the eyes pursue an object moving toward the observer. (Some people can volitionally look "cross-eyed.") Either reflex or volitional convergence automatically triggers pupilloconstriction and lens thickening.

b. **Pupilloconstriction** blocks off the more peripheral rays that strike the cornea and iris, reducing spherical and chromatic aberration and thus promoting visual acuity.

c. **Lens thickening** follows contraction of the ciliary muscle, an intraocular sphincter (see Fig. 10-1).

(1) Reduction of the sphincter diameter relaxes the suspensory ligaments of the lens.

(2) The inherent elasticity of the lens causes it to thicken, increasing its refractive power to accommodate for near vision.

2. Supranuclear pathways for accommodation

a. Cortical projection systems for accommodation arise in the occipital and frontal regions, pass through the deep white matter of the cerebrum, and synapse in the pretectal area for relay to the Edinger-Westphal nucleus.

b. In the pretectal region, the fibers for accommodation are thought to run ventral to the retinopretectal pupilloconstrictor tract.

c. Compression of the pretectal area from above, as from a pineal tumor, may abolish the pupillary light reflex, leaving pupilloconstriction in accommodation intact.

E. Carotid sympathetic nerve and central pathways (see Fig. 6-4)

1. The carotid sympathetic nerve innervates the:

a. Superior tarsal muscle

b. Pupillodilator muscle

c. Smooth muscles of the carotid arteries and their intracranial and extracranial branches

d. Sweat glands of the face

e. Mucosal, salivary, and lacrimal glands of the head

2. Supranuclear pathways descend from the hypothalamus (as described in section VI C 1 c).

a. **Preganglionic neurons** are located in the intermediolateral column of the spinal cord gray matter from C8 to T2 or T3 (ciliospinal center of Budge). The axons leave the spinal cord with the T1 to T3 nerve roots to ascend to the cervical ganglia.

b. **Postganglionic neurons** are located in the superior cervical ganglion (see Fig. 6-4).

(1) The neurons are adrenergic except for most axons to sweat glands, which are cholinergic.

(2) The postganglionic axons join the carotid artery to ascend with it.

3. At the level of the ear, some sympathetic axons detour across the eardrum, forming a **caroti-cotympanic plexus** with branches of CN IX. The sympathetic axons then rejoin the carotid artery.

4. The axons leave the carotid artery, enter the orbit through the superior orbital fissure, and reach their terminal smooth muscles in the eye by two routes:
  a. Anastomosis with the nasociliary branch of CN V
  b. Anastomosis with the short ciliary nerves after passing through, but not synapsing in, the ciliary ganglion of the orbit (see Fig. 10-18)

5. Horner's syndrome of sympathetic paralysis. Interruption of the sympathetic excitatory pathway in the central nervous system (CNS) or peripheral nervous system (PNS) results in characteristic signs **ipsilateral** to the lesion:
  a. Miosis (pupilloconstriction)
  b. Ptosis (mild and corrected when the patient uses the intact levator palpebrae muscle to look up)
  c. Anhidrosis of half of the face
  d. Vasodilation of half of the face

6. Ciliospinal or spinociliary reflex. Pinching of the skin of the neck or face results in bilateral pupillodilation. The reflex is mediated through pain afferents of CN V. The reflex arc runs through reticular formation and the descending sympathetic excitatory pathway to the ciliospinal center of Budge.

VII. CENTRAL PATHWAYS FOR THE CONTROL OF EYE MOVEMENTS

A. Basic clinical neurophysiology of eye movements

1. The optomotor systems are designed to aim and align the eyes and control refraction.
  a. Aiming enables each eye to find, fixate on, and pursue visual targets.
  b. Aiming plus binocular alignment produces stereopsis (binocular stereoscopic vision).
    (1) It causes the two eyes to receive the central rays from the visual target upon the fovea centralis and to receive the entire retinal image upon corresponding points of each retina, allowing the mind to fuse the two retinal images into one visual image.
    (2) Conjugate eye movements and fusion. Unless the eyes align when they are still and move conjugately both horizontally and vertically, the retinal images fall upon noncorresponding retinal points. Since the mind cannot then fuse the two retinal images into one visual image, the patient experiences diplopia.
  c. Refraction control insures maximal visual acuity in each eye.

2. Vergences and accommodation. The two eyes **converge** (cross) to accommodate for viewing near objects and **diverge** to be parallel for viewing distant objects. When the eyes align and view a distant object straight ahead, they are in the **primary** or **null position**.

3. Volitional control and the fixation and visual pursuit reflexes
  a. The act of finding a visual target is volitional, depending on the mental set of the person and the attractiveness of the visual target. Volitional movements depend on frontal pathways.
  b. Once a visual target is found, **fixation reflexes** tend to lock the eyes onto the target; however, these reflexes can be overridden volitionally to select another target.

4. Volitional versus reflex control of eye movements and position
  a. If the visual target moves, and the eyes reflexly pursue it from the primary position, **optokinetic reflexes** tend to kick the eyes back to the primary position. Optokinetic reflexes (i.e., pursuit and the kickback therefrom), depend on occipital lobe pathways and occipitofrontal connections.
  b. If the head moves, reflexes tend to counter-roll the eyes against the direction of head movement to keep the eyes on the visual target. Thus, if the head moves to the right, the eyes counter-roll in equal degree to the left, remaining aligned where they were. These **doll's eye reflexes** depend solely on the vestibular system if the person is comatose or on the vestibular system plus fixation reflexes if the person is alert.
  c. Speed of eye movements
    (1) Eye movements are classed as fast or slow. All voluntary eye movements except vergences are fast (saccadic).
    (2) The deviation phase of most reflex eye movements, particularly optokinetic and vestibular reflexes, is slow, but the kickback is saccadic.
    (3) Intact frontal efferent pathways mediate the saccades of volitional movements and are presumed to mediate the kickback saccades of reflexes.

B. **Basic clinical laws of the central and peripheral optomotor systems** (Table 10-4)

1. The **laws of tonic oppositional innervation of intra- and extraocular muscles and of ocular deviation following rotator muscle paralysis** are explained in section IV B 3.

2. **Law of conjugate alignment of the eyes.** The eyes remain conjugate (aligned) at rest and during horizontal and vertical movements, but they angle in or out during vergences.

3. **Law of equal turning (equal innervation or yoking) of corresponding ocular muscles of the two eyes during movement (Hering's law).** The eyes turn conjugately during reflex or volitional horizontal or vertical movements because of the equal activation of the muscles that move the two eyes in the designated direction.

4. **Law of automatic return or kickback of the eyes to the primary position.** The eyes tend to remain in the primary position or automatically return to it if deviated.
   a. Deviation of the eyes vertically, horizontally, or during convergence triggers a kickback reflex, which tends to return them to the primary position (null point).
   b. The return of the eyes to the null point suggests the presence of an eye (and head) centering center.
      (1) No single eye and head centering center exists as such. Tonic innervation originating at various levels of the right half of the brain tends to drive the eyes to the left and is equally opposed by a drive from the left half of the brain.
      (2) Upward vectors counteract downward vectors.
      (3) The resultant of all of these vectors is the maintenance of the tonic oppositional innervation of ocular muscles and the tendency of the eyes to return to the primary position.
   c. An imbalance or instability in the deviation-kickback forces results in a to-and-fro oscillation of the eyes called **nystagmus**.

C. **Preview of central optomotor pathways**

1. **Optomotor hierarchy**
   a. The optomotor system has the same hierarchical plan as other motor systems, with supranuclear, internuclear, nuclear, and infranuclear levels.
   b. **Supranuclear (cortical) pathways** originate in the nonlimbic and limbic cortex.

Table 10-4. Summary of Clinically Important Laws of Ocular Movements

The eyes fixate and move conjugately. **Corollary**: disconjugate eye movements are abnormal; failure of fixation.

The yoke muscles involved in conjugate deviation of each eye receive equal innervation (Hering's law).

The extraocular muscles and pupillomotor muscles are in tonic opposition. **Corollary**: interruption of the nerve to an ocular rotator or pupillomotor muscle causes the eye to deviate in the direction of pull of the muscle that opposes (antagonizes) the paralyzed muscle; or the pupil assumes the size dictated by the pull of the intact pupilloconstrictor or pupillodilator muscle.

The eyes and head tend to return to the primary position because of an active centering mechanism. **Corollary**: persistent (forced) or recurrent conjugate deviation of the eyes from the primary position is abnormal.

The pathways for horizontal and vertical conjugate eye movements take different courses. **Corollary**: CNS lesions may paralyze conjugate eye movements in only one plane or both (horizontal or vertical).

Fast and slow eye movements originate in different sites and are mediated by different pathways. **Corollary**: CNS lesions may affect each form of movement separately.

When the head turns, the vestibular system counter-rolls the eyes against the direction of the turn (doll's eye test). **Corollary**: when unconsciousness negates fixation and volitional eye movements, failure of the eyes to counter-roll means failure of the vestibular system.

Fixation–fusion of the two images, pursuit, and vergences operate reflexly but can also be controlled volitionally. **Corollary**: a competition exists between reflex demand and volitional intent. Volitional movements tend to dominate or inhibit reflex ocular movements (e.g., induced nystagmus); or, if volitional pathways are interrupted, certain optic reflexes become exaggerated.

(1) Stimulation of almost any cortical or brainstem area influences the position or movement of the eyes.

(2) Unilateral stimulation usually causes the eyes to move **contralateral** to the side of stimulation.

(3) Bilateral stimulation of mirror-image points of the right and left cerebral hemispheres, brainstem, or vestibular system produces **vertical** eye movements.

(4) Supranuclear pathways end on intermediate nuclei, which produce internuclear pathways, rather than directly on lower motoneurons (LMNs).

c. Internuclear pathways that influence the position or movement of the eyes arise in the basal ganglia, diencephalon, brainstem tegmentum, cerebellum, and rostral part of the spinal cord.

(1) The major named internuclear pathway is the medial longitudinal fasciculus.

(2) In addition to the reticular formation at large and the paramedian pontine reticular formation, several satellite or accessory nuclei of the pretectum or rostral brainstem tegmentum coordinate eye movements.

d. LMN optomotor nuclei are CN III, CN IV, and CN VI. Their motoneurons provide the only axons to eye muscles and serve as the final common pathway for all reflex and volitional eye movements.

D. Optomotor control systems and their clinical testing. Eye movements result from the action of one of five systems (Table 10-5), each of which can be tested clinically (Table 10-6).

E. Frontotegmental pathway for volitional horizontal conjugate eye movements (Fig. 10-20)

1. Origin and course. Axons from the posterior frontal region cause horizontal conjugate deviation of the eyes and head to the opposite side.

a. The axons descend through the white matter of the hemisphere, through the internal capsule (and perhaps through the zona incerta slightly medial to the capsule), to enter the midbrain tegmentum.

b. The pathway decussates between the caudal part of the midbrain and the rostral part of the pons (see Fig. 10-20).

2. Termination. The decussated axons synapse near the abducens nucleus in the paramedian pontine reticular formation, a region sometimes called the **para-abducens nucleus**.

3. Internuclear pathways

a. From the para-abducens region, internuclear pathways run:

(1) Ipsilaterally to the LMNs of the abducens nucleus for innervation of the lateral rectus muscle

(2) Contralaterally to ascend in the medial longitudinal fasciculus to the LMNs of the medial rectus muscle in the nucleus of CN III (see Fig. 10-20)

b. These two pathways fulfill Hering's law in providing equal innervation to yoked muscles.

4. Syndrome of interruption of the frontal horizontal gaze pathways

a. Following unilateral destruction of one frontal pathway, the eyes and head deviate to the side of the lesion because of the tonic innervation from the contralateral frontal region.

b. Because of the proximity of the frontal eye field to the motor cortex, the patient usually has

Table 10-5. Five Major Eye Movement Systems

System	Function or Characteristics
Saccadic	Produces all volitional movements and the fast phase of reflex eye movements (frontal lobe)
Fixation (position maintenance)	Fixates eyes on target, maintains them on target, and locks the eyes in unison to fuse the two retinal images into one visual image (occipital lobe)
Smooth pursuit	Keeps eyes on moving target (occipital lobe)
Vergence	Converges or diverges eyes for near or distant targets (occipital lobe)
Counter-rolling	Vestibular and neck proprioceptive system; counter-rolls the eyes to keep them fixed on the visual target in compensation for head movement

Table 10-6. Outline of Clinical Tests for Central Eye Movement Disorders

Type of Eye Movement	Method of Examination
Spontaneous and volitional movements that accompany ordinary behavior and ordinary environmental stimuli	Inspection while taking the history
Volitional fixation and volitional movements	The examiner observes steadiness and range of eye movements after requesting the patient to fixate on a distant, straight-ahead object and then to move the eyes right, left, up, and down
Visual reflex ocular movements	
Smooth pursuit	The patient's eyes pursue the examiner's finger as it moves through the full range of ocular movements
Vergences	The examiner directs the patient to look at near and distant objects and to follow the examiner's moving finger in toward the patient's nose
Reflex fixation	The patient fixates straight ahead, and the examiner turns the patient's head to the right, left, up, and down
Alignment lock	As the patient fixates straight ahead, the examiner alternately covers and uncovers first one, then the other eye and looks for deviation in alignment, resulting from monocular occlusion of vision (cover–uncover test)
Optokinetic nystagmus	The examiner rotates a drum or moves a striped strip. The patient's eyes pursue the drum to one side slowly, and then a saccade kicks them back to the primary position
Nonvisual reflex ocular movements	
Caloric nystagmus	Irrigation of the ears with hot or cold water
Positional nystagmus	Placing the patient's head in various positions
Contraversive eye-turning test (doll's eye test, oculocephalic test)	Rapid turning of the patient's head by the examiner's hands
Associated eye movement (Bell's phenomenon)	The examiner holds the patient's eyelids open and observes the upward movement of the eyes that occurs when the patient attempts to close the lids

contralateral hemiplegia. That is, the hemiplegia is contralateral to the lesion, but the eyes and head deviate ipsilaterally. The deviation is corrected quickly in hours or days.

   c. One frontal cortex initiates both volitional and reflex saccades to move the eyes to the opposite side. After deviation of the eyes to the side of a frontal lesion, kickback saccades in response to vestibular stimulation or optokinetic reflexes are usually reduced to the side opposite the cerebral lesion.

   d. After bilateral destruction of the frontal horizontal gaze pathway, the patient cannot move the eyes to either side voluntarily, but the eyes will still deviate in response to vestibular stimulation or reflex pursuit.

   5. Syndrome of the medial longitudinal fasciculus. A unilateral lesion of the medial longitudinal fasciculus (see the arrow in Fig. 10-20) causes a definite syndrome when the patient volitionally looks contralaterally.

   a. Signs on neurologic examination include:

   (1) Paresis or paralysis of **adduction** of the eye ipsilateral to the lesion when the patient attempts to look **contralaterally**

   (2) Monocular nystagmus of the abducting eye, a feature that cannot be deduced from Figure 10-20

   (3) Preservation of volitional eye movements in all other directions including vertical gaze and convergence

   b. Symptoms include diplopia on contralateral gaze (resulting from medial rectus palsy) and oscillopsia (resulting from nystagmus).

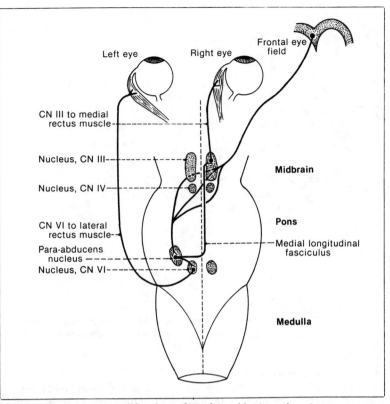

Figure 10-20. Frontotegmental pathway for volitional horizontal conjugate eye movements. Start at the frontal eye field, and trace the pathway to the medial and lateral rectus muscles.

   c. **Neuroanatomical correlation.** Interruption of the frontal pathway through the medial longitudinal fasciculus paralyzes adduction of the medial rectus muscle for volitional horizontal conjugate lateral gaze; however, the muscle acts during convergence because the convergence pathway does not loop down into the pons and back through the medial longitudinal fasciculus.
   d. The most **common causes** are multiple sclerosis, infarcts, and pontine neoplasms.

F. **Supranuclear (cortico-pretecto-midbrain-tegmental) pathway for volitional vertical conjugate eye movements** (Fig. 10-21)

   1. **Origin.** The volitional vertical gaze pathway apparently arises diffusely from the cerebral cortex, mainly from the frontal and occipital lobes.

   2. **Course and termination**
      a. From their diverse cortical origins, the axons converge upon the pretectal region at the junction of the diencephalon and midbrain.
      b. For **vertical upward movements**, the pathway from the pretectal nuclei runs to the appropriate LMNs of CN III.
      c. For **vertical downward movements**, the pathway appears to run through the reticular formation dorsomedial to the red nucleus and thence to the CN III nucleus, directly or through synapses, in other accessory nuclei of the midbrain tegmentum. The periaqueductal gray matter may also be involved.

   3. **Differences in the vertical and horizontal pathways**
      a. The **horizontal gaze pathway** has a recurrent loop down into the pons and back through the medial longitudinal fasciculus to the midbrain (see Fig. 10-20).
      b. The **vertical gaze pathway** runs directly to the pretectal-midbrain region without showing a recurrent loop into the pons (see Fig. 10-21).
      c. Interruption of cortical efferent fibers in the midbrain or pontine basis may cause paralysis of horizontal gaze with complete preservation of vertical gaze. (See the locked-in syndrome in Chapter 8, section XIV D 1).

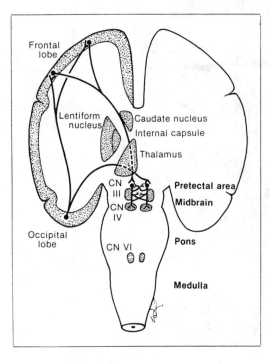

Figure 10-21. Cortico-pretecto-midbrain pathway for volitional vertical conjugate eye movements.

4. Syndromes of vertical gaze paralysis

a. Diffuse cortical or white matter disease will impair volitional vertical eye movements.

b. Downward compression of the pretectal area from above, as by a pineal tumor, initially causes selective paralysis of upward gaze, with downward gaze spared (Parinaud syndrome).

c. Further compression may paralyze downward gaze as well. Lesions dorsomedial to the red nucleus may cause selective paralysis of downward gaze.

G. Occipital pathways for visually mediated optomotor reflexes

1. The visually mediated optomotor reflexes are **fixation, fusion, pursuit, vergences,** and **optokinetic nystagmus**. They require an intact afferent arc through the retino-geniculo-calcarine pathway.

2. From the calcarine cortex, intracortical association pathways connect with the surrounding occipitoparietal cortex, which originates the efferent fibers.

3. The efferents from the occipitoparietal cortex descend through the cerebral white matter to the pretectum or tegmentum, where they probably share the pathways for horizontal and vertical movements already depicted (see Figs. 10-20 and 10-21).

4. Many of the pathways for visually mediated optomotor reflexes are poorly understood. For example, smooth pursuit of a target moving to the patient's right is thought to be mediated by the ipsilateral (i.e., right) hemisphere, with the leftward kickback to the midline mediated by the right frontotegmental pathway. The occipitofrontal connections that would underlie this action are not clearly identified.

H. Comparison of upper motoneuron (UMN) and LMN lesions of the optomotor pathways

1. LMN lesions paralyze both reflex and volitional movements of the individual muscles.

2. UMN lesions (supranuclear lesions) do not paralyze the movements of the individual muscles, but they do affect conjugate movements of the two eyes.

3. Because supranuclear and internuclear pathways arise from several sources, one or more of the pathways will remain intact in the presence of a central lesion and can be used to demonstrate the integrity of the LMNs. Thus, if the patient cannot move the eyes to one side volitionally but can do so reflexly, the lesion has to be in the supranuclear or internuclear pathways, not in the LMNs.

STUDY QUESTIONS

Directions: Each question below contains five suggested answers. Choose the **one best** response to each question.

1. A patient complains of diplopia only when looking up and to the right. The diplopia most likely represents weakness of

(A) the right superior rectus or left inferior oblique muscle
(B) the right superior oblique or left inferior rectus muscle
(C) the right lateral rectus or left medial rectus muscle
(D) the right inferior oblique or left superior rectus muscle
(E) none of the above

2. When a patient cannot adduct the left eye when attempting to look to the right, but the eye adducts on convergence, the lesion is in the

(A) left dorsal longitudinal fasciculus
(B) right medial lemniscus
(C) left medial longitudinal fasciculus
(D) nucleus of CN III
(E) left medial forebrain bundle

3. Contraction of the lateral rectus muscle causes the eyeball to rotate

(A) laterally
(B) medially
(C) upward
(D) downward
(E) inward

4. A patient with unilateral miosis, ptosis, and anhidrosis would most likely have a lesion of

(A) CN III
(B) CN VII
(C) the carotid artery
(D) the ciliary ganglion
(E) the greater superficial petrosal nerve

5. If the other cranial nerves remain intact, interruption of CN III results in rotation of the eyeball

(A) medially and upward
(B) medially and downward
(C) laterally and upward
(D) laterally and downward
(E) upward in the midline

6. A light ray striking the nasal side of the retina causes the person to experience a visual image as if coming from

(A) the opposite eye
(B) the temporal half of space
(C) the midpoint of the horopter
(D) the visual axis
(E) none of the above

7. When a patient voluntarily deviates the eyes to the left, the cortical efferent pathway comes from

(A) the right frontal lobe
(B) the left frontal lobe
(C) the right occipital lobe
(D) the left occipital lobe
(E) the left temporal lobe

8. Ptosis in Horner's syndrome (sympathetic denervation) is characterized by

(A) disappearing or improving when the patient looks up
(B) being more pronounced when the patient looks up
(C) appearing unchanged when the patient looks up
(D) being better after rest
(E) none of the above

9. After CN III enters the subarachnoid space of the interpeduncular fossa, it immediately encounters

(A) CN IV
(B) the infundibular stalk
(C) the posterior cerebral artery
(D) the dura mater
(E) the posterior clinoid process

10. A lesion very likely to affect CN III, CN IV, and CN VI and the ophthalmic division of CN V would most likely be in the

(A) pontine tegmentum
(B) cerebellopontine angle
(C) midbrain tegmentum
(D) cavernous sinus
(E) nasopharynx

11. A large acute destructive lesion of the left posterior frontal region would result in

(A) deviation of the eyes to the left
(B) deviation of the eyes to the right
(C) deviation of the eyes upward
(D) deviation of the eyes downward
(E) no deviation of the eyes

Directions: Each question below contains four suggested answers of which **one or more** is correct. Choose the answer

A   if **1, 2, and 3** are correct
B   if **1 and 3** are correct
C   if **2 and 4** are correct
D   if **4** is correct
E   if **1, 2, 3, and 4** are correct

12. True statements concerning CN IV include which of the following?

(1) It is one of the larger cranial nerves
(2) It innervates the superior and inferior oblique muscles
(3) It courses within the lumen of the cavernous sinus
(4) It wraps around the midbrain

13. In contrast to the pathway for vertical eye movements, the pathway for horizontal eye movements

(1) loops down into the pons and returns back to the nucleus of CN III
(2) causes bilateral nystagmus when interrupted unilaterally
(3) decussates at caudal midbrain or rostral pontine levels
(4) runs just dorsomedial to the red nucleus

14. Correct statements about optic atrophy include which of the following?

(1) After compression of the optic nerve or chiasm, the optic nerve fibers at the optic disk atrophy because of anterograde (wallerian) degeneration
(2) the optic disk appears white
(3) the borders of the disk become elevated
(4) the physiologic cup disappears

15. Which of the following ocular actions or reflexes are mediated through the occipital lobe?

(1) Vergences
(2) Smooth pursuit
(3) Binocular fixation
(4) Saccadic movements

16. The optic nerve contains fibers from which of the following sources?

(1) Lateral geniculate body
(2) Amacrine neurons
(3) Rods or cones
(4) Ganglion cell layer of the retina

17. The sympathetic nervous system innervates which of the following muscles?

(1) Pupillodilator
(2) Levator palpebrae
(3) Superior tarsal
(4) Orbicularis oculi

18. Deficits that result from complete interruption of one optic nerve include which of the following?

(1) Optic atrophy
(2) Ipsilateral loss of the direct pupillary light reflex
(3) Loss of the consensual pupillary light reflex of the contralateral eye
(4) Central scotoma in the affected eye

Directions: The group of questions below consists of lettered choices followed by several numbered items. For each numbered item select the **one** lettered choice with which it is **most** closely associated. Each lettered choice may be used once, more than once, or not at all.

Questions 19–23

Match each lesion listed below with the resultant visual field defect.

(A) Contralateral superior homonymous quadrantanopia
(B) Inferior altitudinal hemianopia (blindness in the inferior half of the visual field of both eyes)
(C) Partial contralateral inferior homonymous quadrantanopia
(D) Complete contralateral homonymous hemianopia without macular sparing
(E) Complete blindness

E 19. Bilateral destruction of the occipital lobes

C 20. Unilateral destruction of the inferior part of one parietal lobe

A 21. Destruction of the anterior to the middle third of the temporal lobe

D 22. Complete destruction of the calcarine cortex of one occipital lobe

B 23. Bilateral destruction of the superior bank of the calcarine fissure

ANSWERS AND EXPLANATIONS

1. The answer is A. [*VII A 1 b (2)*] When the eyes look conjugately in any direction, the muscle that is the prime mover of the leading eye acts in unison with (is yoked to) a muscle of the following eye, which corresponds. Both muscles receive equal innervation in order to move the eyes equally and maintain the visual axes of both eyes on the target, thus avoiding diplopia. On looking upward and to the right, the right superior rectus muscle is yoked to the left inferior oblique muscle.

2. The answer is C. (*VII E 5 a*) When an eye fails to adduct on voluntary horizontal gaze, but it does adduct during convergence, the lesion is in the medial longitudinal fasciculus. This bundle conveys the voluntary pathway from the nucleus of CN VI (or surrounding region in the pons) to the nucleus of CN III. A lesion of the lower motoneurons (LMNs) in the nucleus of CN III would paralyze adduction during volitional movements and convergence.

3. The answer is A. (*IV C 1*) The lateral rectus muscle causes the eyeball to abduct or rotate laterally. No matter which position the eyeball is in, the lateral rectus muscle can only abduct the eye when it contracts. Its antagonist, the medial rectus muscle, can only adduct the eye. Thus, these two muscles have only one action each. The other eye muscles have a variable action, depending upon the position of the eyeball when the muscle contracts.

4. The answer is C. (*VI E 1*) Unilateral miosis, ptosis, and anhidrosis indicate interruption of the sympathetic innervation of that half of the face. Since the sympathetic axons travel along the carotid artery, lesions of that vessel, such as aneurysms, may interrupt the sympathetic axons.

5. The answer is D. (*V B 7 a*) After interruption of CN III, the eyeball turns laterally and down. The tonic contraction of the intact lateral rectus muscle will turn the eyeball laterally, and that of the superior oblique muscle will turn it down and intort it. CN III innervates the muscles that would normally counteract the foregoing two muscles.

6. The answer is B. (*III A 2 a*) The retinal image is inverted in relation to the origin of light rays. Thus, a light ray that comes from the temporal side of the visual field would strike the nasal side of the retina. The person learns to interpret a stimulus on the nasal side of the retina as coming from the temporal half of space.

7. The answer is A. (*VII E 1*) The law of contralateral innervation of movements by the upper motoneuron (UMN) pathways applies to horizontal eye movements. Thus, the right frontal lobe, with its motor area, causes voluntary deviation of the eyes to the left.

8. The answer is A. (*VI E 5; Table 10-3*) Sympathetic denervation paralyzes the superior tarsal muscle. This muscle acts involuntarily to elevate the eyelid. The levator palpebrae muscle acts to elevate the lid further during voluntary elevation of the eyes. Since it receives its innervation from CN III, it will still act to elevate the lid, even though the superior tarsal muscle is paralyzed.

9. The answer is C. (*V B 3 b*) Downward traction on the posterior cerebral artery by herniation of the adjacent temporal lobe may cause the artery to impinge on CN III. The resulting paralysis of the ocular muscles and dilation of the pupil from interruption of the pupilloconstrictor axons constitute important clinical signs of progressing brain herniation, which may kill the patient.

10. The answer is D. (*Figure 10-17*) The cavernous sinus syndrome involves varying combinations of paralysis of CN III, CN IV, and CN VI and sensory loss in the ophthalmic division of CN V. These nerves come into conjunction in the lateral wall of the cavernous sinus. Lesions that would commonly cause the syndrome are aneurysmal dilations of the intracavernous portion of the internal carotid artery or carotid artery–cavernous sinus fistulae. Involvement of the carotid artery might also cause Horner's syndrome due to interruption of the postganglionic sympathetic axons that travel along the artery.

11. The answer is A. (*VII E 4*) A large destructive lesion of the left frontal lobe will result in deviation of the head and eyes to the left. Under normal circumstances, the left side of the brain acts to turn the eyes to the right, and the right side turns the eyes to the left. When a lesion destroys an area of special significance for eye deviation, such as the posterior frontal eye fields, the eyes will deviate to the side of the lesion because the intact, opposite side of the brain acts unopposed. Unilateral cerebral lesions do not paralyze vertical eye movements.

12. The answer is D (4). (*V C 3*) CN IV undergoes complete internal decussation and exits dorsally from the midbrain just caudal to the inferior colliculus. It then wraps around the midbrain before entering the lateral wall of the cavernous sinus.

13. The answer is B (1, 3). [*VII E 1 b, 3 a (2), F 3 a*] The cortical pathway for horizontal eye movement crosses at midbrain and pontine levels to reach the contralateral CN VI nucleus in the pons and then recrosses to go up the medial longitudinal fasciculus to the CN III nucleus. The vertical eye movement pathways run directly into the pretectum and midbrain without looping down through the pons. The pathway for vertical downward eye movements runs just dorsomedial to the red nucleus, with the pathway for vertical upward movements apparently being somewhat more dorsal in the midbrain tegmentum.

14. The answer is C (2, 4). (*II C 3 a–b*) Optic nerve fibers originate in the retina. Following compression of the optic nerve or chiasm, the optic nerve fibers undergo retrograde degeneration rather than anterograde (wallerian) degeneration. Because the axons degenerate back to the retina, they disappear from the optic disk. The capillaries that had given the disk its pink color also disappear. The physiologic cup disappears because it is only a depression in the middle of the ring of nerve fibers that penetrates the optic disk from the retina. The optic disk, denuded of fibers and capillaries, appears flat and has the white color of the lamina cribrosa of the sclera.

15. The answer is A (1, 2, 3). (*VII G 1; Table 10-5*) The ocular movements or actions that require an intact afferent arc from the retina are all mediated through the occipital lobe. These include vergences, smooth pursuit, and binocular fixation. On the other hand, saccadic movements (the normal voluntary movements of the eyes) originate in frontal lobe pathways.

16. The answer is D (4). (*II D 4 b*) The optic nerve contains axons that arise only in the ganglion cell layer of the retina. The rods and cones and amacrine neurons of the retina do not send fibers into the optic nerve, nor does the lateral geniculate body, in which the optic nerve fibers end. Although the optic nerve may contain some efferent fibers, their origin and functional significance are unknown.

17. The answer is B (1, 3). (*VI A 3; Table 10-3*) The muscles within and around the eyes receive their innervation from a variety of different nerves. The sympathetic nerves innervate the pupillodilator and the superior tarsal muscles. The facial nerve innervates the orbicularis oculi muscle; all the rest of the intra- and extraocular muscles receive their innervation from CN III, CN IV, and CN VI.

18. The answer is A (1, 2, 3). (*II C 3 a; VI B 7 a*) A characteristic syndrome follows interruption of one optic nerve. It includes complete ipsilateral optic atrophy, loss of the direct pupillary light reflex ipsilaterally, and loss of the consensual pupillary light reflex of the opposite eye. The patient, of course, is completely blind in the eye rather than having simply a central scotoma.

19–23. The answer are: 19-E, 20-C, 21-A, 22-D, 23-B. (*III C 2 e, F 2 a–c; Figure 10-9*) The topographic representation of the visual fields is very strict. For this reason, lesions affecting particular sites along the optic pathway cause very characteristic and reproducible field defects. Lesions of the parts of the geniculocalcarine pathway as it courses through the hemispheric wall cause different field defects, depending upon the location. Since the geniculocalcarine fibers course deep in the white matter, in the external sagittal stratum (which is a few millimeters lateral to the ventricular wall), the cerebral lesions that cause field defects must be deep within the white matter rather than limited to the cortex or immediately subjacent white matter. A lesion of the most anterior fibers of the geniculocalcarine tract as it loops around the temporal horn causes a contralateral superior quadrantanopia, which is more or less complete, depending upon the number of fibers affected.

As the geniculocalcarine tract proceeds backward, the fibers that represent the inferior visual fields course through the inferior part of the parietal lobe. Hence, lesions of the inferior parietal region that interrupt these fibers give rise to a contralateral inferior homonymous field defect.

Lesions of one occipital lobe likewise cause contralateral defects, which may vary from partial quadrantanopia to a complete contralateral hemianopia. Bilateral occipital lobe destruction causes double hemianopia or, in essence, complete blindness.

Lesions of the superior or inferior banks of the calcarine fissure, either unilateral or bilateral, cause quadrantanopias or hemianopias, depending upon the extent of the tissue destroyed. Destruction of either the superior banks or the inferior banks on both sides causes an altitudinal hemianopia. Destruction of the superior banks causes an inferior altitudinal hemianopia in both eyes; destruction of the inferior banks causes a superior altitudinal hemianopia.

Lesions of the cerebral white matter beyond the actual course of the geniculocalcarine tracts do not cause field defects, nor do lesions of the corpus callosum. The latter lesions interfere with transfer of visual information from one hemisphere to the other but do not cause field defects.

11
Basal Motor Nuclei

I. GROSS ANATOMY OF THE BASAL MOTOR NUCLEI

A. Location. Either coronal or horizontal sections through the base of the cerebrum disclose large nuclear masses consisting of the basal ganglia and thalami (Figs. 11-1 and 11-2).

B. Relationships of the basal nuclei to the internal capsule

1. The basal nuclei cluster on one side or the other of V-shaped zones of white matter called the **internal capsule**. Viewed horizontally, the internal capsule has three parts (see Fig. 11-2):
   a. Anterior limb
   b. Genu (knee)
   c. Posterior limb

2. Medial to the **anterior limb** is the **caudate nucleus**.

3. Medial to the **posterior limb** is the **thalamus**.

4. Lateral to the genu and the **anterior** and **posterior limbs** are the **globus pallidus** and **putamen**.

5. Notice in Figure 11-2 the reciprocity between the V-shape of the capsule and the diameter of the adjacent nuclei.
   a. Going **forward** from the genu, the head of the caudate nucleus increases in size.
   b. Going **backward** from the genu, the thalamus increases in size.
   c. The maximum transverse diameter of the globus pallidus corresponds to the genu. Going forward or backward from the genu, the globus pallidus decreases in diameter.
   d. The transverse plane through the apex of the globus pallidus and the genu falls just behind the foramen of Monro.

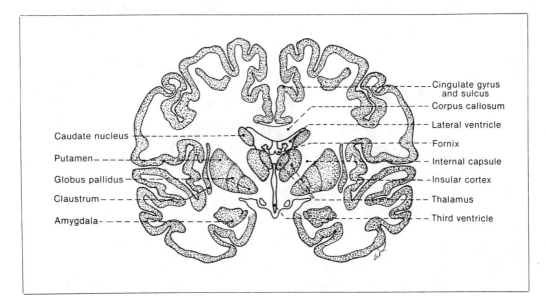

Figure 11-1. Coronal section of the cerebral hemispheres through the level of the basal ganglia. The anterior limb of the internal capsule runs through the crevice between the caudate nucleus and putamen.

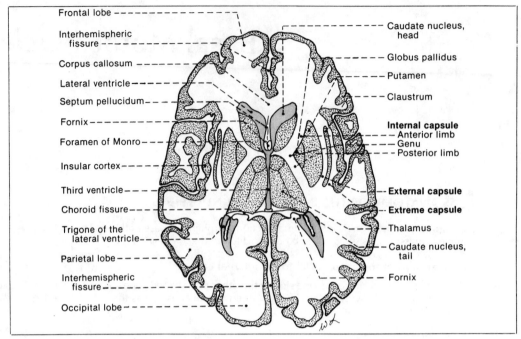

Figure 11-2. Horizontal section of the cerebral hemispheres at the level of the genu of the internal capsule.

C. Gross anatomy of the caudate–putamen

1. The head of the caudate nucleus sits across the anterior limb of the internal capsule from the putamen and globus pallidus.

2. The caudate and putamen are actually one nuclear mass strongly indented by the anterior limb of the capsule. They retain their continuity underneath the crevice for the anterior limb (Fig. 11-3).

3. The **head** and **body** of the caudate nucleus form the ventrolateral wall of the anterior horn of the lateral ventricle (see Fig. 11-1).

4. The **tail** of the caudate nucleus circles the body of the lateral ventricle and proceeds forward in the roof of the temporal horn. It terminates in the amygdala (see Fig. 11-3).

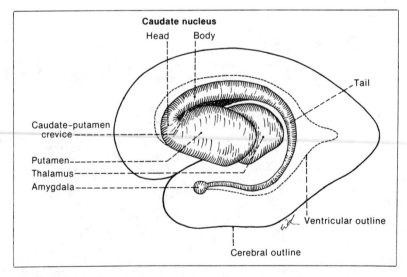

Figure 11-3. Phantom drawing of the caudate nucleus and putamen in situ.

D. Nomenclature of the basal motor nuclei

1. Neuroanatomists originally grouped three nuclei—the corpus striatum, claustrum, and amygdala—as the basal ganglia, before their connections, ontogeny, and functions were understood (Fig. 11-4).

2. Now neuroanatomists assign the amygdala to the limbic system, but the function of the claustrum remains unknown. The caudate–putamen and globus pallidus connect with a number of nearby nuclei to control skeletal muscle activity. These **basal motor nuclei** include **cerebral**, **diencephalic**, and **midbrain** components (Fig. 11-5).

3. The rationale for the concept of the basal motor nuclei is as follows.
   a. They have an anatomical proximity extending from the base of the cerebrum through the diencephalon to the midbrain.
   b. They all modulate somatomotor activity by means of numerous feedback circuits with each other, with the cerebellum, and ultimately with the cerebral motor cortex.
   c. Lesions in these nuclei or their pathways result in predictable motor signs consisting of muscular rigidity and involuntary movements. The involuntary movements include tremors, chorea, ballismus, dystonia, and athetosis, depending on the nucleus affected (see section IV A and Table 11-2).

II. CONNECTIONS OF THE BASAL MOTOR NUCLEI

A. Arrangement of myelinated axons

1. **Capsules**, **laminae**, **bundles**, or **fields** of myelinated axons surround, separate, and interconnect the basal motor nuclei (Fig. 11-6).

2. **Striatopallidal bundles.** Since many feedback loops interconnect the basal motor nuclei with

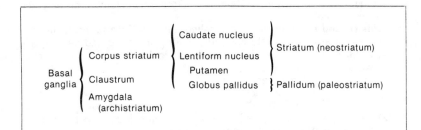

Figure 11-4. Nomenclature of the original basal ganglia.

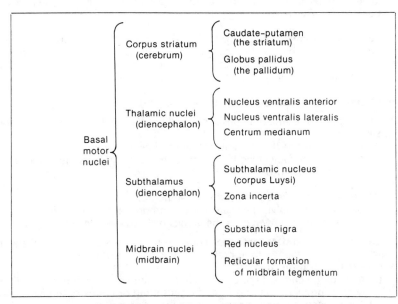

Figure 11-5. Nomenclature of the basal motor nuclei.

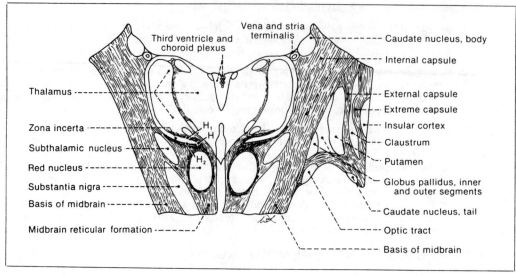

Figure 11-6. Drawing of myelin-stained coronal section through the basal motor nuclei. *H* = field H of Forel.

each other and with the cerebral motor cortex, we can arbitrarily select the striatopallidal fibers as a starting point for a **progressogram** to illustrate the concept (Fig. 11-7).

   3. H fields of Forel and the ansa and fasciculus lenticularis
   a. Field H. From the capsule of fibers around the red nucleus, fibers extend dorsomedially as field H of Forel.
   b. Fields H₁ and H₂. A nuclear plate called the **zona incerta** inserts itself between a dorsal lamina of fibers, called field H_1, and a ventral lamina, called field H_2 (Fig. 11-8).
      (1) Field H_1 is also called the **thalamic fasciculus**. It conveys three major afferent pathways to the thalamus:
      (a) Pallidothalamic tract
      (b) Dentatothalamic tract
      (c) Medial lemniscus
      (2) Field H_2 is also called the **lenticular fasciculus**. It conveys pallidothalamic axons from the globus pallidus of the lentiform nucleus.
   c. The **ansa lenticularis** (ansa means loop) is a stream of pallidal efferents, mainly pallidothalamic. It loops under the internal capsule, rather than penetrating it like the fasciculus lenticularis (see Fig. 11-8).

B. Arrangements of unmyelinated axons. Numerous axons that do not show in standard myelin and silver stains of the basal region course through the previously named nuclei and pathways. These axons, demonstrated by fluorescence microscopy, are described in the discussion of the substantia nigra (section II G) and in Chapter 14.

C. Connections of the caudate–putamen (the striatum)

   1. Neuron types of the striatum consist of small neurons and large neurons in a ratio of 170:1.
   a. Small neurons:
      (1) Receive most of the afferents to the caudate–putamen
      (2) Belong to the Golgi type II category and mostly synapse within the caudate–putamen and globus pallidus
   b. Large neurons:
      (1) Receive their afferents from the small neurons
      (2) Belong to the Golgi type I category and produce the bundles of myelinated striatopallidal axons that converge on the globus pallidus (see Fig. 11-8).

   2. Afferents to the caudate–putamen come from the cerebral cortex, thalamus, substantia nigra, and median raphe of the brainstem reticular formation.
   a. Corticostriatal projections
      (1) Most of the cerebral cortex, including the limbic cortex, projects to the striatum. The densest projection comes from the sensorimotor cortex of the paracentral region.
      (2) The projection from the general cortex remains mainly ipsilateral, but the sensorimotor

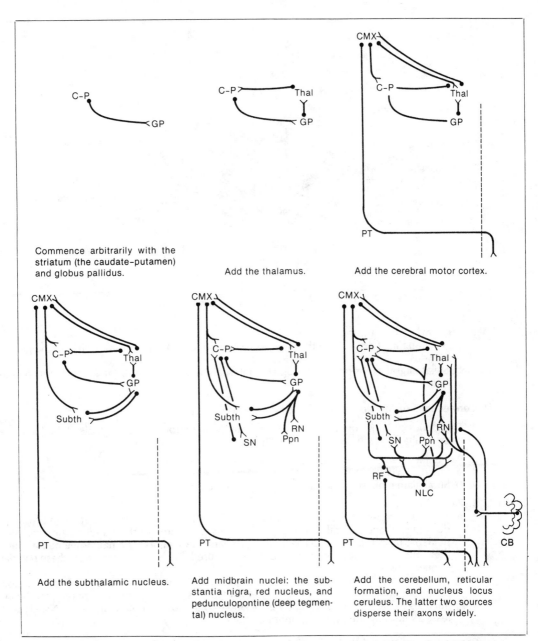

Commence arbitrarily with the striatum (the caudate–putamen) and globus pallidus.

Add the thalamus.

Add the cerebral motor cortex.

Add the subthalamic nucleus.

Add midbrain nuclei: the substantia nigra, red nucleus, and pedunculopontine (deep tegmental) nucleus.

Add the cerebellum, reticular formation, and nucleus locus ceruleus. The latter two sources disperse their axons widely.

Figure 11-7. Progressogram for the conceptual understanding of basal motor circuitry. *CB* = cerebellum; *CMX* = cerebral motor cortex; *C–P* = caudate–putamen; *GP* = globus pallidus; *NLC* = nucleus locus ceruleus; *Ppn* = pedunculopontine nuclei of the reticular formation; *PT* = pyramidal tract; *RN* = red nucleus; *SN* = substantia nigra; *Subth* = subthalamic nucleus; *Thal* = thalamus.

cortex and limbic cortex project bilaterally. The axons cross in the corpus callosum (see Fig. 13-29).

b. Thalamostriatal afferents. Intralaminar nuclei of the thalamus and centrum medianum send striatal afferents across the internal capsule. Probably the ventrolateral and ventral anterior parts of the thalamus also project to the striatum.

c. Nigrostriatal afferents. Unmyelinated dopaminergic axons from the pars compacta of the substantia nigra travel to the striatum via the internal capsule and field H, and as fibers of passage through the medial part of the globus pallidus.

d. Raphe–striatal afferents. The raphe nuclei of the reticular formation send serotonergic axons to the striatum (see Chapter 14, section III).

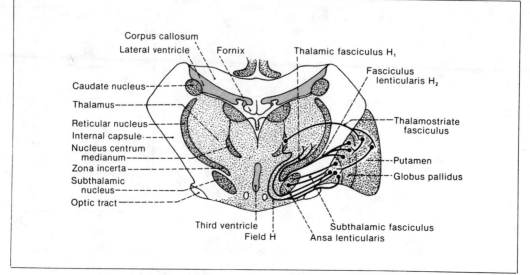

Figure 11-8. Diagram of connections of the globus pallidus.

3. Efferents of the striatal neurons

a. Striatopallidal axons from the large, and some small, striatal neurons project to the globus pallidus.

b. Striatonigral axons project through the internal capsule to the substantia nigra, pars reticulata.

D. Connections of the globus pallidus (the pallidum)

1. The globus pallidus contains large, typical multipolar motoneurons. Its "pale globe" appearance results from the number of myelinated axons that enter and leave it.

2. Pallidal afferents. Two known major afferent sources are the:
a. Striatum, via the striatopallidal fibers
b. Subthalamic nucleus, via the subthalamic fasciculus

3. Pallidal efferents

a. The pallidum issues four major bundles of fibers. They depart from its apex and from its dorsomedial and ventral aspects. Figure 11-8 shows three of the bundles: the **ansa lenticularis, fasciculus lenticularis**, and **subthalamic fasciculus**. The **pallidotegmental bundle** to the pedunculopontine nucleus is not pictured. Table 11-1 summarizes these pallidal connections.

b. We can state, as a very crude oversimplification, that the pallidum acts as a final common pathway from the basal motor nuclei to the thalamus. The thalamus in turn relays these influences to the motor cortex and hence down to the lower motoneurons (LMNs). This at least is clinically the most important circuit.

E. Connections of the subthalamic nucleus (corpus Luysi)

1. Afferents come from the pallidum and a somatotopic projection from the motor cortex.

2. Efferents of the subthalamic nucleus run to the ipsilateral pallidum via the subthalamic fasciculus. Some cross to the contralateral pallidum in the dorsal supraoptic commissure of the hypothalamus.

F. Connections of the red nucleus

1. Neuronal types

a. Small neurons comprise the bulk of the red nucleus (**parvocellular part**).

b. Large neurons comprise only a small part of the nucleus (**magnocellular part**) and are less prominent in man than in lower animals.

2. Afferents come from two main sources: the cerebral cortex and cerebellum.

a. Corticorubral fibers come from the ipsilateral precentral gyrus via the internal capsule.

Table 11-1. Pallidal Efferent Pathways*

Pathway	Course	Destination
Ansa lenticularis	Loops ventromedially under the internal capsule to enter fields H and H_1	Thalamus, nuclei ventralis lateralis and ventralis anterior
Fasciculus lenticularis	Cuts directly through the internal capsule to join field H_2 before recurving dorsally into field H_1	Thalamus, as above
Pallidosubthalamic fasciculus	Cuts directly through the internal capsule	Subthalamic nucleus of Luysi; this pathway also conveys subthalamopallidal fibers
Pallidotegmental tract	Runs dorsomedially past the subthalamic nucleus and descends into the midbrain tegmentum near the ventrolateral border of the red nucleus	Pedunculopontine nucleus of reticular formation of midbrain tegmentum

*See Figure 11-8.

   b. Dentatorubral fibers come via the contralateral rostral cerebellar peduncle. The tract decussates in the midbrain tegmentum just caudal to the red nucleus.
   3. Efferents from the red nucleus consist of two large pathways and several of lesser size.
      a. The two major pathways are the rubro-olivary and rubrospinal tracts.
         (1) The **rubro-olivary tract** descends ipsilaterally in the central tegmental tract.
         (2) The **rubrospinal tract** decussates in the ventral tegmental decussation and enters the spinal cord on the ventral border of the crossed lateral corticospinal tract.
      b. Smaller rubral efferent pathways run to the lateral reticular nucleus of the medulla, which, like the inferior olivary nucleus, relays to the cerebellum.
      c. Recent work has not confirmed the existence of a rubrothalamic tract, suggested by older studies.

   G. Connections of the substantia nigra
      1. The substantia nigra contains large multipolar neurons, which accumulate large amounts of melanin as the brain matures and ages. The neurons form two groups.
         a. The **pars compacta** is located dorsally, and its perikarya are relatively closely packed. This zone originates most of the efferents.
         b. The **pars reticulata** is located ventrally, between the pars compacta and the cortical efferent fibers of the midbrain basis. This zone receives most of the afferents.
      2. Afferents to the substantia nigra come from the striatum and, to a lesser extent, the thalamus. No known projections come from the cerebral cortex, cerebellum, or spinal cord.
      3. Efferents from the substantia nigra arise mainly in the pars compacta. They pass dorsally over the subthalamic nucleus and traverse the globus pallidus to end in the striatum and, to a lesser extent, in the nucleus ventralis lateralis and the nucleus ventralis anterior of the thalamus.
         a. Some may reach basal forebrain structures and the frontal cortex.
         b. The nigral efferent axons are dopaminergic (see Chapter 14, section II B).

III. PYRAMIDAL/EXTRAPYRAMIDAL DICHOTOMY

   A. Definition of the extrapyramidal motor system
      1. As traditionally described, the extrapyramidal system includes all motor pathways of the brain that influence LMNs but do not send their axons directly into the pyramidal tract— namely, the circuitry of the basal motor nuclei and the reticulospinal, rubrospinal, olivospinal, vestibulospinal, and tectospinal tracts. Some authors include a cortical extrapyramidal component.
      2. Because of the diversity of extrapyramidal components and the difficulty in extrapolating the results of animal experiments on the two systems to humans, many authors have argued, often contentiously, in favor of abolishing the pyramidal/extrapyramidal concept altogether.
      3. Clinicians, however, retain the concept because distinctive pyramidal and extrapyramidal syndromes (see Tables 7-5 and 11-2) serve to localize lesions and separate disease entities [e.g., familial spastic paraplegia (pyramidal) versus Parkinson's disease (extrapyramidal)].

B. **Resolution of the pyramidal/extrapyramidal controversy by phylogeny and clinicopathologic correlation**

1. In **submammalia**, all movements are extrapyramidal because these animals have no cerebral cortex as such and no pyramidal tract.

2. In **lower mammals**, such as marsupials, the cortex appears but the pyramidal tract is short and relatively expendable.

3. In **lower primates**, the cortex and pyramidal tract increase in importance, but the extrapyramidal system can compensate considerably for pyramidal tract interruption.

4. In **humans**, complete unilateral interruption of the pyramidal tract paralyzes most contralateral voluntary movements, particularly of the hand.
   a. Clinicopathologic correlation at autopsy or by computed tomography (CT) and magnetic resonance imaging (MRI) shows that complete bilateral interruption of the pyramidal tract paralyzes all volitional movements of the body parts caudal to the lesion (see Chapter 8, section XIV D 1).
   b. Furthermore, total pyramidal tract destruction in humans paralyzes not only all volitional movements but also those involuntary movements that result from lesions of the basal motor nuclei. In addition, the paralysis masks the ataxia resulting from cerebellar lesions.

5. Thus, the phylogenetic series illustrates a gradual increase in the dependence of movement on the pyramidal tract. Somatomotor activity originating in the forebrain or brainstem is extrapyramidal in submammalia, mixed pyramidal/extrapyramidal in subhuman mammalia, and essentially pyramidal in humans.

6. **Pyramidal funnel concept**
   a. In humans, movement has become corticalized and pyramidalized, as it were.
   b. Various afferent pathways, originating in the reticular formation, cerebellum, basal motor nuclei, and sensory systems, feed through the thalamus and to the motor cortex to modulate its activity. The motor cortex in turn feeds back to many of these sources.
   c. Lesions of the various afferent pathways result in dysmodulation of the motor cortex, which is expressed through an intact pyramidal tract by predictable clinical signs (e.g., chorea, ataxia) and has predictable laterality.
   d. Thus, we can view the motor cortex as an internuncial neuronal pool that acts as a funnel, as the final common motor pathway to the LMNs from diverse sources (Fig. 11-9).

7. **Caveats**
   a. The previous statements apply to patients who have an acquired lesion in a relatively mature, previously normal nervous system.
   b. Congenital malformations or prenatal lesions may destroy the cerebral cortex and cause complete absence of the pyramidal tracts, as in hydranencephaly, anencephaly, or holoprosencephaly. Affected infants may indeed move their extremities, obviously through "extrapyramidal" pathways, but the movements would appear to be "reflexive," automatic, and nonadaptive, rather than "volitional," in origin. Given the same degree of destruction of a normal postnatal brain, the previously stated rules apply.
   c. Some patients will show considerable recovery of volitional movements following severe, but incomplete, unilateral interruption of the pyramidal tract. Recovery in these patients might be because the pyramidal system can function with relatively few remaining crossed axons, or volitional control might develop through extrapyramidal pathways or through uncrossed fibers of the ipsilateral pyramidal tract.

IV. PATHOGENESIS AND TREATMENT OF INVOLUNTARY MOVEMENTS

A. **Pathoanatomical basis of clinical signs**

1. The individual basal motor nuclei show selective vulnerability to various toxins, medications, viruses, and heredofamilial diseases and to anoxia. The ensuing syndromes of rigidity and involuntary movements differ, depending on the particular nucleus affected (Table 11-2).

2. Most pathogens act bilaterally, causing **bilateral** signs. Unilateral lesions, such as hemorrhages or infarcts, cause **contralateral** signs. Following a unilateral lesion of the basal motor nuclei, the dysmodulation of the ipsilateral thalamus and, in turn, of the ipsilateral motor cortex is expressed by **contralateral** involuntary movement due to the crossing of the pyramidal tract (see Fig. 11-9).

B. **Treatment of involuntary movements**

1. **Medical treatment**
   a. Various medications can substitute for neurotransmitters lacking after destruction of their

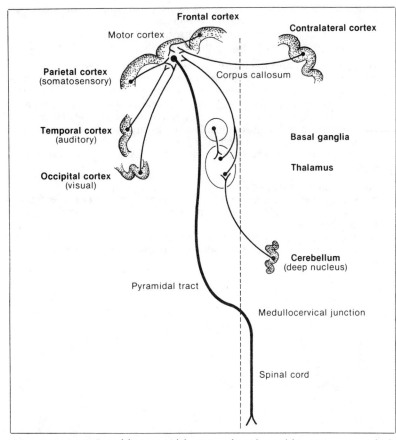

Figure 11-9. Depiction of the pyramidal tract as a funnel out of the motor cortex, which is internuncial for the motor and sensory systems that modulate its activity.

Table 11-2. Clinicopathologic Correlations between Movement Disorders and Lesions of the Basal Motor Nuclei

Movement Disorder	Lesion
Chorea: multiple quick, random movements (the "fidgets"), usually most prominent in the appendicular muscles	Atrophy of the striatum, as in Huntington's chorea
Athetosis: slow writhing movements, usually more severe in the appendicular muscles	Diffuse hypermyelinization (status marmoratus) of the corpus striatum and thalamus, as in cerebral palsy
Dystonia: long sustained twisting movements, predominantly of axial muscles	Various genetic, acquired, or pharmacologic lesions of the basal motor nuclei; however, in classic hereditary dystonia, the lesion site is unclear
Hemiballismus: wild flinging movements of half of the body	Hemorrhagic destruction of the contralateral subthalamic nucleus, most commonly seen in hypertensive patients
Parkinsonism (paralysis agitans): pill-rolling tremor (5–6 cycles per second) of the fingers at rest, lead-pipe rigidity, and akinesia	Degeneration of the substantia nigra
Terminal, **postural**, or **rubral tremor**	Interruption of the dentatothalamic pathway, as in multiple sclerosis

neurons; medications also can block neurotransmission by the neurons in the overactive circuits that drive the abnormal movements.

b. Levodopa (L-dopa), a dopamine precursor, effectively counteracts the loss of the dopaminergic nigrostriatal tract following degeneration of the substantia nigra in parkinsonism.

2. Stereotaxic surgery and the theory of the countervailing lesion

a. If a lesion interrupts one part of the maze of inhibitory and excitatory basal motor circuits, another part may become overactive, resulting in rigidity and involuntary movements. In such cases, a countervailing lesion of the overactive circuit may reduce or eliminate the involuntary movements. That is, one lesion counteracts the effects of the other.

b. Neurosurgeons, using anatomical landmarks on x-ray films and stereotaxic coordinates, can selectively direct a needle into a nucleus or tract designated for destruction, since the positions of these structures are well-known. Dystonia responds best, athetosis least, to stereotaxic surgery.

3. Destruction of the pyramidal tract

a. Neurosurgeons have tried to relieve disabling involuntary movements by partially interrupting the pyramidal tract, either in the motor cortex or by pedunculotomy (sectioning of the cerebral peduncles).

b. Although these operations reduce involuntary movements, the concomitant loss of voluntary movements limits their value to a trade-off between paralysis and movement disorder.

STUDY QUESTIONS

Directions: Each question below contains five suggested answers. Choose the **one best** response to each question.

1. All of the following pathways contribute to the H fields of Forel EXCEPT

(A) the fasciculus lenticularis
(B) the ansa lenticularis
(C) the fornix
(D) the dentatothalamic tract
(E) the medial lemniscus

2. An elderly hypertensive patient experiences the sudden onset of violent, flinging involuntary movements of the left extremities. His lesion most likely involves the

(A) left pontine tegmentum
(B) left caudate nucleus
(C) right subthalamic nucleus
(D) left dentate nucleus
(E) right inferior olivary nucleus

3. A coronal section through the plane of the genu of the internal capsule would almost exactly bisect which structure?

(A) Caudate nucleus
(B) Putamen
(C) Globus pallidus (posture)
(D) Thalamus
(E) Subthalamic nucleus

4. The pallidothalamic axons would be interrupted by transection of each of the following structures EXCEPT

(A) the pyramidal tract
(B) the ansa lenticularis
(C) the fasciculus lenticularis
(D) field H of Forel
(E) field H_2 of Forel

Directions: Each question below contains four suggested answers of which **one or more** is correct. Choose the answer

A if **1, 2, and 3** are correct
B if **1 and 3** are correct
C if **2 and 4** are correct
D if **4** is correct
E if **1, 2, 3, and 4** are correct

5. Major components of the thalamic fasciculus include which of the following?

(1) The medial lemniscus
(2) The dentatothalamic tract
(3) Pallidal efferent fibers
(4) Corticothalamic fibers

6. The term "striatum" includes the

(1) caudate nucleus
(2) claustrum
(3) putamen
(4) globus pallidus

7. The striatum receives significant numbers of afferent fibers from which of the following sources?

(1) Cerebral cortex
(2) Substantia nigra
(3) Nucleus centrum medianum
(4) Subthalamic nucleus

8. Pallidothalamic fibers run in significant numbers to which of the following thalamic nuclei?

(1) Ventralis posterolateralis
(2) Ventralis lateralis
(3) Medialis dorsalis
(4) Ventralis anterior

9. Which of the following nuclei receive well-established efferent axons from the striatum?

(1) Red nucleus
(2) Globus pallidus (Pallidum)
(3) Nucleus pulvinaris of the thalamus
(4) Substantia nigra

10. Correct statements relating the basal motor nuclei to the internal capsule include the

(1) caudate nucleus is medial to the posterior limb
(2) globus pallidus is lateral to the anterior and posterior limbs
(3) subthalamic nucleus is medial to the anterior limb
(4) putamen is lateral to the anterior and posterior limbs

ANSWERS AND EXPLANATIONS

1. The answer is C. *(II A 3)* Numerous pathways run through the laminae of myelinated fibers designated as H fields of Forel. These include afferents to the thalamus from the pallidum, cerebellum, and somatosensory systems. The fornix arches over the thalamus and runs in the hypothalamus, ventral to the H fields of Forel.

2. The answer is C. *(IV A 2; Table 11-2)* Lesions of the various basal motor nuclei tend to cause characteristic syndromes. One such characteristic syndrome, hemiballismus (wild flinging movements of the extremities on one side), results from a lesion of the contralateral subthalamic nucleus. Since the lesion is usually a hemorrhage, the hemiballismus will have an abrupt onset. If the patient later becomes hemiplegic, the movements disappear.

3. The answer is C. *(I B 5 c; Figure 11-1)* A coronal section through the plane of the genu will almost exactly bisect the globus pallidus. The globus pallidus has a triangular shape, with the apex fitting into the genu of the internal capsule.

4. The answer is A. *(II D 3; Figure 11-8)* The globus pallidus provides the efferent pathway from the corpus striatum. The major target is the thalamus. Two pallidal efferent pathways reach the thalamus: the ansa lenticularis, which loops under the internal capsule, and the fasciculus lenticularis, which runs directly across the posterior limb of the internal capsule into field H_2 and then recurves through fields H and H_1.

5. The answer is A (1, 2, 3). *[II A 3 b (1)]* Field H_1 of Forel, also known as the thalamic fasciculus, is a composite tract consisting mainly of fibers from the medial lemniscus, the dentatothalamic tract, and the pallidothalamic tracts. The ansa lenticularis from the pallidum loops under the internal capsule to enter fields H and H_1, and the fasciculus lenticularis cuts through the capsule to enter field H_2 and to curve dorsally through field H and then laterally through field H_1 to disperse to the ventral–anterior region of the thalamus.

6. The answer is B (1, 3). *(I D 1; Figure 11-4)* Unfortunately, the basal ganglia are overladen with redundant terminology. The term "striatum" refers to the caudate nucleus and putamen together. "Lentiform nucleus" refers to the putamen and the globus pallidus. The term "corpus striatum" includes all three masses—the caudate nucleus, the putamen, and the globus pallidus. The striate appearance of the region is caused by the interdigitations of the fascicles of myelinated fibers of the internal capsule that run through the crevice between the caudate nucleus and putamen.

7. The answer is A (1, 2, 3). *(II C 2 a, b, c)* The striatum, which is a huge nuclear mass, receives significant numbers of afferents from the cerebral cortex and from the nucleus centrum medianum of the diencephalon. Its best-known afferent pathway comes from the substantia nigra. The subthalamic nucleus has strong to-and-fro connections with the globus pallidus, but few if any demonstrated connections with the striatum.

8. The answer is C (2, 4). *(II D 3 a; Table 11-1)* The pallidothalamic fibers mainly terminate in nuclei ventralis lateralis and ventralis anterior. These nuclei relay to the cerebral motor cortex, which in turn sends efferents to the caudate nucleus. These connections link the cortex and basal ganglia into feedback circuits.

9. The answer is C (2, 4). *(II C 3)* The striatum sends numerous efferents to the pallidum and substantia nigra. The pallidum reconnects with the striatum indirectly through the thalamus and cerebral cortex, while the substantia nigra connects directly via a nigrostriatal dopaminergic pathway. Interruption of the latter causes parkinsonism, characterized by tremor at rest and rigidity.

10. The answer is C (2, 4). *(I B)* The internal capsule sharply demarcates some of the basal motor nuclei. The caudate nucleus and thalamus are medial to the anterior and posterior limbs, respectively. The globus pallidus is lateral to the genu and the anterior and posterior limbs. The putamen is lateral to the pallidum and hence to both the anterior and posterior limbs.

I. EMBRYOLOGY OF THE DIENCEPHALON AND BASAL GANGLIA

A. Diencephalic development is characterized by:

1. Evagination of the pineal body, neurohypophysis, and optic bulbs (see Fig. 3-5)

2. Retention of the diencephalic cavity as the third ventricle, with a membranous roof (Fig. 12-1)

3. Elaboration of four longitudinal nuclear zones in the diencephalic wall on each side

B. Nuclear zones of the diencephalon

1. Masses of neuroblasts proliferate in the periventricular matrix zone and condense into **four longitudinal zones** of nuclei (Table 12-1; see Fig. 12-1).

2. The subthalamic nucleus and globus pallidus both arise from the hypothalamus (see Table 12-1). Their common origin may explain their similar fiber connections and similar susceptibilities to pathogens. For example, in kernicterus, bilirubin leaks through the blood–brain barrier and stains these nuclei yellow. The neuronal damage may account for the ballistic or choreiform hyperkinesias that ensue.

3. The caudate nucleus and putamen arise from the ganglionic hillock of the telencephalon (see Fig. 3-10). The amygdala and the claustrum of the four original basal ganglia also arise from the telencephalon.

II. THALAMUS DORSALIS

A. Gross anatomy

1. Definition. The thalamus is an egg-shaped, small egg-sized mass of diencephalic neurons arranged into nuclei. It develops on each side as the second and by far the largest of the four longitudinal nuclear zones of the diencephalic wall (see Fig. 12-1).

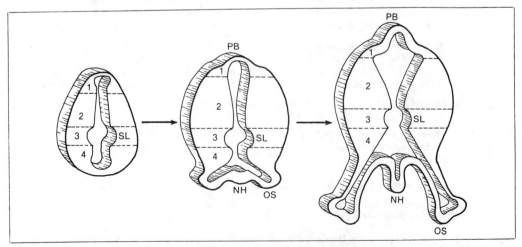

Figure 12-1. Cross section of the diencephalic part of the neural tube, showing four nuclear zones on each side: *1* = epithalamus; *2* = thalamus dorsalis; *3* = thalamus ventralis; *4* = hypothalamus. *NH* = neurohypophysis; *OS* = optic stalk; *PB* = pineal body; *SL* = sulcus limitans (hypothalamic sulcus), in the wall of the third ventricle.

Table 12-1. Embryonic and Adult Derivatives of the Diencephalon

Embryonic Subdivision (Dorsal-to-Ventral Order)	Adult Derivative
Epithalamus	Habenular nuclei and commissure and the stria medullaris and taenia tectae, which suspend the membranous roof of the third ventricle, and an evagination, which forms the pineal body
Thalamus dorsalis	Large nuclear bulk known as the "thalamus" and the metathalamus, consisting of the medial and lateral geniculate bodies
Thalamus ventralis	Zona incerta and nucleus reticularis thalami
Hypothalamus	Evaginations: neurohypophysis and optic bulbs, nerves, and chiasm
	Dorsal nuclear group: globus pallidus, subthalamic nucleus, interstitial nuclei of the inferior thalamic peduncle, and entopeduncular nucleus
	Ventral nuclear group: nuclei of the hypothalamus proper

2. Location

    a. Each thalamus is **medial** to the posterior limb of the internal capsule. (Observe this fact in the horizontal section in Figure 11-2 and in the coronal section in Figure 12-2.)

    b. The two thalami form the lateral walls of the third ventricle, superior to the hypothalamic sulcus (see Fig. 12-2).

B. Boundaries of the thalamus. Each thalamus has **rostral** and **caudal poles** and **dorsal, ventral, medial,** and **lateral surfaces**.

    1. Rostral and caudal thalamic poles

        a. The **rostral** pole commences just behind the plane of the foramen of Monro and the genu of the internal capsule (see Fig. 11-2).

        b. The **caudal** pole—the **pulvinar** ("cushioned seat")—overhangs the geniculate bodies and superior colliculi (Fig. 12-3).

    2. Dorsal boundary of the thalamus

        a. Dorsolaterally, the thalamus borders on the body and tail of the caudate nucleus and on the vena and stria terminalis (see Fig. 12-2).

        b. Dorsomedially, the thalamus forms the floor of the body of the anterior horn of the lateral ventricle. The tela choroidea covers the dorsomedial aspect of the thalamus and bridges the lumen of the third ventricle as its roof. The tela choroidea consists of an inner lining of ependyma and an outer layer of pia, enclosing blood vessels of the choroid plexus.

    3. Medial boundary of the thalamus

        a. Medially, the lumen of the third ventricle bounds the thalamus.

        b. A nuclear mass, the **massa intermedia**, may connect the two thalami across the lumen of the third ventricle (see Fig. 12-2). It is inconstant in size and is sometimes missing.

    4. Ventral boundary of the thalamus. Ventrally, the thalamic fasciculus (field H_1) separates the thalamus from the zona incerta of the subthalamus.

    5. Lateral boundary of the thalamus. Laterally, an extension of the zone incerta, called the **nucleus reticularis thalami**, separates the thalamus proper from the posterior limb of the internal capsule.

C. Capsules and laminae of myelinated axons that delineate the thalamus and some of its nuclei

    1. The medial thalamic wall, bordering on the third ventricle, consists of a myelin-free zone of **midline thalamic nuclei** (see Fig. 12-2).

    2. Then, on the dorsal border of the myelin-free zone, a continuous myelinated capsule commences with the **stria terminalis**. The myelinated capsule extends **laterally**, **ventrally**, and

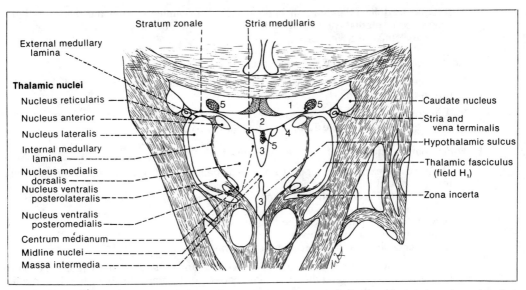

Figure 12-2. Myelin-stained coronal section of the thalamus and surrounding structures. *1* = Lateral ventricle; *2* = cavum veli interpositi; *3* = third ventricle; *4* = tela choroidea; *5* = choroid plexus.

medially, surrounding the thalamus in the shape of a C. In sequence, it consists of the following regions (see Fig. 12-2).

  a. The **stria medullaris**, a tiny bundle of axons, extends longitudinally along the dorsomedial margin of the thalamus.

  b. The **stratum zonale**, a thin myelinated sheet, extends over the dorsum of the thalamus as far as the caudate nucleus.

  c. The **stria** and **vena terminalis** overlie the lateral extent of the stratum zonale.

  d. The **external medullary lamina**, a thin myelinated sheet, extends lateroventrally from the stratum zonale to the thalamic fasciculus.

  e. The **thalamic fasciculus** extends ventromedially from the external medullary lamina. It ends at the midline thalamic nuclei in the plane of the hypothalamic sulcus.

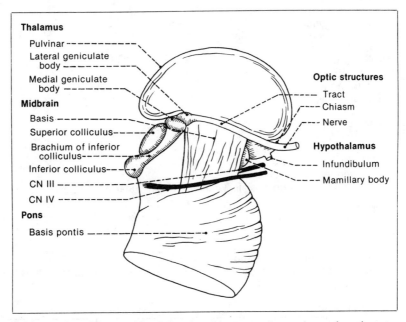

Figure 12-3. Lateral view of the thalamus and brainstem dissected away from the cerebrum.

3. Internal medullary lamina. An internal medullary lamina cleaves the thalamus into two roughly equal **medial** and **lateral** nuclear groups. It splits dorsally around the anterior nucleus of the thalamus (see Fig. 12-2).

D. Anatomical classification of thalamic nuclei

1. The internal medullary lamina separates the thalamic nuclei into obvious **medial**, **lateral**, and **dorsal** nuclear groups.

2. Anterior and posterior nuclear groups occupy the anterior and posterior poles of the thalamus, respectively. (Relate Table 12-2 to Figure 12-4C and *D*.)

E. Functional classification of the thalamic nuclei

1. Thalamic nuclei censor or modulate almost all neural activity into and out of the cerebral cortex. The **nuclei receive and relay**:
    a. The **great afferent pathways** (lemnisci and optic tract) from the sensory receptors (olfaction excepted)
    b. Somatomotor pathways of the basal motor nuclei
    c. Reticular formation pathways
    d. Rhinencephalic and limbic system pathways

2. By means of to-and-fro (reciprocal) thalamocortical and corticothalamic circuits, the thalamus influences the cortex and the cortex influences the thalamus. In short, the thalamic nuclei mediate the functions dictated by their subcortical and cortical connections. The five functional nuclear groups are:
    a. Sensory relay nuclei
    b. Motor relay nuclei
    c. Ascending reticular activating system relay nuclei

Table 12-2. Topographic Grouping of Thalamic Nuclei*

Anterior group
    N. anterior dorsalis
    N. anterior ventralis (largest component)
    N. anterior medialis

Posterior group
    N. pulvinaris
    N. corpus geniculati lateralis
    N. corpus geniculati medialis

Medial group
    N. medialis (n. medialis dorsalis, n. dorsomedialis)
    Centrum medianum (n. medialis centralis; center median Luysi)
    N. parafascicularis

Lateral group
    N. ventralis
        N. ventralis anterior
        N. ventralis lateralis
        N. ventralis posterolateralis
        N. ventralis posteromedialis (arcuate, or semilunar n.)

    N. lateralis
        N. lateralis dorsalis
        N. lateralis posterior

Intralaminar group and midline group
    Centrum medianum may be included here and, arguably, n. reticularis thalami

Pretectal group

N. and n. = nucleus.
*Partial listing.

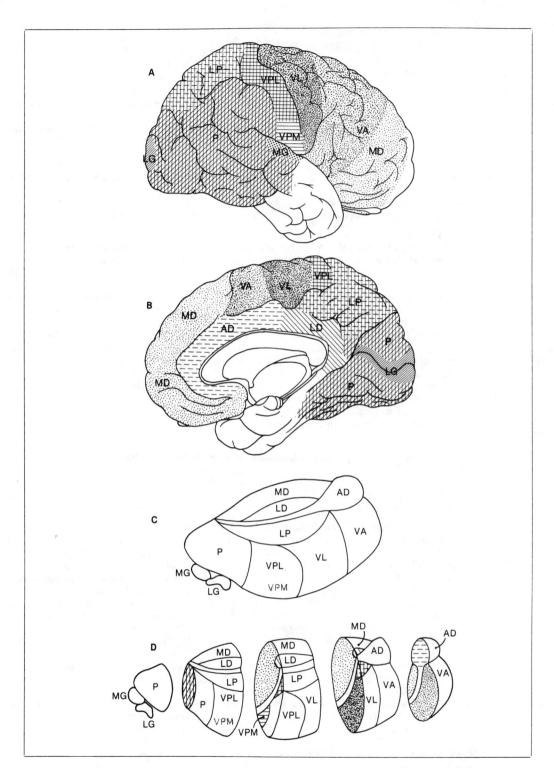

Figure 12-4. Pattern of projection of the thalamic nuclei to the cerebral cortex. (A) Lateral view of the right cerebral hemisphere showing the cortical areas to which the thalamic nuclei project. (B) Medial view of the right cerebral hemisphere showing the cortical areas to which the thalamic nuclei project. (C) Lateral view of the right thalamus. (D) Exploded view of the right thalamus. AD = nucleus anterior dorsalis; LD = nucleus lateralis dorsalis; LG = lateral geniculate body; LP = nucleus lateralis posterior; MD = nucleus medialis dorsalis; MG = medial geniculate body; P = nucleus pulvinaris; VA = nucleus ventralis anterior; VL = nucleus ventralis lateralis; VPL = nucleus ventralis posterolateralis; VPM = nucleus ventralis posteromedialis.

      d. Limbic system relay nuclei

      e. Association (ectocortical) relay nuclei

F. Overview of thalamic connections (see Fig. 12-4)

  1. Ventral (ventrolateral) tier of thalamic nuclei. Nuclei of the ventrolateral underbelly of the thalamus relay **somatomotor, general somatosensory,** and **special somatosensory pathways** in an orderly anterior-to-posterior sequence.

    a. Nucleus ventralis anterior and **nucleus ventralis lateralis** receive somatomotor pathways from the basal motor nuclei and cerebellum. These nuclei project to the cerebral motor cortex and receive reciprocal connections from it.

    b. Nucleus ventralis posterior receives the general somatic afferent (GSA) pathways via lemnisci and forms reciprocal connections with the somatosensory cortex of the postcentral gyrus.

    c. The **medial** and **lateral geniculate bodies** receive the auditory and visual pathways and project to the transverse temporal gyri and calcarine cortex, respectively.

  2. Dorsal tier of thalamic nuclei

    a. Anteriorly, nucleus anterior caps **nucleus anterior ventralis.** It receives afferents via the mamillothalamic tract from the mamillary body of the hypothalamus, which in turn receives the fornix from the hippocampus. Nucleus anterior has reciprocal connections with the part of the cingulate gyrus overlying it.

    b. Nucleus lateralis dorsalis, just behind nucleus anterior, receives connections from the amygdala and fornix. It has reciprocal connections with the part of the cingulate gyrus overlying it.

    c. Nucleus lateralis posterior and **nucleus pulvinaris** cover the ventral tier of thalamic nuclei, including the geniculate bodies posteriorly. They belong to the association nuclei. Infracortical afferents to these nuclei are not as well understood as are those to the ventral tier. Some are thalamic in origin.

      (1) Nucleus lateralis posterior forms reciprocal connections with the parietal lobe behind the somatosensory receptive cortex.

      (2) Nucleus pulvinaris forms reciprocal connections with the remaining cortex of the parietal lobe and with the occipital and temporal lobes.

  3. Medial group

    a. Nucleus medialis forms most of the thalamic bulk medial to the internal medullary lamina.

    b. It receives subcortical afferents from basal olfactory structures, the hypothalamus, periventricular fiber systems, the striatum, and the cerebellum.

    c. It forms reciprocal circuits with the general cortex of the frontal lobe anterior to the motor region and with the orbitoinsular limbic cortex.

  4. Midline and intralaminar nuclei and nucleus reticularis thalami

    a. The **midline nuclei** are diffuse groups in the periventricular region resembling reticular formation. These periventricular nuclei belong to the visceral control system consisting of the periaqueductal gray matter, the hypothalamus, and basal rhinencephalic structures.

    b. The **intralaminar nuclei** occupy a split in the internal medullary lamina. The largest, **centrum medianum,** is thought to connect with the striatum and other basal motor nuclei.

    c. Physiologic evidence indicates that the **ascending reticular activating system** connects diffusely with the cerebral cortex through the foregoing and perhaps other thalamic nuclei. The exact synaptic connections have been notably difficult to define.

      (1) These connections mediate the sleep–wake cycle, the alerting responses, and consciousness in general.

      (2) This diffusely acting system is called nonspecific to contrast it with the very discrete, highly organized, and specific connections mediated through the lemniscal and optic pathways.

    d. Nucleus reticularis thalami is a wafer of neurons continuing upward between the external medullary lamina and the internal capsule from the zona incerta. Its axons point toward the thalamus, but its function is unknown.

G. Mnemonic exercise for the cortical projection zones of the thalamic nuclei

  1. In general, the thalamic nuclei connect with the cortex that is most convenient to them and that mirrors the location of the nucleus in the thalamus.

  2. Start with **nucleus medialis dorsalis** as the cornerstone of the mnemonic exercise. The nucleus projects to the frontal lobe anterior to the motor strip of the precentral gyrus (see Fig. 12-4). Its zone extends around to the orbital and medial surfaces (see Fig. 12-4).

3. Consider next the **lateral nuclear group, ventral tier**.

    a. Nuclei ventralis anterior and **lateralis** project to the overlying motor area of the precentral gyrus.

    b. Nucleus ventralis posterior projects to the overlying sensory receptive cortex of the postcentral gyrus.

4. Consider next the **dorsal tier of thalamic nuclei**.

    a. Nucleus anterior projects conveniently to the part of the cingulate gyrus just above and medial to it.

    b. Nucleus lateralis dorsalis, which is just posterior to nucleus anterior, projects to the cingulate gyrus just posterior to the zone of nucleus anterior.

    c. Nucleus lateralis posterior projects to the parietal lobe immediately overlying it, posterior to the postcentral gyrus.

    d. Nucleus pulvinaris projects to the shell of parietal, occipital, and temporal cortex that surrounds or mirrors it.

5. Finally, recall the projection of the **medial** and **lateral geniculate bodies** to their respective temporal and occipital cortices.

6. It is debatable whether the frontal and temporal poles receive thalamic connections.

H. Anatomical types of pathways to and from the thalamus

1. The grossly visible, named pathways are arranged into bundles, laminae or capsules, and thalamic peduncles (Table 12-3).

2. The **bundles** consist of **lemnisci, fasciculi, tracts, striae**, and the **fornix**. These bundles mostly connect the thalamus with subcortical structures.

3. The **laminae** or **capsules** convey fibers directly entering from the other sources or exiting from the thalamus.

4. The thalamic **peduncles** or **radiations** mostly convey axons that fan out to or converge down from various parts of the cerebral cortex. These axons pass through the various parts of the internal capsule and the cerebral white matter.

I. Sensory pathways to the thalamus

1. The thalamus receives all lemnisci: spinal, trigeminal, medial, and lateral. It also receives the optic lemniscus, if we choose to call the optic tract a lemniscus (see Table 12-3).

2. Each lemniscus ends in a specific thalamic sensory relay nucleus. That thalamic nucleus has

Table 12-3. Named Pathways to and from the Thalamus

Bundles	Laminae or capsules
Lemnisci	Internal medullary lamina
Spinal	External medullary lamina
Medial	Stratum zonale
Lateral	Internal capsule
Trigeminal	
Fasciculi and ansae	**Peduncles or radiations**
Lenticular fasciculus	Anterior (frontal)
Thalamic fasciculus	Superior (centroparietal)
Ansa peduncularis	Posterior (occipital and optic)
Temporothalamic fascicle of Arnold	Inferior (temporal)
Tracts	
Dentatothalamic tract	
Mamillothalamic tract	
Optic tract	
Geniculocalcarine tract	
Striae	
Stria medullaris	
Stria terminalis	
Fornix	

Table 12-4. Pathways through Various Parts of the Internal Capsule

Subdivision of the Internal Capsule	Pathway

Anterior limb
  Lenticulocaudate part of
  the internal capsule
	Anterior thalamic peduncle
	Frontopontine tract
	Corticostriatal projections

Genu	Anterior part of superior (centroparietal thalamic) peduncle Corticobulbar tract and frontal eye field projections, according to dogma

Posterior limb
  Lenticulothalamic part
  (posterior limb per se)
	Posterior part of superior thalamic peduncle
	Corticospinal tract
	Corticostriatal, corticorubral, and corticoreticular projections
	Parietopontine tract

Sublenticular part	Inferior thalamic peduncle
	  Temporothalamic radiations
	  Auditory radiations
	  Origin of optic radiations (geniculocalcarine tract)
	  Ansa peduncularis

Retrolenticular part	Posterior thalamic peduncle Occipitopretectal and occipitotegmental tracts Temporopontine tract

the same topographic organization as its afferent lemniscus. The thalamic projection then preserves that topography through to the cortex.

3. A thalamocortical relay apparently is necessary for full conscious appreciation of sensation.

4. Of the senses, only the olfactory sense has no direct, known lemniscal pathway unless the medial forebrain bundle is an analog.

5. The vestibular system a priori ought to have a lemniscus, but its route and connections are uncertain.

J. Motor pathways to the thalamus

1. The thalamic somatomotor nuclei are nucleus ventralis anterior, nucleus ventralis lateralis, and centrum medianum.

2. Major somatomotor afferent pathways arrive from the cerebral motor cortex, reticular formation, the dentatothalamic tract, and the ansa and fasciculus lenticularis.

K. Limbic pathways to the thalamus come from the limbic cortex, periventricular system, hypothalamus (especially the mamillothalamic tract), fornix, and striae.

L. Internal capsule and thalamic peduncles

1. The internal capsule requires visualization in **vertical** and **horizontal** sections. (Compare Figures 12-5 and 11-2.)

2. The bulk of the fibers in the internal capsule belong to two systems:
   a. Cortical efferent fibers, mostly motor, which go to the brainstem and spinal cord
   b. Thalamic peduncles, whose fibers convey the thalamocortical/corticothalamic circuits

3. The fiber systems of the internal capsule tend to converge into its **longitudinal** (superior–inferior) axis (see Fig. 12-5) or to cut across it **transversely** (see Fig. 12-6).
   a. The mainly longitudinal fibers, that is, those radiating to or from the cerebral cortex, consist of:
   (1) Corticobulbar and corticospinal fibers
   (2) Corticopontine fibers
   (3) The majority of the corticothalamic/thalamocortical fibers

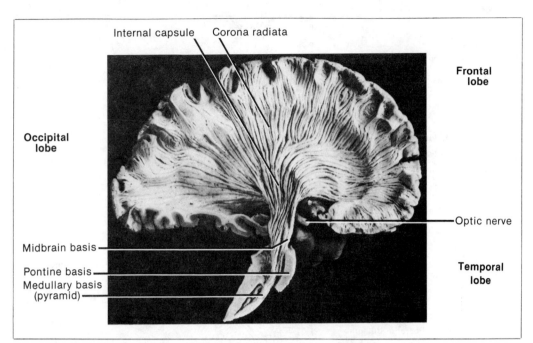

Internal capsule   Corona radiata

Frontal
lobe

Occipital
lobe

Optic nerve

Midbrain basis

Temporal
lobe

Pontine basis
Medullary basis
(pyramid)

Figure 12-5. Gross photograph of the medial aspect of the left cerebral hemisphere dissected to show the fiber bundles of the thalamic peduncles, corona radiata, internal capsule, and basis of the brainstem. (Reprinted with permission from Gluhbegovic N, Williams TH: *The Human Brain: A Photographic Guide*. Philadelphia, Harper and Row, 1980, p 123.)

    b. The bundles that mainly run transversely across the internal capsule consist of:
        (1) A minority of the corticothalamic/thalamocortical connections; however, these do include the auditory and optic radiations
        (2) Fasciculus lenticularis
        (3) Subthalamic fasciculus
        (4) Connections with the claustrum and insular cortex
    c. Table 12-4 summarizes the components of the internal capsule (relate it to Figure 12-6).

4. Location of corticobulbar and corticospinal fibers (pyramidal tract) within the internal capsule
    a. As the pyramidal tract descends through the internal capsule, the fibers migrate toward the back part of the posterior limb before entering the midbrain basis (Fig. 12-7).
    b. Older texts erroneously show the fibers more anteriorly in the posterior limb, near the genu. This anterior position holds only for the superior part of the capsule.
    c. Because of the restricted location of the pyramidal tract in the internal capsule, a small infarct can cause a pure contralateral hemiplegia, sparing the sensory radiations entering from the thalamus.

M. Thalamic peduncles (thalamic radiations). The fibers connecting the thalamus and cerebral cortex present a continuous, fan-like arrangement as they radiate out from or return to the thalamus (Fig. 12-8 and Table 12-5; see Fig. 12-5).

N. External and extreme capsules

    1. These two thin laminae of white matter form a sandwich, with the external capsule medial, the claustrum (a lamina of neurons) in the middle, and the extreme capsule lateral. The insula is lateral to the extreme capsule (see Fig. 11-2).

    2. They convey axons from the longitudinal fasciculi of the cerebrum and the cingulum, connecting the insular cortex and the rest of the cerebrum.

    3. Transversely crossing axons interconnect the thalamus and basal ganglia with the claustrum and insula.

    4. No known clinical syndrome results from lesions of the external and extreme capsules and the claustrum.

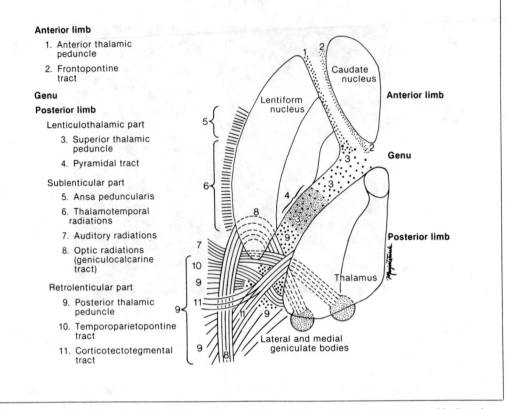

Anterior limb

  1. Anterior thalamic peduncle

  2. Frontopontine tract

Genu

Posterior limb

  Lenticulothalamic part

    3. Superior thalamic peduncle

    4. Pyramidal tract

  Sublenticular part

    5. Ansa peduncularis

    6. Thalamotemporal radiations

    7. Auditory radiations

    8. Optic radiations (geniculocalcarine tract)

  Retrolenticular part

    9. Posterior thalamic peduncle

    10. Temporoparietopontine tract

    11. Corticotectotegmental tract

Figure 12-6. Horizontal section of the right internal capsule (cut at right angles to its vertical axis and looking down on its cut surface) [See Fig. 11-2]. *Dots* represent pathways that run in the vertical axis of the capsule or that run radially (see Fig. 12-8). *Lines*, solid or interrupted, represent pathways that run transversely across the vertical axis of the capsule. (Adapted from Crosby E, Humphrey T, Lauer E: *Correlative Anatomy of the Nervous System.* New York, Macmillan, 1962.).

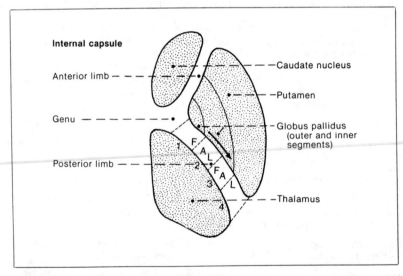

Figure 12-7. Horizontal section of the internal capsule. At superior levels, the face (*F*), arm (*A*), and leg (*L*) fibers of the pyramidal tract are located anteriorly, in sections *1* and *2* of the posterior limb; while at inferior levels, before the fibers enter the midbrain, they have migrated posteriorly to sections *3* and *4*.

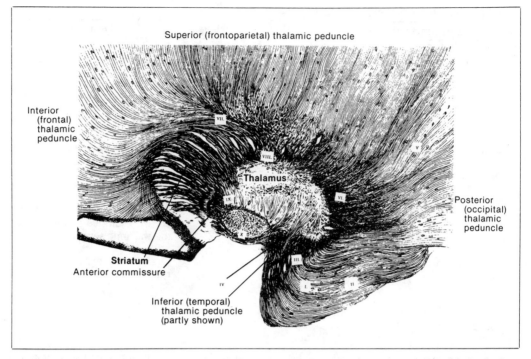

Superior (frontoparietal) thalamic peduncle

Interior
(frontal)
thalamic
peduncle

Thalamus

Posterior
(occipital)
thalamic
peduncle

Striatum
Anterior commissure

Inferior (temporal)
thalamic peduncle
(partly shown)

Figure 12-8. Drawing of a parasagittal section of a cerebral hemisphere demonstrating the fan of fibers that radiate to and from the thalamus. A continuous arc of 300 degrees, the fan is more or less arbitrarily divided into peduncles. *I, II,* and *III* = geniculocalcarine tract of the occipital peduncle (see Fig. 10-11); *IV* = transversely cut auditory radiation of the inferior peduncle; *V* and *VI* = superior part of the occipital peduncle; *VII* = subcallosal fasciculus of the frontal peduncle; *VIII* = fibers of the stria terminalis; *IX* and *X* = fibers approaching and surrounding the subthalamic nucleus. (Reprinted with permission from Rosett J: A study of the cerebral fibre systems by means of a new modification of anatomical methods. The lateral wall of the thalamus and the sagittal portion of its cerebral fibre system. *Brain* 45:357–384, 1922. Labels have been added; Roman numerals are original author's.)

O. Clinical syndromes resulting from lesions of the thalamus dorsalis

1. Since the functions of the thalamus reflect the functions of the entire cerebrum, thalamic lesions may impair any of the three great categories of cerebral function: mental, motor, and sensory.

2. Unilateral thalamic lesions

a. The functions of the left thalamus reflect the functions of the left cerebral hemisphere. Lesions of the left thalamus tend to cause deficits in language production, syntax, word production, prosody, voice volume, and interpretation and expression of words as symbols for communication, a condition known as **thalamic aphasia.**

b. The functions of the right thalamus reflect the functions of the right cerebral hemisphere. Lesions of the right thalamus cause difficulties with spatial relationships. The patient neglects tactile, visual, and auditory stimuli from the left half of space and gets lost in going from one place to another. Language functions and mentation are preserved.

c. A unilateral lesion of nucleus ventralis posterior causes contralateral loss of sensation. Since the lesion is usually an infarct, the condition is called "pure thalamic sensory stroke."

   (1) Sometimes, along with the loss of sensation, the patient also experiences intense pain in the affected extremities, the classic thalamic syndrome of anesthesia dolorosa known as the Dejerine-Roussy syndrome.

   (2) Because the lateroventral region of the thalamus shares its blood supply with the internal capsule, the patient with thalamic sensory stroke may also have mild or transient hemiparesis.

d. Lesions of the lateral geniculate body cause contralateral homonymous hemianopia, which may also accompany thalamic sensory stroke or capsular infarction.

e. Interruption of the thalamic connections with basal motor nuclei may lead to some types of tremor or other involuntary movements of choreiform or athetoid type.

Table 12-5. Thalamic Peduncles (Radiations)*

Thalamic Peduncle and Course	Thalamic Nucleus	Destination
Anterior thalamic peduncle (through anterior limb of the internal capsule)	N. medialis dorsalis	Frontal granular cortex (prefrontal cortex rostral to motor area)
	N. anterior	Anterior part of cingulate gyrus
	N. ventralis anterior and lateralis	Area 6 (all fibers from n. ventralis are sometimes grouped with superior peduncle) Area 4
Superior (centroparietal) peduncle (through genu and posterior limb per se of the internal capsule)	N. ventralis posterolateralis	Body and extremity area of postcentral gyrus
	N. ventralis posteromedialis	Face area of somesthetic cortex
	N. pulvinaris	Parietal, occipital, and temporal cortex, exclusive of areas served by the thalamic sensory relay nuclei
Posterior peduncle (through retrolenticular part of the internal capsule)	N. pulvinaris	Occipital cortex, exclusive of calcarine cortex
Inferior thalamic peduncle (through sublenticular part of the internal capsule)		
Anterior component (ansa peduncularis)	Rostromedial thalamic nuclei (exact origin unsettled)	Medial-basal part of temporal lobe: amygdala, piriform lobe, and orbital surface of frontal lobe
Posterior component	Medial geniculate body body	Transverse temporal gyri (auditory receptive area)
	Lateral geniculate body (geniculatocalcarine tract)	Calcarine cortex of occipital lobe (Area 17, visual receptive area)

N. and n. = nucleus.
*Most of the connections are thalamocortical/corticothalamic circuits.

3. **Bilateral thalamic lesions** impair consciousness and higher mental functions.
   a. The patient becomes demented, amnestic and emotionally labile and loses orientation to person, time, and place.
   b. The patient may display various degrees of hypokinesia, mutism, or permanent loss of consciousness.
   c. Bilateral destruction of the nucleus medialis, of its frontal connections through the anterior thalamic peduncle, or of the frontal cortex anterior to the motor region results in a loss of drive and initiative and a general indifference to stimuli. For this reason, neurosurgeons may transect the anterior thalamic peduncle (prefrontal leukotomy or lobotomy) in moribund cancer patients to reduce their reaction to pain.

III. HYPOTHALAMUS AND PITUITARY BODY

A. **Gross anatomy of the hypothalamus**

1. **Definition.** The hypothalamus is the most ventral of the four longitudinal nuclear zones of the diencephalon (see Fig. 12-1). It comprises the floor and that portion of the wall of the third ventricle ventral to the hypothalamic sulcus (see Fig. 12-1).

2. **Functional significance.** Although weighing only a few grams, the hypothalamus is essential to life because it controls the viscera, endocrine system, and homeostasis in general (fluid balance, body temperature, and so forth). Its limbic lobe connections involve it in the experience of emotion and in the control of instinctive behaviors such as mating, feeding, and fright/flight responses.

3. **Visualization** of the hypothalamus requires:
   a. A **ventral view** of the base of the brain to see its external aspect
   b. **Sagittal section** through the lumen of the third ventricle to see its medial aspect
   c. **Coronal sections** to see its transverse extent

4. **Ventral aspect of the hypothalamus.** Locate the following (Fig. 12-9):
   a. Optic chiasm and tract
   b. Infundibular stalk (neurohypophysis cutoff)
   c. Median and lateral eminences (the tuber cinereum or tuberal region)
   d. Mamillary bodies (the postmamillary sulcus separates the hypothalamus from the midbrain basis)

5. **Medial aspect of the hypothalamus** (Fig. 12-10)
   a. The **rostral** boundary of the hypothalamus is the junction of the lamina terminalis with the anterior commissure of the telencephalon.
   b. Trace the hypothalamus ventrally and caudally in Figure 12-10 from the lamina terminalis through the optic chiasm, median eminence, and mamillary body region to its midbrain junction.
   c. The **dorsal** boundary of the hypothalamus is the hypothalamic sulcus, running longitudinally in the wall of the third ventricle.
   d. The **caudal** boundary of the hypothalamus is the plane of a line drawn from the posterior edge of the mamillary body to the lip of the posterior commissure.

6. **Lateral boundary of the hypothalamus in transverse section** (Fig. 12-11)
   a. **Rostrally**, the hypothalamus is bounded laterally by the:
      (1) Ventromedial edge of the internal capsule
      (2) Medial tip of the globus pallidus and the ansa lenticularis
      (3) Substantia innominata of the anterior perforated substance and diagonal band, which are part of the telencephalon (see Fig. 12-9)
   b. **Caudally**, the lateral hypothalamic area continues to follow roughly the ventromedial edge of the internal capsule as it descends into the midbrain basis.

7. Giving the hypothalamus a name and formal boundaries may obscure a more important fact—its anatomical and functional continuity. It is an upward continuation of the periaqueductal gray matter and reticular formation and continues rostrally into rhinencephalic structures, namely the anterior perforated substance, substantia innominata (just ventral to the caudate nucleus), and septal region.

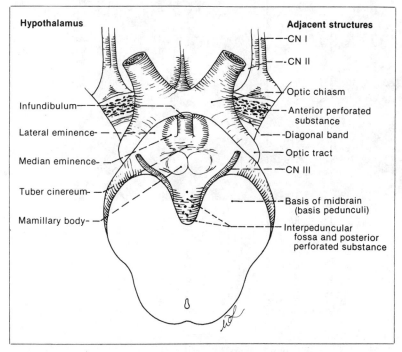

Figure 12-9. Gross anatomy of the ventral surface of the hypothalamus.

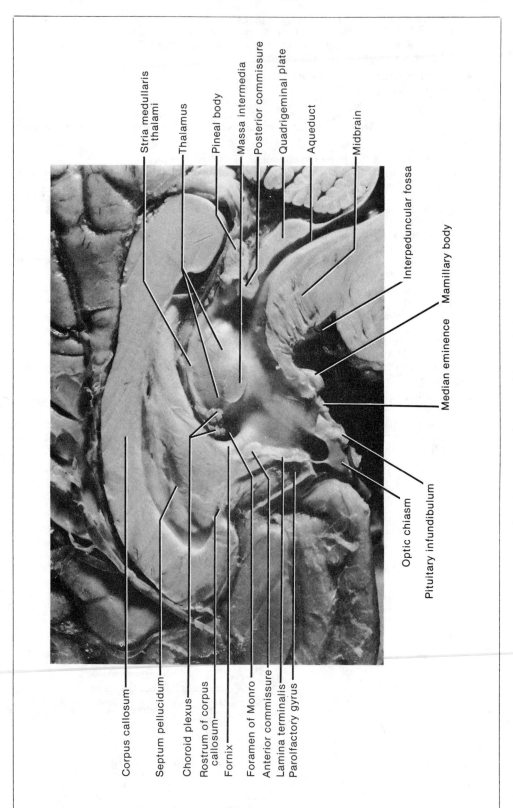

Figure 12-10. Saggital section of the cerebrum.

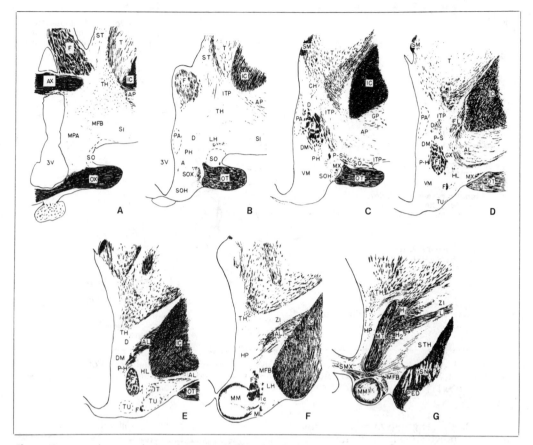

Figure 12-11. Myelin-stained atlas of coronal sections of the hypothalamus, anterior to posterior levels (A)–(G). A = anterior hypothalamic area; AL = ansa lenticularis; AP = ansa peduncularis; AX = anterior commissure; CH = corticohabenular fibers; D = dorsal hypothalamic area; DM = dorsomedial hypothalamic nucleus; F = fornix; FL = fasciculus lenticularis; GP = globus pallidus; GX = dorsal supraoptic commissure, pars dorsalis; H_1, H_2 = fields of Forel; HL and LH = lateral hypothalamic area; HP = posterior hypothalamic area; IC = internal capsule; Ic = nucleus intercalatus; IT = fibers of nucleus tuberalis; ITP = inferior thalamic peduncle; MFB = medial forebrain bundle; ML = lateral mamillary nucleus; MM = medial mamillary nucleus; MPA = medial preoptic area; MT = mamillothalamic tract; MX = dorsal supraoptic commissure, pars ventralis; OT = optic tract; OX = optic chiasm; PA = paraventricular nucleus; PED = cerebral peduncle; PH = paraventriculohypophyseal fibers; P-H = pallidohypothalamic fibers; P-S = paraventriculosupraoptic fibers; PV = periventricular system; SI = substantia innominata; SM = stria medullaris; SMX = supramamillary commissure; SN = substantia nigra; SO = supraoptic nucleus; SOH = supraopticohypophyseal tract; SOX = supraoptic commissures; ST = stria terminalis; STH = subthalamic nucleus; T = thalamus; TH = thalamohypothalamic fibers; TU = nucleus tuberis laterale; VM = ventromedial hypothalamic nucleus; ZI = zona incerta; 3V = third ventricle. (Reprinted with permission from Raven Press, NY. Originally from Ingram WR: Nuclear organization and chief connections of the primate hypothalamus. In *Proceedings of the Association for Research in Nervous and Mental Disease*, 1939.)

B. Nuclei and regions of the hypothalamus

    1. The hypothalamus displays some well-delineated nuclei and others with obscure boundaries, referred to as groups or areas (Fig. 12-12). Table 12-6 lists the nuclei; only a few will be discussed.

    2. Anterior group of hypothalamic nuclei
        a. The **preoptic area** is at the junction of the hypothalamus and the telencephalon.
        b. The **paraventricular** and **supraoptic** nuclei have fairly large neurons, which are sharply grouped (see Fig. 12-11B and C).
            (1) The **paraventricular nucleus** forms a plate of neurons along the wall of the third ventricle.
            (2) The **supraoptic nucleus** drapes over the optic tract.

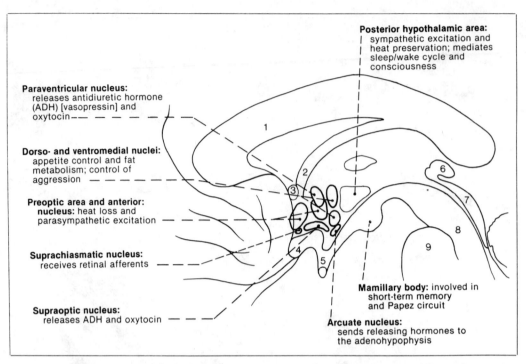

Posterior hypothalamic area: sympathetic excitation and heat preservation; mediates sleep/wake cycle and consciousness

Paraventricular nucleus: releases antidiuretic hormone (ADH) [vasopressin] and oxytocin

Dorso- and ventromedial nuclei: appetite control and fat metabolism; control of aggression

Preoptic area and anterior: nucleus: heat loss and parasympathetic excitation

Suprachiasmatic nucleus: receives retinal afferents

Supraoptic nucleus: releases ADH and oxytocin

Mamillary body: involved in short-term memory and Papez circuit

Arcuate nucleus: sends releasing hormones to the adenohypophysis

Figure 12-12. Nuclear regions of the hypothalamus as superimposed on a sagittal section of the cerebrum (compare with Fig. 12-10). *1* = Corpus callosum; *2* = fornix; *3* = anterior commissure; *4* = optic chiasm; *5* = infundibulum; *6* = pineal body; *7* = quadrigeminal plate; *8* = midbrain; *9* = pons.

3. **Middle group of hypothalamic nuclei.** The plane of the fornix splits the hypothalamus into roughly **medial** and **lateral** nuclear areas (see Fig. 12-11*C–E*).
   a. The **medial** hypothalamic region contains two large nuclei, the **ventromedial** and **dorsomedial**, at the midhypothalamic level. A small arcuate nucleus (infundibular nucleus) and several small, vaguely defined nuclear groups occupy the tuberal region.
   b. The **lateral** hypothalamic area extends into the posterior hypothalamus.

4. **Posterior group of hypothalamic nuclei** (see Fig. 12-11*F*)
   a. The **mamillary nucleus** has two distinct parts.
      (1) The **medial** part sends mamillary efferents to the thalamus and brainstem tegmentum.
      (2) The **lateral** part receives the fornix.
   b. The posterior hypothalamic nuclei merge with similar neurons of the posterior part of the lateral nucleus.

C. **Connections of the hypothalamus**

   1. **Preview**
      a. Highlighting its role in the rhinencephalic, limbic, autonomic, and endocrine systems, the strongest afferent and efferent connections of the hypothalamus are with basal rhinencephalic structures of the telencephalon, including the:
         (1) Amygdala and adjacent temporal lobe cortex
         (2) Hippocampus
         (3) Limbic nuclei and midline nuclei of the thalamus
         (4) Reticular formation and periaqueductal gray matter of the brainstem
      b. To focus on the sources of hypothalamic afferents, note where **they do not come from**:
         (1) Most of the general cortical surface
         (2) Striatum
         (3) Lemniscal systems (medial, lateral, spinal, and trigeminal)
         (4) Cerebellum
      c. Frontohypothalamic and retinohypothalamic connections, well established in lower animals, are not known to exist in man.
      d. In general, the hypothalamus will return efferents to its afferent sources, either directly or by feedback circuits.

Table 12-6. Hypothalamic Nuclei*

Dorsal group
   N. subthalamicus
   N. globus pallidus

Anterior group
   Preoptic area
   N. paraventricularis
   N. supraopticus (n. tangentialis of Cajal)
   N. praeopticus lateralis (interstitial n. of the medial forebrain bundle)
   N. hypothalamicus anterior

Middle group
   N. hypothalamicus lateralis
   N. hypothalamicus ventromedialis
   N. hypothalamicus dorsomedialis

Posterior group
   N. hypothalamicus posterior
   N. corporis mamillaris medialis, pars medialis and pars lateralis
   N. corporis mamillaris lateralis (n. intercalatus of Le Gros Clark)

N. and n. = nucleus.
*Partial listing.

 e. The hypothalamus has numerous short, multisynaptic connections within itself and with neighboring structures, as well as several conspicuous, named long tracts.

2. Fiber systems of the hypothalamus
 a. Medial forebrain bundle
   (1) The medial forebrain bundle runs longitudinally from the medial basal rhinencephalic structures through the lateral part of the hypothalamus and into the brainstem tegmentum and periaqueductal gray matter (see Fig. 12-11A and F).
   (2) The bundle conveys afferent and efferent fibers, receiving and paying them out along its course. It is laden with interstitial neurons, forming numerous short, polysynaptic pathways, resembling reticular formation in this regard.
   (3) Edinger named it the **medial** forebrain bundle to contrast it with the **lateral** forebrain bundle, which is composed of the internal capsule and the pallidal efferents.
      (a) The **lateral forebrain bundle** is the highway for somatic motor and sensory events and willed movements, as related to external space.
      (b) The **medial forebrain bundle** is the highway for automatic visceral control, as related to internal space.
 b. Three arching systems of fibers
   (1) Three arching fiber systems serve the depths of the cerebrum: the **stria terminalis**, **stria medullaris**, and **fornix** (Figs. 12-13 and 12-14).
   (2) These bundles interchange axons in complicated pathways. They connect the amygdala, rhinencephalon, and hippocampus of the telencephalon with the hypothalamus, thalamus, and epithalamus (habenula) of the diencephalon.
 c. The **stria terminalis** arises in the amygdala and follows the tail of the caudate nucleus around the roof of the inferior horn to occupy the thalamostriate seam in the floor of the body of the lateral ventricle (see Fig. 12-13). The stria terminalis decussates in part at the anterior commissure. At this site, the fibers are distributed to the:
   (1) Opposite stria terminalis and amygdala
   (2) Preoptic area and anterior hypothalamus
   (3) Thalamus dorsalis and habenula of the epithalamus via the stria medullaris
 d. The **stria medullaris** of the thalamus runs along the dorsomedial edge of the thalamus, where it marks the line of suspension of the roof of the third ventricle (see Figs. 12-13 and 12-14). Its fiber systems are more closely related to the habenula than to the hypothalamus.
 e. The **fornix** arises in the hippocampus.
   (1) Proceeding dorsally, it forms a commissure with its mate and arches over the roof of the third ventricle to reach the anterior commissure (see Figs. 12-13 and 12-14).
   (2) At the anterior commissure, it splits into **precommissural** and **postcommissural bundles**.

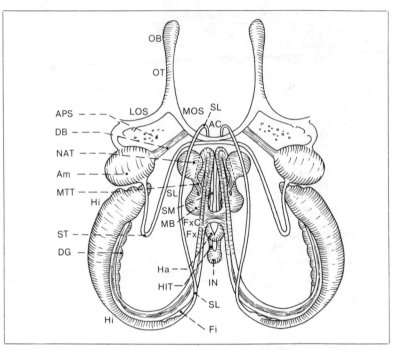

Figure 12-13. Dorsal stereoscopic view of the arching fiber systems related to the hypothalamus. *AC* = anterior commissure; *Am* = amygdala; *APS* = anterior perforated substance; *DB* = diagonal band; *DG* = dentate gyrus; *Fi* = fimbria; *Fx* = fornix; *FxC* = fornix commissure; *Ha* = habenula; *Hi* = hippocampus; *HIT* = habenulointerpeduncular tract; *IN* = interpeduncular nucleus; *LOS* = lateral olfactory stria; *MB* = mamillary body; *MOS* = medial olfactory stria; *MTT* = mamillothalamic tract; *NAT* = nucleus anterior of the thalamus; *OB* = olfactory bulb; *OT* = olfactory tract; *SL* = stria lancisii; *SM* = stria medullaris; *ST* = stria terminalis.

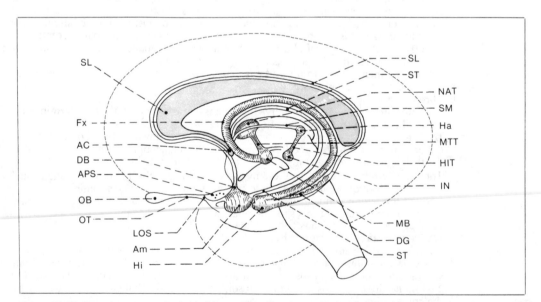

Figure 12-14. Lateral stereoscopic view of the arching fiber systems related to the hypothalamus. *AC* = anterior commissure; *Am* = amygdala; *APS* = anterior perforated substance; *DB* = diagonal band; *DG* = dentate gyrus; *Fx* = fornix; *Ha* = habenula; *Hi* = hippocampus; *HIT* = habenulointerpeduncular tract; *IN* = interpeduncular nucleus; *LOS* = lateral olfactory stria; *MB* = mamillary body; *MTT* = mamillothalamic tract; *NAT* = nucleus anterior of the thalamus; *OB* = olfactory bulb; *OT* = olfactory tract; *SL* = stria lancisii; *SM* = stria medullaris; *ST* = stria terminalis.

    (a) Precommissural fornix fibers enter the basal rhinencephalic region, septum, and anterior region of the hypothalamus.

    (b) Postcommissural fibers, the bulk of the fornix, turn caudally through the hypothalamus to synapse in the lateral part of the mamillary nucleus and the lateral and posterior hypothalamic areas.

  (3) Some fornix axons reach the thalamus, particularly nucleus medialis dorsalis, and may even reach the midbrain.

f. The **mamillary fasciculus** arises in the medial nucleus of the mamillary body. It divides into two components.

  (1) The **mamillothalamic tract** runs to nucleus anterior, one of the limbic nuclei of the thalamus (see Fig. 12-11G).

  (2) The **mamillotegmental tract** turns caudally to enter the midbrain tegmentum just ventral to the medial lemniscus. It ends in the reticular formation. Efferents return through the mamillotegmental tract to the mamillary nucleus from the reticular formation.

g. The **ansa peduncularis** originates in the amygdala and adjacent cortex of the temporal lobe (see Fig. 12-11A–C). It divides into two parts: One part connects with the thalamus through the inferior thalamic peduncle, and the other enters the medial forebrain bundle for the hypothalamus.

h. The **dorsal longitudinal fasciculus** (of Schutz) runs the length of the brainstem, in the periaqueductal gray matter, ventral to the lumen of the aqueduct and fourth ventricle. It interconnects the hypothalamus with the periaqueductal gray matter and with the dorsal motor nucleus of CN X.

i. Commissures. Several commissural pathways run through the supraoptic area, midportion, and mamillary region of the hypothalamus. They interconnect the hypothalamus, basal motor nuclei, reticular formation, and pretectal and tectal areas of the two sides of the cerebrum.

j. Chemically specified tracts. The brainstem sends catecholaminergic and serotonergic pathways to the hypothalamus and much of the rest of the forebrain (see Chapter 14, sections II and III).

k. Function of the hypothalamus as an auto- or self-receptor

  (1) In addition to receiving axons from the foregoing pathways, the hypothalamus acts as its own receptor, in part because of the selective permeability of the blood–brain barrier in certain hypothalamic nuclei.

  (2) Intrinsic mechanisms sample body temperature and osmolality of the blood and cerebrospinal fluid (CSF).

  (3) Various hormones and drugs become affixed to hypothalamic neurons and alter the endocrine activity and general behavior of the individual by neuronal excitation or inhibition.

D. Pituitary body (of Vesalius)

1. The pituitary body is only 0.5 cm high, 1.0 cm long, and 1.5 cm wide, yet it controls the endocrine system under the direction of the hypothalamus.

2. The pituitary body consists of the **pituitary stalk**, the **adenohypophysis**, and the **neurohypophysis** (Fig. 12-15).

3. Embryologically, the pituitary body has a dual origin.

a. The **neurohypophysis** is an evagination from the hypothalamus, thus originating from and remaining neural tissue.

b. The **adenohypophysis**, which is glandular tissue, evaginates from oral ectoderm. Its cells manufacture and store a number of major hormones: thyrotropin (thyroid-stimulating hormone; TSH), adrenocorticotropic hormone (ACTH), luteinizing hormone (LH), follicle-stimulating hormone (FSH), growth hormone (GH), and prolactin.

4. The hypothalamus controls the release of pituitary hormones by direct axonal endings and by portal systems (Fig. 12-16).

a. A **tuberoinfundibular tract** conveys axons from the ventromedial, infundibular, and tuberal nuclei to the portal blood system of the pituitary stalk.

  (1) The neuronal perikarya manufacture releasing factors that travel down the axons by axoplasmic flow.

  (2) The releasing factors empty into the portal system, which conveys them to the glandular cells of the adenohypophysis (see Fig. 12-16A). The glandular cells then release their trophic hormones directly into the bloodstream, which distributes them to tissues and endocrine glands elsewhere in the body.

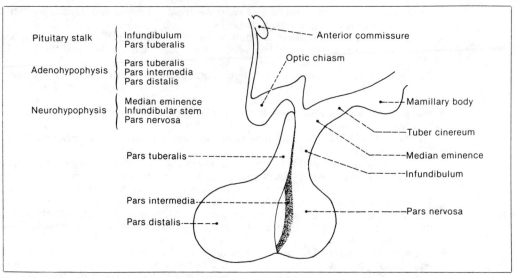

Figure 12-15. Sagittal section of the hypothalamus and pituitary body, showing the three divisions of the pituitary body.

    b. A **supraopticohypophyseal tract** conveys axons from the supraoptic and paraventricular nuclei to the portal system of the neurohypophysis (see Fig. 12-16*B*). The axons release two neurosecretory hormones: antidiuretic hormone (ADH; vasopressin) and oxytocin.

        (1) **ADH** increases the absorption of water from the distal tubule of the kidney; thus, it conserves water. The supraoptic nucleus mainly produces ADH.

            (a) The release of ADH is governed in part by the osmolality of the blood circulating through the supraoptic nucleus.

            (b) Increased filling of the heart by an overload of fluid causes inhibition of ADH secretion by way of vagal afferents.

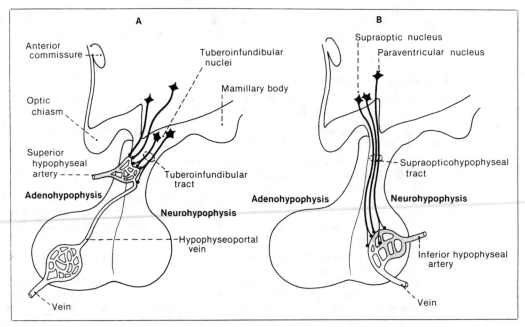

Figure 12-16. Sagittal section of the hypothalamus and pituitary body. (*A*) System of portal blood vessels for the transport of hormone-releasing factors from the hypothalamus to the adenohypophysis. (*B*) Supraopticohypophyseal tract and paraventricular–hypophyseal tract for the release of antidiuretic hormone and oxytocin into the systemic circulation.

(2) Oxytocin causes contraction of smooth muscle of the uterus and breast. The paraventricular nucleus mainly produces oxytocin.

E. Functions and clinical syndromes of the hypothalamus

  1. A review of the adult derivatives of the hypothalamus will emphasize its extreme structural and functional diversity (Table 12-7).

  2. To emphasize further the diverse functions of the hypothalamus, we may cite the diametric syndromes that occur when lesions upset the balances it maintains:
  a. Hyperthermia/hypothermia
  b. Anorexia/hyperphagia leading to cachexia/obesity
  c. Oliguria/polyuria
  d. Precocious puberty/delayed puberty
  e. Gigantism/dwarfism
  f. Lethargy/aggression
  g. Hyperpituitarism/hypopituitarism

  3. Role in control of autonomic function. The anterior and posterior areas of the hypothalamus contain centers that coordinate the activities of the sympathetic and parasympathetic nervous systems.
  a. Parasympathetic control
    (1) The anterior and medial hypothalamus tend to produce parasympathetic discharges.
    (2) Stimulation of certain sites causes pupilloconstriction, bradycardia, vasodilation, and a tendency for reduced blood pressure, and increased motility of the gut and bladder.
    (3) Destruction of the anterior hypothalamus results in irreversible hyperthermia. Normally it acts as the heat loss center.
  b. Sympathetic control
    (1) Stimulation of the posterior and lateral hypothalamus produces a fright/flight response manifested by pupillodilation, increased heart rate and blood pressure, increased breathing, and reduced gut motility.
    (2) Destruction of this hypothalamic region results in lethargy, sleepiness, and decreased body temperature. Normally it acts as a heat conservation center.

  4. Control of appetite
  a. Hypothalamic lesions may cause hyperphagia or aphagia. The most critical region appears to be the midhypothalamus. Destruction of the ventromedial nucleus in rats causes hyperphagia, with obesity and aggressive behavior.
  b. In the diencephalic syndrome of infancy, which is usually caused by a glioma of the hypothalamus, the patient shows extreme cachexia and emotional lability.

  5. Water balance
  a. Damage to the infundibular stalk or neurohypophysis results in failure of release of ADH. The individual has polyuria (diabetes insipidus).

Table 12-7. Derivatives of the Thalamus Ventralis

Adult Derivative	Function
Retina and optic stalk	Receptor for vision
Globus pallidus and subthalamic nucleus	Somatomotor control
Neurohypophysis (including median eminence)	Secretes antidiuretic hormone and oxytocin
	Controls release of adenohypophyseal trophic factors for endocrine glands, influencing growth and body proportions
Hypothalamus proper	Integrates autonomic nervous system and limbic lobe
	Controls instinctive and cyclic behaviors and the expression of emotion: appetite for food and water, sexual development and mating, maternal responses, expression of aggression, sleep
	Role in memory and maintenance of consciousness

b. Certain forms of injury to the region result in excessive or inappropriate release of ADH, resulting in oliguria and water retention.

c. The hypothalamus also acts to control water balance by mediating the release of ACTH, which controls adrenal secretions.

6. Role in affective expression and sexuality

a. Stimulation or lesions of the hypothalamus may elicit behavioral reactions resembling fear and rage. The animal will snarl, hiss, bite, and claw in response to trivial stimuli, such as a puff of air. If the hypothalamus remains intact, removal of the cerebral hemispheres rostral to the diencephalon also results in these reactions, termed sham rage.

b. Small tumors of the hypothalamus may cause gelastic epilepsy, in which eipileptiform discharges, as documented by electroencephalography, are associated with outbursts of laughter.

c. Hypothalamic or neighboring tumors may cause precocious puberty with adult sexual drives or delayed puberty with lack of sexual development.

7. Role in mental processes and memory

a. Korsakoff's syndrome. The patient, usually a severe alcoholic, has hallucinations and shows delirium, disorientation to time and place, loss of recent memory, and confabulation.

  (1) The brain shows hemorrhagic, necrotic foci in the hypothalamus, particularly in the mamillary bodies; in the thalamus, particularly in nucleus medialis dorsalis; and in the periaqueductal gray matter and tegmentum of the midbrain.

  (2) The midbrain lesion may cause palsy of CN III and pupillary abnormalities.

b. Drug addiction. The presence of opioid receptors in the hypothalamus and its relationship to affective states such as satiety and euphoria make it a prime region for the action of addictive and mood-altering drugs (see Chapter 14, section V).

IV. EPITHALAMUS

A. The epithalamus is the most dorsal of the four longitudinal nuclear zones of the diencephalon (see Fig. 12-1).

B. The epithalamus consists of the:

1. Roof of the third ventricle and stria medullaris

2. Habenular nuclei and commissure

3. Pineal body

C. Connections of the habenula

1. The habenular nuclei receive afferents from the stria medullaris, the periventricular neurons of the third ventricle, the periaqueductal gray matter, reticular formation, and interpeduncular nucleus of the midbrain.

2. The habenula sends efferents to the interpeduncular nucleus by the habenulointerpeduncular tract (fasciculus retroflexus of Meynert), the reticular formation, and the periaqueductal gray matter.

3. A habenular commissure connects the habenular nuclei of the two sides.

D. Functions of the habenula. The function of the habenular complex is uncertain. It may link the rhinencephalic, hypothalamic, and limbic control mechanisms with the rostral part of the brainstem. It is presumed to mediate olfactory stimuli and feeding behavior.

E. Pineal body. The pineal body manufactures melatonin. This hormone has a cyclic release and is thought to mediate some cyclic functions, such as the sleep cycle, and to control reproductive cycles and puberty.

STUDY QUESTIONS

Directions: Each question below contains five suggested answers. Choose the **one best** response to each question.

1. In addition to blindness, a lesion that destroys the optic chiasm and the immediately related overlying part of the hypothalamus would most likely cause

(A) diabetes insipidus
(B) hypertension
(C) hypothermia
(D) hyperphagia
(E) precocious puberty

2. A single lesion that interrupts axons of the fornix, stria terminalis, and stria medullaris would involve the

(A) roof of the third ventricle
(B) floor of the third ventricle
(C) genu of the corpus callosum
(D) midregion of the anterior commissure
(E) habenula

3. A lesion of which of the following thalamic nuclei would be most likely to cause a syndrome of apathy, reduced drive, and reduced reactions to stimuli such as pain?

(A) Nucleus medialis
(B) Nucleus pulvinaris
(C) Nucleus ventralis posterior
(D) Nucleus ventralis anterior
(E) Nucleus reticularis

4. As the pyramidal tract descends through the internal capsule, it shifts

(A) from the genu into the anterior limb
(B) into the external capsule
(C) posteriorly in the posterior limb
(D) from the posterior limb into the genu
(E) from the posterior limb to the inferior thalamic peduncle

5. The most important structure for describing the location of the various thalamic nuclei is the

(A) nucleus pulvinaris
(B) nucleus reticularis
(C) stratum zonale
(D) zona incerta
(E) internal medullary lamina

6. The region of the brain most important for regulation of body temperature is the

(A) hippocampus
(B) hypothalamus
(C) globus pallidus
(D) cingulate gyrus
(E) thalamus dorsalis

7. Each of the following senses is relayed to the cortex through a specific thalamic nucleus EXCEPT

(A) sight
(B) hearing
(C) smell
(D) touch
(E) pain

Directions: Each question below contains four suggested answers of which **one or more** is correct. Choose the answer

    A if **1, 2, and 3** are correct
    B if **1 and 3** are correct
    C if **2 and 4** are correct
    D if **4** is correct
    E if **1, 2, 3, and 4** are correct

8. All of the sensory relay nuclei of the thalamus share which of the following characteristics?

(1) They have a strict topographic organization
(2) They receive a discrete afferent pathway
(3) They project in a topographic way to the cerebral cortex
(4) They overlap each other in their location in the thalamus

9. The nuclei that project strongly to the limbic lobe include which of the following?

(1) Nucleus pulvinaris
(2) Nucleus anterior
(3) Centrum medianum
(4) Nucleus lateralis dorsalis

10. Correct statements about the medial forebrain bundle include which of the following?

(1) It interconnects the basal telencephalic olfactory region with the hypothalamus and brainstem
(2) It consists mainly of rapidly conducting, myelinated axons
(3) It occupies the lateral part of the hypothalamus
(4) It conducts mainly ascending impulses

11. Major pathways through the internal capsule consist of which of the following?

(1) Corticofugal pathways to the brainstem and spinal cord
(2) Superior thalamic (frontoparietal) peduncle
(3) Geniculocalcarine tract
(4) Auditory radiations

Directions: The group of questions below consists of lettered choices followed by several numbered items. For each numbered item select the **one** lettered choice with which it is **most** closely associated. Each lettered choice may be used once, more than once, or not at all.

Questions 12–16

Match the thalamic boundary with the structure to which it is immediately related.

(A) Third ventricle
(B) Anterior limb of the internal capsule
(C) Thalamic fasciculus and zona incerta
(D) Stratum zonale and body of the lateral ventricle
(E) None of the above

12. Caudal pole
13. Dorsal border
14. Lateral border
15. Ventral border
16. Medial border

ANSWERS AND EXPLANATIONS

1. The answer is A. [*III D 4 b (1), E 5 a*] The infundibular stalk conveys the axons that release antidiuretic hormone from the posterior pituitary gland. Absence of this hormone due to interruption of the hypophyseal stalk will result in diabetes insipidus with excessive water loss.

2. The answer is D. (*III C 2 c, d, e; Figures 12-13 and 12-14*) A number of pathways come together at the anterior part of the third ventricle. The anterior commissure crosses the midline at the dorsal part of the lamina terminalis. The fornix, which arches over the roof of the third ventricle, splits into an anterior and a posterior component around the anterior commissure; the stria medullaris and the stria terminalis partially decussate across the midportion of the anterior commissure. A single lesion at that site would interrupt all of these fiber tracts.

3. The answer is A. (*II F 3 c, O 3 c*) In the 1930s, it was found that lesions of the frontal lobe white matter caused a syndrome consisting of apathy, reduced drive, and reduced responsivity. Further investigations disclosed that such lesions interrupted the thalamocortical circuit between the nucleus medialis and the frontal cortex anterior to the motor area. Lesions of this circuit at either the nuclear, white matter, or cortical level tend to produce a similar behavioral result.

4. The answer is C. (*II L 4 a, b*) Recent investigations have shown that as the pyramidal tract descends through the internal capsule, it shifts posteriorly from the region of the genu into the posterior part of the posterior limb. The older textbooks show the fibers as located only in the anterior part of the posterior limb. This relationship holds only in the superior part of the capsule.

5. The answer is E. (*II C 3*) Gross cuts through the thalamus disclose that a lamina of medullated fibers —the internal medullary lamina—roughly divides it into medial and lateral halves. This gross subdivision corresponds with the histologic and functional separation of the medial and lateral groups of thalamic nuclei.

6. The answer is B. [*III A 2, E 3 a (3), b (2)*] The hypothalamus maintains the constancy of the internal environment by controlling temperature, circulation, and metabolism through its influence on the pituitary gland and endocrine system. The hypothalamus acts through connections with the limbic system of the cerebrum and the reticular formation of the brainstem, as well as the pituitary gland.

7. The answer is C. (*II E 1 a, I 4*) The thalamus serves as a relay center interposed between almost all of the major sensory systems and the cerebral cortex. The only major sensation known to bypass the thalamus is the sense of smell. The olfactory nerve synapses directly on the olfactory bulb, making it unique among all of the sensory pathways in bypassing the thalamus.

8. The answer is A (1, 2, 3). (*II I 1, 2*) The thalamic relay nuclei have a strict topographic organization: Each has a discrete afferent pathway, and each projects in a topographic way to the cerebral cortex. They do not overlap each other. In fact, these nuclei provide one of the strongest proofs for the topographic separation of sensory pathways.

9. The answer is C (2, 4). (*II F 2 a, b*) The various thalamic nuclei can be divided on the basis of their efferent connections. When they are so divided, two of the nuclei have primarily limbic lobe connections—the nucleus anterior and nucleus lateralis dorsalis, which project in an orderly anterior/posterior way to the overlying parts of the cingulate gyrus.

10. The answer is B (1, 3). (*III C 2 a*) The medial forebrain bundle contrasts with the lateral forebrain bundle. The lateral bundle consists of myelinated fibers that form the "capsules" (internal and external) and mainly convey somatosensory and somatomotor pathways. The medial forebrain bundle is, in analogy, a pathway of the visceral system. It consists of poorly myelinated fibers running to-and-fro from the basal telencephalic olfactory region, through the hypothalamus and periventricular region of the third ventricle, to the periaqueductal gray matter and reticular formation of the brainstem.

11. The answer is E (all). (*II L 2, 3; Table 12-4; Figure 12-6*) The internal capsule conveys virtually all thalamocortical and corticothalamic connections, including the auditory and optic radiations from the geniculate bodies. Another large component is the corticofugal motor system that runs in the long or longitudinal axis of the capsule. Fibers running transversely through the capsule connect the basal motor nuclei with each other and with the thalamus.

12–16. The answers are: 12-E, 13-D, 14-E, 15-C, 16-A. (*II B*) The thalamus is bordered laterally by the posterior limb of the internal capsule, medially by the third ventricle, ventrally by the thalamic fasciculus and zona incerta, and dorsally by the stratum zonale and body of the lateral ventricle. Thus, the thalamus borders on the lateral ventricle dorsally and on the third ventricle medially. Its dorsomedial border is the stria medullaris thalami. The stria medullaris marks the junction of the dorsal and medial boundaries of the thalamus. The choroid plexus of the third ventricle is suspended between the stria. The thalamus ends posteriorly in the tip of the pulvinar that projects over the superior colliculus. The pineal body rests between the pulvinars of the two thalami. The anterior limit of the thalamus is the tip of nucleus ventralis anterior or the shell formed by nucleus reticularis, depending upon one's viewpoint as to the classification of these structures. The anteromedial limit of the thalamus is also the posterolateral border of the foramen of Monro. The anteromedial boundary of the foramen is the fornix.

13
Cerebrum

I. GROSS EXTERNAL ANATOMY OF THE CEREBRUM

A. Review these facts before starting this chapter.

1. Definition of the cerebrum (see Fig. 1-3)

2. Lobes of the cerebrum (see Fig. 1-4A and B)

3. Four components of a cerebral hemisphere as seen in coronal section (see Fig. 1-6)

4. Origin of the two cerebral hemispheres by evagination from a median connecting stalk (see Fig. 3-6)

B. Three facies, three poles, and three margins of a hemisphere (Fig. 13-1)

1. Each hemisphere has **three facies: lateralis, medialis,** and **inferior (inferomedial)**.
   a. Facies lateralis is strongly **convex** because it conforms to the curve of the skullcap (calvaria).
   b. Facies medialis is completely **flat** because it conforms to the cerebral falx, a stiff, flat fold of dura mater inserted into the interhemispheric fissure.
   c. Facies inferior of the frontal lobe is **concave** because it conforms to the convex orbital plate of the floor of the frontal fossa.
   d. Facies inferior of the temporo-occipital lobe is faintly convex because it conforms to the floor of the middle fossa and cerebellar tentorium.

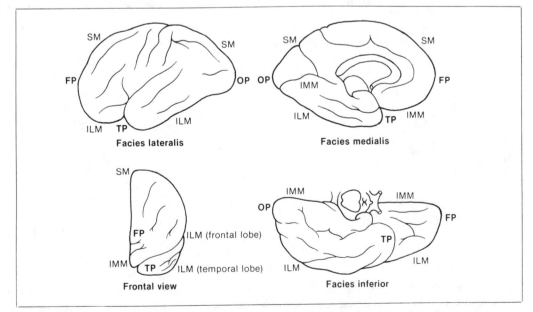

Figure 13-1. The three facies, poles, and margins of a cerebral hemisphere. *ILM* = inferolateral margin; *IMM* = inferomedial margin; *SM* = superior margin; *FP* = frontal pole; *OP* = occipital pole; *TP* = temporal pole.

2. Three margins—superior, inferolateral, and **inferomedial**—divide the three facies.

3. Each hemisphere has **three poles: frontal, occipital,** and **temporal.**

C. Lobes of the cerebrum are reviewed in Figure 1-4.

D. External crevices (fissures and sulci)

   1. Fissures versus sulci

   a. Fissures differ from sulci because they form by evagination or invagination of the entire cerebral wall and thus alter the ventricular contour.

   b. The sulci merely indent the outer surface of the cerebrum but do not, in general, alter the ventricular contour. Only the calcar avis of the calcarine sulcus significantly indents the ventricle.

   c. Nomenclature note. Some authors refer to some sulci as fissures; thus, for example, the calcarine sulcus may be called the calcarine fissure. However, the major fissures, such as the sylvian, are never called sulci.

   2. Fissures

   a. The **interhemispheric fissure** separates the two cerebral hemispheres as they evaginate (see Fig. 1-6).

   b. The **sylvian,** or **lateral, fissure** separates the frontal and parietal lobes above from the temporal lobe below as it evaginates (see Fig. 13-3).

   c. The **transverse cerebral fissure** forms by invagination of the forebrain roof plate, separating the fornix, fornix commissure, and corpus callosum above from the roof of the third ventricle below (see Fig. 13-19).

   d. The **choroid fissure** is an extension of the invaginated transverse cerebral fissure. It forms as the parahippocampal gyrus and hippocampal formation roll inward (see Fig. 13-19).

   3. Timetable for sulcus formation

   a. After the fissures appear, the cerebral surface remains otherwise completely smooth until sulcation commences in the fifth to sixth months of gestation.

   b. From the timetable of sulcation, the pathologist can estimate the gestational age of a premature infant at autopsy (Fig. 13-2).

   4. Final pattern of sulci and gyri (Figs. 13-3, 13-4, and 13-5)

E. Sylvian fissure, insular region, and opercula

   1. Course of the sylvian fissure

   a. The sylvian fissure begins at the **vallecula** (vallecula means little valley). This space, which admits a fingertip, is located just lateral to the angle formed by the optic nerve, optic chiasm, and optic tract (see Fig. 13-9). The roof of the vallecula is the anterior perforated substance.

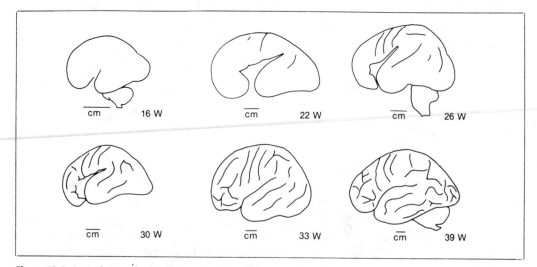

Figure 13-2. Lateral view of a cerebral hemisphere showing the progressive timetable of sulcation. At 16 weeks gestation, the cerebrum lacks sulci. By 39 weeks, sulcation is nearly complete. See Figures 13-3 through 13-5 for the names of the sulci. W = weeks of gestation. (Reprinted with permission from Chi JG, Dooling EC, Giles FH: Gyral development of the human brain. *Ann Neurol* 1:86–93, 1977.)

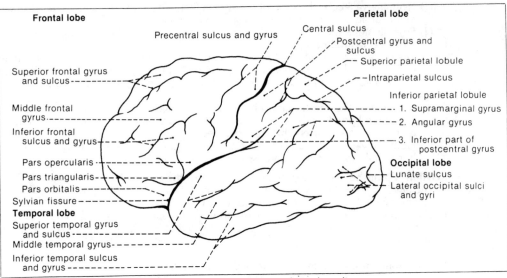

Figure 13-3. Sulci and gyri on facies lateralis.

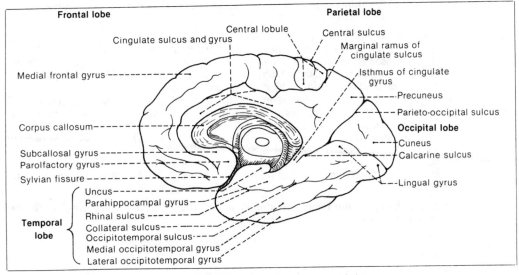

Figure 13-4. Sulci and gyri on facies medialis.

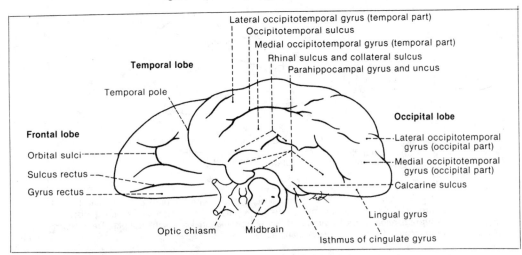

Figure 13-5. Sulci and gyri on facies inferior.

(1) From the vallecula, the **stem** of the sylvian fissure extends laterally. It separates the inferior surface of the frontal lobe from the temporal pole (Fig. 13-6).

(2) From its stem, the sylvian fissure continues on facies lateralis as the **anterior** and **posterior horizontal rami**.

(3) The posterior horizontal ramus separates the frontal and parietal lobes from the temporal lobe. It ends in an upcurved tip, surrounded by the supramarginal gyrus. The superior temporal sulcus often ends in a similar upcurved tip, surrounded by the angular gyrus.

b. Relationship of the carotid and middle cerebral arteries to the sylvian fissure

(1) The carotid artery ends at the vallecula by bifurcating into its terminal branches: the **middle** and **anterior cerebral arteries** (see Fig. 15-9).

(2) From the vallecula, the middle cerebral artery courses laterally through the stem and horizontal rami of the sylvian fissure to ramify over facies lateralis.

2. Relationship of the insular region and opercula to the sylvian fissure

a. The largest infolded cortical region—the insula (island of Reil)—can be reexposed by dissecting off the **frontal** and **parietal opercula** (Fig. 13-7).

b. The dissection shows a circular sulcus around the insula and a **radial pattern of insular gyri**. Also exposed are the transverse temporal gyri of Heschl, which receive the auditory radiations from the medial geniculate body.

F. Surface anatomy of the rhinencephalon and basal forebrain

1. Definition of rhinencephalon (rhin means nose, and encephalon means brain; therefore, nose–brain). The rhinencephalon is that part of the basal forebrain that mediates olfaction (the sense of smell) [Figs. 13-8 and 13-9].

2. Phylogenetic primacy of the rhinencephalon

a. The cerebrum in lower vertebrates consists largely of rhinencephalon (Fig. 13-10).

b. In comparison to the bulk of our cerebral hemispheres, our olfactory bulbs seem to be unimportant dependencies. In fact, phylogeny indicates that the cerebral hemispheres developed as dependencies of the rhinencephalon.

c. Olfaction and its closely allied sense of taste put the organism in **chemical** contact with its environment. The other senses all deal with aspects of **physics**: light, sound, mass, gravity, heat, texture, position, and contour.

d. We need only to smell and taste our food and smell our mates to survive and perpetuate our kind. Since a blind, deaf rat feeds, mates, and mothers better than one without olfaction, chemistry serves better than physics for these instinctual behaviors, which remain much more closely linked to our nose–brain and its limbic derivatives than to our rational brain.

3. Rhinencephalon as the hemispheric pedicle and the three concentric rings of the hemispheric wall

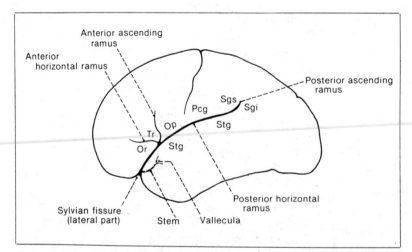

Figure 13-6. Lateral view of cerebral hemisphere with the parts of the sylvian (lateral) fissure labeled. *Op* = pars opercularis; *Or* = pars orbitalis; *Pcg* = postcentral gyrus; *Sgi* = supramarginal gyrus, superior part; *Sgs* = supramarginal gyrus, inferior part; *Stg* = superior temporal gyrus; *Tr* = pars triangularis.

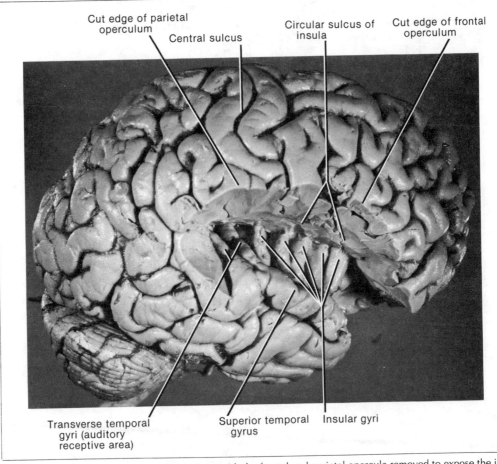

Cut edge of parietal operculum

Central sulcus

Circular sulcus of insula

Cut edge of frontal operculum

Transverse temporal gyri (auditory receptive area)

Superior temporal gyrus

Insular gyri

Figure 13-7. Lateral view of cerebral hemisphere with the frontal and parietal opercula removed to expose the insular region.

    a. The cerebral hemispheres and olfactory bulbs evaginate bilaterally from a median rhinencephalic stalk (see Fig. 3-5).

    b. A sagittal cut through the rhinencephalic stalk discloses it to consist of **commissures**, connecting **nervous tissue**, and a **membrane**.

    c. Connecting commissures consist of:

        (1) Corpus callosum (great cerebral commissure)

        (2) Fornix commissure (hippocampal commissure)

        (3) Anterior commissure (rhinencephalic, temporal lobe, and amygdalar commissures) [see Fig. 13-30].

        (4) Optic chiasm and **hypothalamic commissures**

        (5) Habenular commissure (commissure of habenular nuclei)

        (6) The posterior commissure, located just beneath the habenular commissure, belongs to the midbrain, not to the foregoing group of forebrain commissures.

    d. Connecting nervous tissue consists of:

        (1) Lamina terminalis

        (2) Hypothalamic floor

        (3) Massa intermedia (variably present)

    e. Connecting membrane. The tela choroidea, the connecting roof plate of the cerebrum, bridges the ventricles (see Fig. 13-19).

  4. Stretching of the rhinencephalic stalk by the corpus callosum. Huge numbers of callosal axons connect the cerebral cortex of the two hemispheres by growing through the original median rhinencephalic stalk, stretching its wall out thin. Although thinned out, rhinencephalic rudiments still form a topologically complete **inner hemispheric ring**, the first of three such concentric rings (Fig. 13-11).

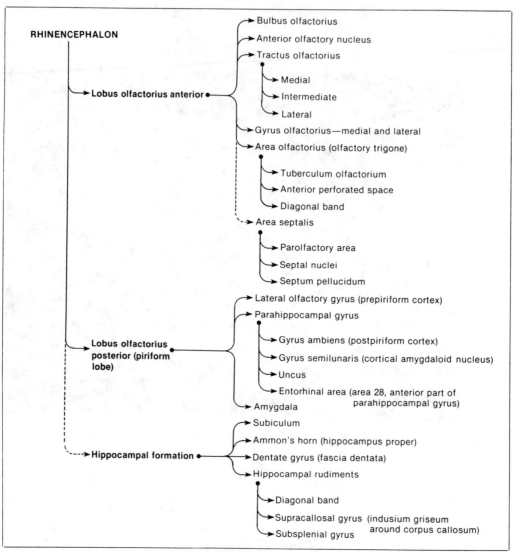

RHINENCEPHALON

- **Lobus olfactorius anterior**
  - Bulbus olfactorius
  - Anterior olfactory nucleus
  - Tractus olfactorius
    - Medial
    - Intermediate
    - Lateral
  - Gyrus olfactorius—medial and lateral
  - Area olfactorius (olfactory trigone)
    - Tuberculum olfactorium
    - Anterior perforated space
    - Diagonal band
  - Area septalis
    - Parolfactory area
    - Septal nuclei
    - Septum pellucidum

- **Lobus olfactorius posterior (piriform lobe)**
  - Lateral olfactory gyrus (prepiriform cortex)
  - Parahippocampal gyrus
    - Gyrus ambiens (postpiriform cortex)
    - Gyrus semilunaris (cortical amygdaloid nucleus)
    - Uncus
    - Entorhinal area (area 28, anterior part of parahippocampal gyrus)
  - Amygdala

- **Hippocampal formation**
  - Subiculum
  - Ammon's horn (hippocampus proper)
  - Dentate gyrus (fascia dentata)
  - Hippocampal rudiments
    - Diagonal band
    - Supracallosal gyrus (indusium griseum around corpus callosum)
    - Subsplenial gyrus

Figure 13-8. Dendrogram of nomenclature for the rhinencephalon. Some authors exclude the hippocampal formation from the olfactory lobe per se as indicated by the interrupted line.

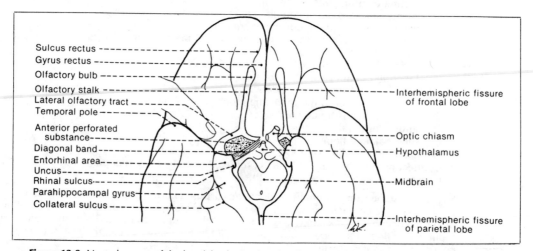

Sulcus rectus
Gyrus rectus
Olfactory bulb
Olfactory stalk
Lateral olfactory tract
Temporal pole
Anterior perforated substance
Diagonal band
Entorhinal area
Uncus
Rhinal sulcus
Parahippocampal gyrus
Collateral sulcus

Interhemispheric fissure of frontal lobe
Optic chiasm
Hypothalamus
Midbrain
Interhemispheric fissure of parietal lobe

Figure 13-9. Ventral aspect of the basal forebrain showing the external landmarks of the rhinencephalon.

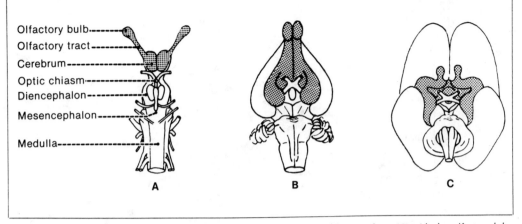

Olfactory bulb
Olfactory tract
Cerebrum
Optic chiasm
Diencephalon
Mesencephalon
Medulla

A   **B**   **C**

Figure 13-10. Ventral view of the brain of the shark (A), rodent (B), and human fetus (C) with the *olfactory lobe* shaded. (Reprinted with permission from DeMyer W: *Technique of the Neurologic Examination: A Programmed Text*, 3rd ed. New York, McGraw-Hill, 1980, p 268.)

> **a. Olfactory lobe** (olfactory ring; rhinencephalon proper)
> **b. Limbic lobe** (limbic ring)
> **c. Supralimbic ring**

G. External anatomy of the limbic lobe

1. The external surface of the limbic lobe consists of a ring of gyri (Table 13-1; see Fig. 13-11).

2. An **inner ring** of sulci separates the limbic lobe proper from the olfactory lobe. An **outer ring** of sulci roughly separates the limbic lobe from the supralimbic (ectocortical) ring (see Table 13-1).

3. The infolding of the cortex along the sylvian fissure indents the limbic ring and distorts its contour. Similarly, evagination of the olfactory bulbs and invasion of their median connection by the corpus callosum distort the olfactory ring (Fig. 13-12).

Table 13-1. Surface Anatomy of the Limbic Ring*

Inner ring of sulci (separates limbic gyri from rhinencephalon)
   Pericallosal sulcus
   Hippocampal sulcus (medial boundary of parahippocampal gyrus)
   (Orbital limbus has no inner sulcus—it borders on medial and lateral olfactory stria)

Ring of limbic gyri
   Paraterminal gyrus (parolfactory gyrus of Broca)
   Subcallosal gyrus
   Cingulate gyrus
   Isthmus (connection between cingulate and parahippocampal gyri)
   Parahippocampal gyrus
   Uncus
   Gyrus ambiens (joins entorhinal area of parahippocampal gyrus to insula)
   Insula
   Orbital limbus (posterior inferior frontal cortex), which extends to paraterminal and subcallosal gyri

Outer ring of sulci (roughly separates limbic gyri from supralimbic gyri)
   Anterior parolfactory sulcus
   Cingulate sulcus
   Subparietal sulcus
   Collateral sulcus
   Rhinal sulcus
   Circular sulcus of insula
   (Orbital limbus has no external sulcal boundary)

*Compare to Figures 13-4 and 13-11.

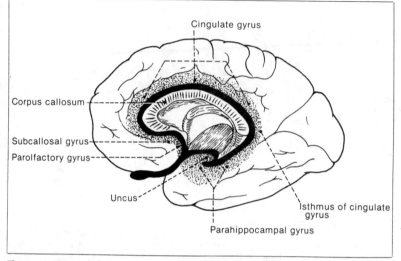

Figure 13-11. Medial view of a cerebral hemisphere showing the three fundamental concentric rings, with the gyri of the limbic ring labeled. *Black area* = olfactory lobe; *dotted area* = limbic lobe; *white area* = supralimbic lobe.

II. CONNECTIONS OF THE OLFACTORY AND LIMBIC LOBES

A. Olfactory lobes

1. After the primary olfactory axons synapse on the olfactory bulb, olfactory pathways disperse to a number of structures of the basal forebrain that bound the vallecula and its roof, the anterior perforated substance (Fig. 13-13).

2. Numerous pathways connect the basal forebrain around the vallecula with the septal region, hypothalamus, and hippocampal formation. Although once devoted to olfaction, many of these pathways assume diverse roles in the limbic system.

3. **Nucleus basalis of Meynert of the anterior perforated substance**
   a. **Histologic sections** through the anterior perforated substance disclose a plate of large, cholinergic neurons oriented tangential to the vallecular surface.
   b. **Afferents** arrive from many of the adjacent rhinencephalic/limbic structures.
   c. **Efferents** go to the superficial layers of the cerebral cortex, particularly of the frontal and parietal lobes, hippocampus, and brainstem.
   d. **Functions of nucleus basalis**
      (1) Because it projects diffusely to the cortex, nucleus basalis, unlike many of its phylogenetically regressive neighbors, increases in size in higher animals.
      (2) Once dismissed in textbooks as a phylogenetic curiosity, nucleus basalis is now known to undergo severe degeneration in Alzheimer's disease, the most common dementing disease of the middle and later years of life.
      (3) The diffuse cholinergic projection of this nucleus, comparable to that of the catecholaminergic and serotonergic brainstem nuclei (see Chapter 14, sections II and III), suggests some type of augmenting or modulating action rather than a specific function.
      (4) Nucleus basalis is thought to augment learning, memory, consciousness, and attention span, all of which are impaired in dementia.

B. Amygdala

1. **Definition**. The amygdala is a large nuclear mass located in the temporal pole at its transition to the posterior inferior surface of the frontal lobe (see Fig. 11-1). Formerly classed with the basal ganglia, it is now assigned to the limbic lobe.

2. The amygdala receives **afferents** from the:
   a. Anterior olfactory lobe
   b. Piriform, temporal, and prefrontal cortex
   c. Hypothalamus
   d. Nucleus medialis dorsalis of the thalamus
   e. Brainstem tegmentum

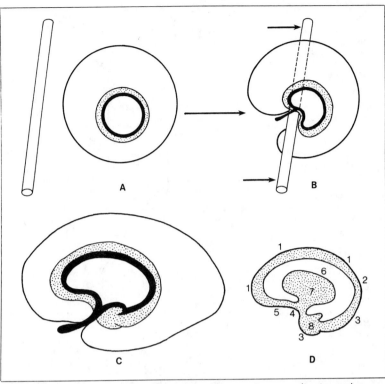

Figure 13-12. Medial view of a cerebral hemisphere. (A) Conceptualization as three geometrically perfect concentric rings. (B) Indentation of the rings and evagination of the olfactory bulbs and tracts. (C) Final configuration of medial hemispheric wall. (D) Limbic ring dissected out of the hemisphere to show its final geometry and the expansion ventrally at the uncus (8) and laterally to include the insula (7). *Black area* = olfactory lobe; *dotted area* = limbic lobe; *white area* = supralimbic lobe. Limbic ring components are: *1* = cingulate gyrus; *2* = isthmus of cingulate gyrus; *3* = parahippocampal gyrus; *4* = parolfactory gyrus; *5* = subcallosal gyrus; *6* = insula (island of Reil).

3. The amygdala sends **efferents** to the:
   a. Medial preoptic area, septal region, hypothalamus, and opposite amygdala, via the stria terminalis
   b. Nucleus medialis dorsalis
   c. Prefrontal cortex
   d. Brainstem tegmentum
   e. Hypothalamus, via the ventral amygdalofugal pathway

4. **Functions of the amygdala**
   a. Like many brain centers, the amygdala augments or modulates several functions rather than being a single center with a single function.
   b. Destruction may result in passive or aggressive behavior.
   c. Stimulation may cause changes in mood.
   d. Through its hypothalamic connections, the amygdala modulates endocrine activity, sexuality, and reproduction.

C. **Hippocampal formation**

1. **Definition.** The hippocampal formation is primitive cortex, most of which, the hippocampus proper (see Fig. 13-8), is rolled into the floor of the temporal horn along the choroid fissure.
   a. The hippocampal formation consists of three major regions: **subiculum, hippocampus proper** (Ammon's horn), and **dentate gyrus** (Figs. 13-14 and 13-15).
   b. Both the hippocampus and dentate gyrus have a three-layered cortex. The subiculum is the transition zone from the three- to the six-layered cortex of the temporal lobe.

2. Phylogenetically, the hippocampal formation originates as rhinencephalic cortex. It retains the primitive arrangement of a superficial layer of white matter, the **alveus**, rather than deep white matter.

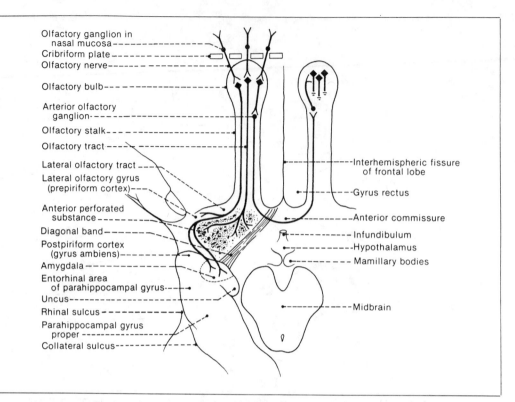

Figure 13-13. Basal aspect of the cerebrum showing the axonal pathways from the olfactory bulb.

3. The hippocampal formation receives **afferents** from the:
   a. Entorhinal and limbic cortex via the cingulum, uncinate fasciculus, and temporoammonic tracts
   b. Nucleus basalis of Meynert (cholinergic)
   c. Noradrenergic and serotonergic pathways from the reticular formation (see Chapter 14, sections II C and III)
   d. Contralateral hippocampus via the hippocampal commissure

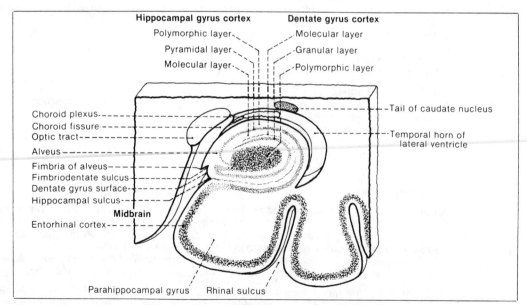

Figure 13-14. Coronal section through the hippocampal formation, as seen in Nissl stain, to show neuronal peri-karya (cytoarchitecture).

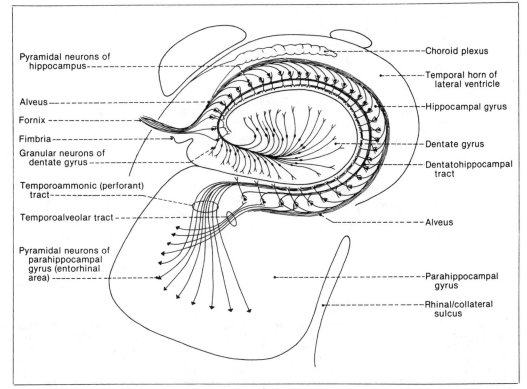

Pyramidal neurons of
  hippocampus

Alveus

Fornix

Fimbria

Granular neurons of
  dentate gyrus

Temporoammonic (perforant)
  tract

Temporoalveolar tract

Pyramidal neurons of
  parahippocampal
  gyrus (entorhinal
  area)

Choroid plexus

Temporal horn of
  lateral ventricle

Hippocampal gyrus

Dentate gyrus

Dentatohippocampal
  tract

Alveus

Parahippocampal
  gyrus

Rhinal/collateral
  sulcus

Figure 13-15. Coronal section of the hippocampal formation showing the axonal connections, as seen in Golgi and other silver impregnations.

    4. Efferents from the hippocampal formation
        a. The granular neurons of the dentate cortex synapse on the pyramidal neurons of the hippocampal cortex (see Fig. 13-15).
        b. The hippocampal pyramidal axons, joined by axons from the subiculum and adjacent temporal lobe cortex (temporoammonic tract of Cajal), form the **alveus** on the surface of the hippocampus.
        c. The alveus separates from the hippocampal cortex as the fimbria. Its axons then continue through the fornix to the hypothalamus (see Figs. 12-13 and 12-14). Some axons cross to the opposite hippocampus in the hippocampal commissure.

    5. Functions of the hippocampus
        a. The hippocampus is part of the circuitry involved in learning and recent memory (see section VI K). It may also have a chemoreceptor–endocrine function.
        b. The hippocampus has a low seizure threshold and may be involved in the pathogenesis of epilepsy.

  D. Limbic lobe connections: Papez circuit

    1. In 1937, James Papez (pronounced Papes, as in grapes) suggested that certain rhinencephalic and limbic pathways provided the anatomical basis for emotions and their expression through visceral and instinctual actions such as those involved in feeding, mating, mothering, and aggression (Fig. 13-16).

    2. The Papez circuit, like the basal motor nuclei, consists of feed-in/feed-out pathways between cortical and subcortical centers, with a major connecting bundle in the cerebral white matter, the cingulum (see section IV E).

    3. Functions of the limbic lobe
        a. Lesions or electrical stimulation of the limbic lobe cause principally visceral/autonomic and complex behavioral responses. Various sites may be excitatory or inhibitory with regard to a particular function.
        b. Visceral/autonomic responses include changes in pupillary size, blood pressure, pulse, gastrointestinal peristalsis, and bladder contraction.
        c. Stimulation of the cingulate gyrus can arrest breathing. Conversely, breathing may be increased by stimulation of other sites.

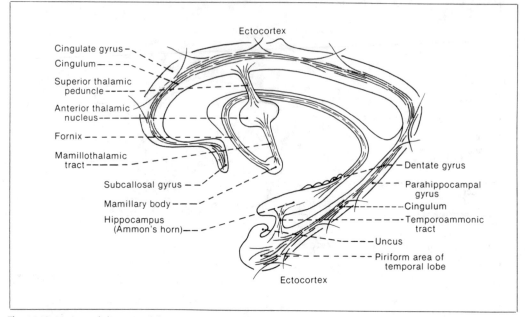

Figure 13-16. Lateral diagram of the circuit proposed by Papez as the anatomical basis of emotion. The cingulate gyrus connects with the parahippocampal gyrus and piriform area of the temporal lobe via the cingulum. The temporal lobe connects with the hippocampus (Ammon's horn) via the temporoammonic tract. The hippocampus connects with the mamillary body via the fornix. The mamillary body connects with the anterior nucleus of the thalamus via the mamillothalamic tract. The anterior nucleus of the thalamus connects with the cingulate gyrus via the superior thalamic peduncle, completing the circuit. Papez also included feed-in pathways to the circuit from the septal and olfactory regions and amygdala.

    d. Stimulation of limbic structures may also cause a generalized arrest of activity, often accompanied by positive viscera-related actions, such as chewing, swallowing, licking the lips, or grooming.

        (1) In man, psychomotor seizures, which originate in or propagate through limbic connections, are characterized by an aura of fear or visceral sensation, loss of consciousness, and performance of automatic acts such as chewing or picking at the clothes.

        (2) The patient may show an arrest in behavior or may walk around and even drive a car and carry on a limited conversation. However, the patient does not remember the episode.

        (3) The complex behavioral reactions resulting from limbic stimulation contrast with the relatively simple contractions or twitches of the contralateral muscles following stimulation of the precentral motor cortex.

    e. Reward behavior and pleasurable sensation also seem to have a limbic basis.

        (1) Animals with electrodes implanted in the septal region and connected to a bar will press the bar compulsively thousands of times, yet the only reward triggered by the bar is the electrical stimulus to the limbic structure.

        (2) Paul Yakovlev suggested that the posterior cingulate gyrus contains a **cenesthesic center,** a "feeling good" center, which might control moods of elation.

    f. Midline gliomas of the septum pellucidum and corpus callosum extend laterally into the limbic structures in a symmetrical, butterfly pattern.

        (1) The patient shows changes in mood, affect, drive, and general behavior but shows no overt motor, sensory, or visual signs upon neurologic examination.

        (2) The lesion is one of many organic disorders that may be mistaken for a functional mental illness.

III. PHYLOGENETIC–ONTOGENETIC THEORY OF CEREBRAL MORPHOGENESIS

A. Encephalization

    1. Animals can be arranged in a series of increasing intelligence in rough proportion to the increasing number of neurons in their cephalic ganglion or cerebrum. The phylogenetic process leading to increased neurons in the brain is called **encephalization**.

2. Two evolutionary developments increase the number of cerebral neurons tremendously yet keep the head circumference down to a manageable size:

    a. Cortex formation, which coats the spherical cerebral surface with layers of neurons

    b. Fissuration/sulcation, which enfolds the spherical surface to increase its area relative to its circumference, enabling the greatest area to fit into the smallest possible space

B. Phylogeny of the semicircular shape of the cerebral hemispheres

    1. The cerebral hemispheres fundamentally have a semicircular shape externally and internally and medially and laterally (Fig. 13-17).

    2. As seen **laterally**, a side-by-side series of animal brains show the gradual evolution of the semicircular shape by the downward and forward evagination of the temporal lobe (Fig. 13-18).

        a. Evagination of the temporal pole extends the temporal horn of the ventricle and lengthens and increases the depth of the sylvian fissure.

        b. Similar but less extensive evagination of the frontal and occipital poles extends the ventricles in their directions (see Fig. 1-7). Hence, growth vectors expand all three cerebral poles.

    3. As seen medially, the cerebral wall invaginates.

        a. Figure 13-19 conceptualizes the cerebrum before invaginating as showing a:

            (1) Fully exposed roof plate

            (2) Fully exposed hippocampal formation, still in its primordial dorsal position, before it migrates downward and forward with the temporal lobe

        b. The initial evagination of the hemispheres creates an **interhemispheric fissure**.

        c. Then, **invagination** medially of the roof plate and rolling in of the hippocampal formation creates the **transverse cerebral fissure** (see Fig. 13-19).

            (1) Growth vectors in the cerebral wall force the hippocampal formation back, down, and forward in a semicircular arc (Fig. 13-20), extending the transverse cerebral fissure as the **choroid fissure**.

            (2) Thus, the backward, downward, and forward semicircular migration of the hippocampal formation medially matches the similar configuration of the temporal lobe laterally.

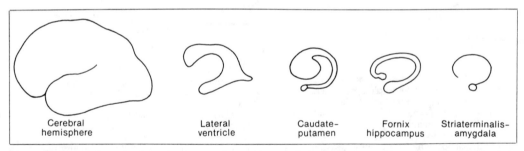

| Cerebral hemisphere | Lateral ventricle | Caudate-putamen | Fornix hippocampus | Striaterminalis-amygdala |

Figure 13-17. Lateral aspect of a cerebral hemisphere with exploded view of its internal structures showing the fundamental semicircular configuration.

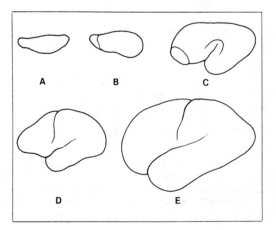

Figure 13-18. Lateral view of the left hemispheres of a series of animals showing the progressive phylogenetic increase in the evagination of the temporal lobe and increasing length of the sylvian fissure. (*A*) Salamander. (*B*) Rodent. (*C*) Dog. (*D*) Monkey. (*E*) Human.

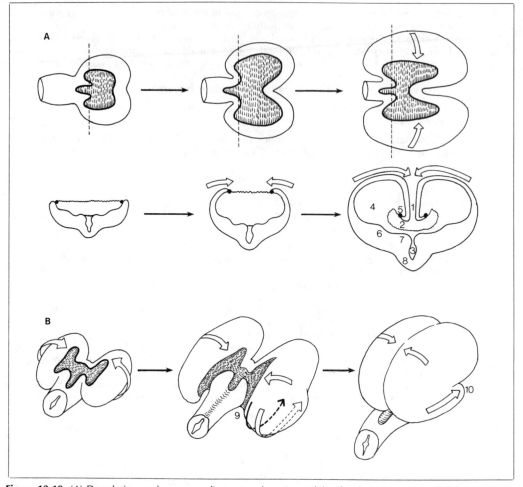

Figure 13-19. (A) Dorsal view and corresponding coronal sections of the developing prosencephalon. (B) Dorsal perspective view of developing prosencephalon. The drawing depicts the infolding of the roof plate (*shaded membrane*) along the interhemispheric fissure and the creation of the transverse fissure by inrolling of the hippocampal formation. The corpus callosum is not shown. *1* = interhemispheric fissure; *2* = transverse fissure; *3* = third ventricle; *4* = lateral ventricle; *5* = hippocampal formation (*black region*); *6* = ganglionic hillock of corpus striatum; *7* = thalamus; *8* = hypothalamus; *9* = transverse fissure extending as the choroid fissure as the hippocampus, originally in a dorsal position, undergoes its backward, downward, and forward migration into the evaginating temporal horn (*thin interrupted arrow*); *10* = completed evagination of the temporal lobe.

    d. The same process draws out the tail of the caudate nucleus (see Fig. 13-17).

C. Formation of cavum veli interpositi and cavum septi pellucidi

    1. The transverse cerebral and interhemispheric fissures are extracerebral spaces originally in free communication with each other.

    2. The backward hump created by the growth of the corpus callosum, with the fornix and fornix commissure clinging to its underbelly, separates the two fissures.

        a. The space beneath the corpus callosum, fornix, and fornix commissure, in the plane of the transverse cerebral fissure, is now called the **cavum veli interpositi.**

        b. The **velum interpositum,** which is the roof of the third ventricle, reflects backward at the foramen of Monro (Fig. 13-21).

    3. As the two anterior pillars of the fornix stretch away from the undersurface of the genu of the corpus callosum, they pull out a thin membrane, the **septum pellucidum,** on each side. The cavity between the two leaves of the septum pellucidum, the **cavum septi pellucidi,** is an entirely separate space from the cavum veli interpositi, and both caves are topologically separate from the ventricles.

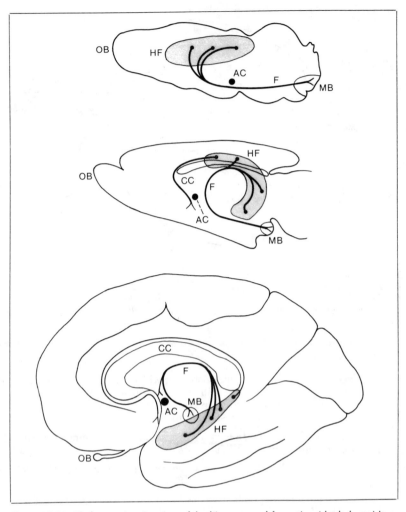

Figure 13-20. Phylogenetic migration of the hippocampal formation (*shaded area*) in a semicircular arc. From its primitive dorsal position, it undergoes a backward, downward, and forward migration, in keeping with the phylogeny of the temporal lobe (see Fig. 13-18). The fornix strings out along the pathway of migration of the hippocampal formation, retaining its anchor to the anterior commissure and hypothalamus. *AC* = anterior commissure; *CC* = corpus callosum; *F* = fornix; *HF* = hippocampal formation; *MB* = mamillary body; *OB* = olfactory bulb.

D. Review of cerebral organogenesis. In summary, the major events of cerebral organogenesis are:

1. **Closure** of the neural tube and the **transverse segmentation** of the prosencephalon into a telencephalon and a diencephalon

2. **Evagination**
   a. Evagination converts the holospheric prosencephalon into a hemispheric organ (see Fig. 3-5).
   b. Evagination produces the three hemispheric poles, particularly the temporal. The temporal lobe evagination creates the sylvian fissure, and opercularization along the fissure buries the insula.
   c. The olfactory bulbs and tracts also evaginate.

3. **Invagination** of the medial hemispheric wall, which creates the transverse fissure, a lateral extension of the interhemispheric fissure that resulted from evagination of the cerebral hemispheres
   a. Then, backward, downward, and forward arching of the hippocampal formation extends the transverse fissure as the choroid fissure.

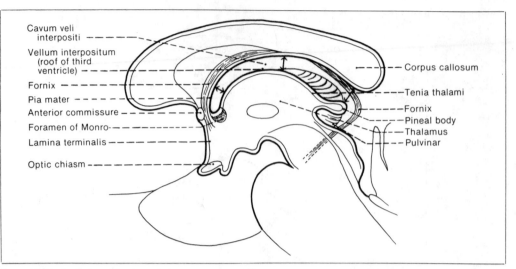

Figure 13-21. Sagittal section through the cavum veli interpositi (*shaded area* delineated by *arrows*). The cavum is a subarachnoid space, outside of the brain proper, created by the backward growth of the corpus callosum over the thalami and the roof of the third ventricle. The pial portion (*dark line*) of the velum interpositum, which is the roof of the third ventricle, reflects backward on the undersurface of the fornix after bridging the foramen of Monro.

   b. The corpus callosum enlarges backward as a hump, forming a roof over the cavum veli interpositi.

 E. Holoprosencephaly is a striking malformation in which the cerebrum bears an uncanny resemblance to the diagrammatic representation of the prosencephalon shown in Figure 13-19*A*. Holoprosencephaly (Fig. 13-22) can be interpreted as a total arrest in the process of evagination and invagination of the forebrain described above.

  1. The prosencephalon remains **holospheric** rather than proceeding to evaginate its walls laterally to become hemispheric (see Fig. 3-5).

  2. The cerebrum lacks all three poles, in particular a fully evaginated temporal pole, and, therefore, lacks an infolded insula and sylvian fissure.

  3. If we consider the olfactory bulb as the pole of the olfactory lobe, then all four lobes of the cerebrum fail to evaginate in holoprosencephaly.

  4. The prosencephalic cavity remains as a single holoventricle without a subdivision into lateral and third ventricles connected by a Y-shaped foramen of Monro.
   a. The foramen of Monro remains as a gaping communication, which occupies the anterior–posterior diameter of the ventricle, rather than narrowing to a small aperture under the two columns of the fornix.
   b. Since the thalami fail to hemispherize by separating in the midline, they do not form a cleft for the third ventricle.

  5. The roof plate remains totally exposed—everted, as it were—because of failure of infolding of the medial hemispheric wall to create an interhemispheric fissure and transverse cerebral fissure.

  6. The corpus callosum fails to grow back over the ventricular roof.

  7. The hippocampal formation remains exposed in its primordial dorsal position because it fails to roll into the choroid fissure and migrate backward, downward, and forward.

  8. The limbic lobe occupies its familiar position as a concentric ring around the hippocampal formation and rhinencephalon of the inner ring (see Figs. 13-11 and 13-19).

  9. The ectocortex of the supralimbic lobe forms and sulcates because histogenesis is governed by laws different from those governing organogenesis.

IV. WHITE MATTER OF THE CEREBRUM

 A. Composition. White matter consists of:

  1. Axons, which run in organized tracts

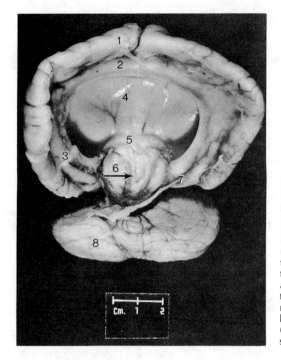

Figure 13-22. Dorsal view of a human brain showing holoprosencephaly (compare with Fig. 13-19). *1* = gyrated ectocortex covering the prosencephalic holosphere, which has failed to evaginate (cleave) into hemispheres; *2* = limbic mesocortex; *3* = archicortex (hippocampal formation) with fimbria–fornix bordering monoventricle; *4* = cavity of holoventricle (monoventricle); *5* = ganglionic hillock of corpus striatum; *6* = thalamus, uncleft from its neighbor; hence the two thalami are not divided by a third ventricle; *7* = cut edge of the greatly expanded roof plate, which covered the monoventricle intra vitam. The roof plate should have been folded into the transverse and choroid fissures (see Fig. 13-19*B*); *8* = normally sulcated and hemispherized cerebellum.

    2. Glia, including oligodendrocytes, which provide myelin, and astrocytes with processes, which provide scaffolding

    3. Blood vessels

B. Timetable for development of cerebral white matter. The various tracts to and from the cerebral cortex invade the cerebral wall in a definite sequence (Table 13-2) and then myelinate in a definite sequence (see Fig. 3-23).

C. Connections of cortical efferent fibers

    1. Cortical axons may synapse on other **cortical neurons** or on **infracortical neurons**.
        a. Since both the cortical target neuron and the infracortical target neuron may be ipsilateral or contralateral, the developing axon has four possible destinations.
        b. Depending on their destinations, cortical efferent axons are classed as **association fibers, commissural fibers**, or **projection fibers**.

    2. Association fibers. The axons of cortical neurons, which synapse on **ipsilateral** cortical neurons, associate these neurons functionally, hence the name association fibers (Fig. 13-23).

    3. Commissural fibers
        a. Cortical axons that cross the midline to synapse on **contralateral** cortical neurons are called commissural fibers.
        b. Commissures differ from decussations because commissural fibers cross the midline to connect mirror-image points, whereas decussating fibers cross to connect nonmirror-image points.

    4. Projection fibers
        a. Cortical axons, which synapse on infracortical neurons, "project" the cortical influence onto the lower centers. Hence, they are called projection fibers.
        b. Projection fibers may end ipsilaterally or contralaterally. In the latter case, they are decussations.
        c. The term "projection fiber" may also apply to infracortical connections. Thus, the cerebellum "projects" to the thalamus.

    5. Any given axon may branch to provide a fiber to association, commissural, or projection pathways (see Fig. 13-23).

D. Association pathways of the cerebral white matter

    1. Short association fibers

Table 13-2. Approximate Times during Gestation When Various Tracts Appear

End of first month	Spinal trigeminal tract
	Fasciculus solitarius
	Medial longitudinal fasciculus
During second month	Mamillotegmental tract
	Olfactory nerve
	Posterior commissure
	Transverse fibers of hindbrain
	Fasciculus retroflexus
	Crossed olivary fibers
	Thalamic peduncles
	Stria medullaris thalami
	Inferior cerebellar peduncle
	Internal capsule
During third month	Anterior commissure
During fourth month	Columns of fornix
	Corpus callosum
	Pontine fibers
During fifth month	Pyramidal fibers

a. Many association axons synapse close to their neuron of origin. They remain intracortical and do not enter the deep white matter.
b. These association axons, which travel for short distances around the depth of a sulcus, form a visible U-shaped lamina on the undersurface of the cortex, called an **arcuate bundle** (Fig. 13-24).
c. The **uncinate** (U-shaped) **fasciculus** is one of the largest arcuate bundles (Figs. 13-25 and 13-26).
d. As the intercortical association fibers of one hemisphere travel longer distances, they laminate in a peripheral-to-central manner.

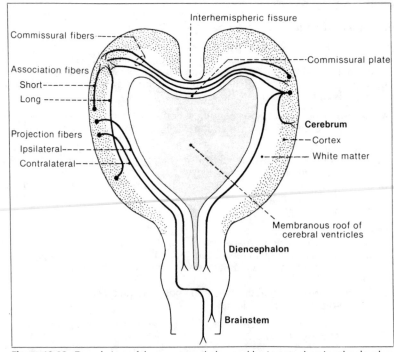

Figure 13-23. Dorsal view of the prosencephalon and brainstem showing the development of commissural, association, and projection fibers.

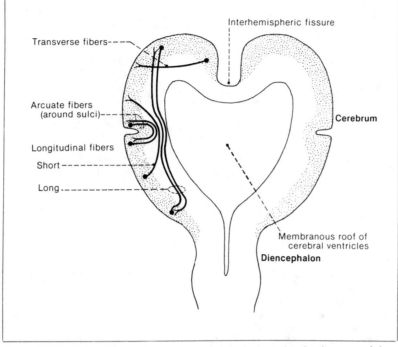

Figure 13-24. Dorsal view of the prosencephalon showing the development of the short, arcuate association fibers and the lamination of the long association fibers deep to them. Transverse and vertical association fibers of intermediate length crisscross the deep white matter.

(1) In the cerebral white matter, the short fibers, the arcuate bundle, laminate on the **inner** surface of the cortex and the long fibers laminate deeper in the white matter.

(2) In the spinal cord, in contrast, the short axons or ground bundles laminate on the **outer** surface of the gray matter and the long fibers laminate on the periphery of the ground bundles.

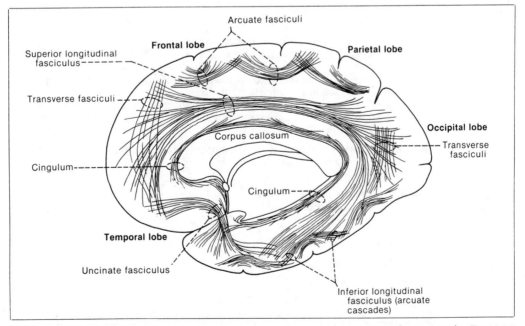

Figure 13-25. Sagittal section of a cerebral hemisphere showing several association pathways (see also Fig. 13-26).

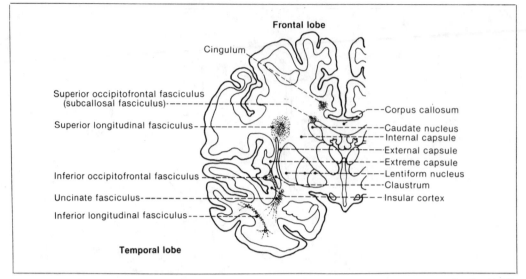

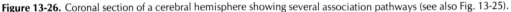

Figure 13-26. Coronal section of a cerebral hemisphere showing several association pathways (see also Fig. 13-25).

2. Long association fibers
a. The long association fibers accumulate into more or less distinctive bundles that stand out on gross dissection (Table 13-3).

b. The bundles continually pay out and receive axons along their course. In fact, recent studies confirm that a series of arcuate cascades, rather than a single inferior longitudinal fasciculus, connects the temporal and occipital regions.

c. In addition to the **longitudinally** running long bundles, pathways of intermediate length crisscross **vertically** and **transversely** between facies medialis and facies lateralis or in a superior to inferior direction in all of the lobes.

d. Lesions of the long pathways disconnect one part of the cerebrum from another and from infracortical centers, leading to varying degrees of motor and sensory deficits and dementia.

e. Certain demyelinating diseases preferentially attack the long pathways, sparing the arcuate bundles.

E. Cingulum

1. The cingulum is the long and short association pathway of the limbic lobe. It girdles the hemisphere from the parolfactory and subcallosal regions of the frontal lobe around to the parahippocampal gyrus and temporal pole (see Figs. 13-16, 13-25, and 13-26).

a. A limbic component of the uncinate fasciculus then completes the limbic ring by connecting the temporal lobe to the inferior frontal region.

b. The temporal cortex that receives the limbic connections of the cingulum and uncinate fasciculus sends axons to the hippocampus (Ammon's horn) as the temporoammonic tract (of Cajal) as part of the Papez circuit (see Fig. 13-16).

2. In addition to its cortical connections, the cingulum distributes axons from the limbic nuclei of the thalamus and to the corpus striatum (Fig. 13-27).

Table 13-3. Long Association Bundles of the Cerebral Hemisphere Arranged in Medial-to-Lateral and Dorsal-to-Ventral Order*

Cingulum (supracallosal fasciculus)
Superior occipitofrontal fasciculus (subcallosal fasciculus)
Superior longitudinal fasciculus
Inferior occipitofrontal fasciculus
Inferior longitudinal fasciculus (occipitotemporal fasciculus)—now regarded as a series of arcuate cascades rather than a single bundle

*Compare to Figures 13-25 and 13-26.

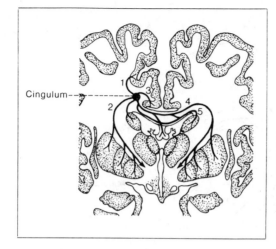

Figure 13-27. Coronal section through the cerebrum at the level of the body of the corpus callosum and the genu of the internal capsule showing the distribution of axons by the cingulum. Fibers of the cingulum form the dorsal and ventral lamina of the corpus callosum. The core of the corpus callosum transmits cortical commissural fibers. See also Figure 13-29. *1* = corticocortical fibers; *2* = lateral fibers; *3* = corticoperforant fibers; *4* = dorsal transcallosal fibers; *5* = ventral transcallosal fibers.

3. Cingulotomy by stereotaxic surgery may reduce the reaction of the chronically ill patient to pain and may reduce the intensity of obsessive-compulsive neuroses.

F. Cortical commissures (Table 13-4)

  1. Corpus callosum

    a. Development (see section III C and Fig. 13-20).

    b. Gross subdivisions. The corpus callosum, the largest commissure in the central nervous system (CNS), has a **rostrum, genu, body,** and **splenium** (Fig. 13-28).

    c. Fiber connections. Through its middle lamina, the corpus callosum connects mirror-image areas of the cortex of the two hemispheres. Its dorsal and ventral lamina convey axons of the cingulum (see Fig. 13-27).

      (1) Those axons that curve around the interhemispheric fissure anteriorly comprise the **forceps minor;** they form the **genu**. Those curving around posteriorly comprise the **forceps major;** they form the **splenium** (Fig. 13-29).

      (2) Some regions lack transcallosal connections, including:

        (a) Primary sensory areas 1,2, and 17 and part of the primary auditory receptive area (area 41)

        (b) Those parts of the motor cortex (area 4) serving the upper and lower extremities (in contrast, the motor areas for the face, shoulder, and pelvic girdle and trunk do have callosal connections)

        (c) Anterior superior frontal region

Table 13-4. Cortical Commissures

Corpus callosum*
Gross subdivisions: rostrum, genu, body, and splenium
Radiatio corporis callosi
Tapetum
Anterior forceps (forceps minor)
Posterior forceps (forceps major)
Anterior commissure[†]
Interbulbar and intertubercular components from olfactory bulb and olfactory tubercle
Prepiriform, interamygdaloid, and interparahippocampal gyrus components
Ectocortical components
Small contingent from the superorostral frontal cortex
Intertemporal component connecting the temporal gyri (the largest component in primates)
Hippocampal commissure (psalterium)

*See Figure 13-29.
[†]See Figure 13-30.

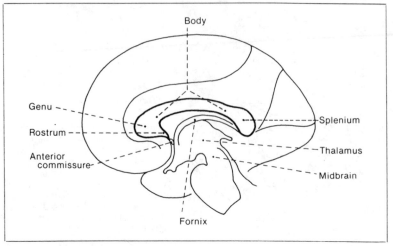

Figure 13-28. Sagittal section of the corpus callosum showing the division into four parts: rostrum, genu, body, and splenium.

2. Hippocampal commissure (psalterium, lyre of David)

    a. The hippocampal commissure connects the hippocampal formations of the two hemispheres.

    b. Moved backward by the growth of the corpus callosum and the migration of the hippocampal formations, the hippocampal commissure crosses beneath the posterior part of the body of the corpus callosum. It is part of the rhinencephalic underwall of that structure.

3. Anterior commissure

    a. The anterior commissure crosses in the commissural plate ventral to the corpus callosum (Fig. 13-30; see Fig. 12-10).

    b. Phylogenetically, it originates as a noncortical or rhinencephalic commissure, linking the olfactory bulbs, the amygdala, and other basal forebrain neurons.

    c. In higher animals, ectocortical fibers linking the frontal and temporal cortex predominate. The fibers laminate in the same manner as the corpus callosum (see Table 13-4 and Fig. 13-30).

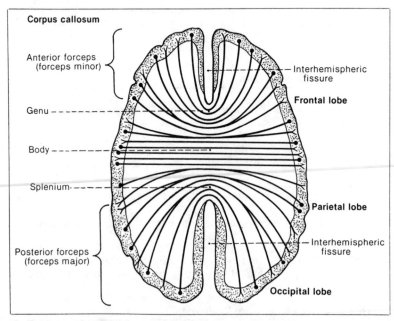

Figure 13-29. Horizontal section through the cerebral hemispheres and corpus callosum showing the pattern of the crossing of the nerve fibers.

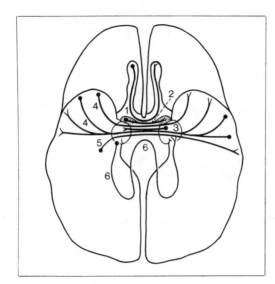

Figure 13-30. Ventral view of the cerebral hemispheres showing the fibers of the anterior commissure. *1* = interbulbar component; *2* = intertubercular (interanterior perforated substance) component; *3* = interamygdaloid component; *4* = ectocortical component; *5* = interparahippocampal gyrus component; *6* = stria terminalis (interamygdaloid component).

4. Clinical effects of cerebral commissurotomy: the split brain

    a. Sagittal section of the corpus callosum, anterior commissure, and optic chiasm disconnects the two cerebral hemispheres. The individual has a "split brain" (actually a split cerebrum) and cannot transfer information from one hemisphere to the other. Specific tests are required to demonstrate the deficits.

        (1) If blindfolded, the individual cannot match an item held in one hand or seen in one visual field with what is felt or seen on the other side.

        (2) A right-handed patient can execute a verbal command with the right hand because the left motor cortex remains connected to the language centers of the left hemisphere. The patient cannot execute the command with the left hand because the right hemisphere, disconnected from the left, does not understand language.

    b. Agenesis of the corpus callosum. The fibers of the corpus callosum may fail to cross during development. The fibers then accumulate along the ipsilateral ventricular wall (Probst's bundle), rather than crossing in the commissural plate.

G. Noncortical commissures of the diencephalon

    1. The **hypothalamic commissures** connect the globus pallidus and the subthalamus, the pretectal nuclei, the medial geniculate bodies, and the hypothalamic nuclei themselves.

    2. The **habenular commissure** links the habenular nuclei of the epithalamus and anchors the dorsal lip of the evagination that produces the pineal body.

    3. The **posterior commissure**, technically part of the midbrain, anchors the ventral lip of the evagination that produces the pineal body. It connects the pretectal and collicular areas of the two sides and the satellite optomotor nuclei around the nucleus of CN III.

H. Table 13-5 summarizes the cortical projection pathways of the cerebral white matter.

Table 13-5. Subcortical Projection Pathways from Cortical Neurons

Corticobulbar and corticospinal projections of the pyramidal system
Corticoextrapyramidal projections to basal motor nuclei
Corticotegmental optomotor projections to the reticular formation and accessory nuclei for control of volitional eye movements
Corticopretectal–tectal projections, mainly from the occipital lobe for reflex eye movements based on vision
Corticopontine projections
Corticohypothalamic projections (existence uncertain in humans)
Corticoreticular projections

I. **Summary of all of the pathways comprising the cerebral white matter**

    1. Short (arcuate), intermediate, and long association bundles (see Table 13-3)

    2. Commissures (see Table 13-4)

    3. Cortical projection fibers (see Table 13-5)

    4. Thalamic peduncles (see Table 12-5)

    5. Internal (see Table 12-4), external, and extreme capsules

V. CEREBRAL CORTEX

A. **Definition**. The cerebral cortex consists of thin horizontal layers of neurons and nerve fibers, forming a gray–brown sheet on the surface of the cerebral hemispheres.

B. **Ontogeny of cortical lamination**

    1. Ontogenetically, the cerebral wall consists of three zones: **periventricular (germinal), intermediate**, and **marginal**.

    2. The cortical neuroblasts start migrating from the germinal zone into the marginal zone in the second month of gestation (see Fig. 3-10).

        a. After migrating to the cerebral surface, the vast majority of cortical neuroblasts direct their axons inward, into the intermediate zone, expanding it to form the deep white matter.

        b. Successive waves of cortical neuroblasts leave the germinal zone at later and later times.

        c. The neurons for the outer layers migrate outward through the inner layers to reach their terminal positions. Thus, the four outer layers develop after the inner two in an inside-out manner.

        d. By the eighth month of gestation, the cortex shows its final six lamina.

C. **Phylogeny of the cerebral cortex: paleocortex, archicortex, and neocortex**

    1. Paleocortex

        a. In **primitive animals**, the cerebral neurons have a nucleate–reticulate pattern throughout the entire cerebral wall. This nucleate–reticulate pattern, with a hint of lamination, persists as paleocortex in all subsequent animals, including humans, in the olfactory region around the vallecula of the basal forebrain.

        b. In **higher submammalia**, particularly reptiles, more and more neurons migrate to the surface, where they commence to laminate (see Fig. 3-10).

        c. In **mammalia**, the cortex thence has three or six distinct layers, called **archicortex** and **neocortex**, respectively (Fig. 13-31).

    2. Archicortex

        a. The three-layered archicortex, phylogenetically more recent than paleocortex, is found in the hippocampal formation. Its efferent axons are directed **outwards**, into the **alveus**, which forms a superficial rather than a deep layer of white matter (see Figs. 13-14 and 13-15).

        b. Archicortex, along with paleocortex and the pericallosal rudiment (indusium griseum), is the cortex of the inner of the three concentric rings of the hemispheric wall (see Fig. 13-11), the ring that is perforated and expanded by the corpus callosum.

    3. Neocortex, consisting of **mesocortex** and **ectocortex**, is six-layered.

        a. Mesocortex is the six-layered cortex that covers the limbic lobe, the second of the three concentric cerebral rings (see Fig. 13-11).

        b. Ectocortex is the six-layered **supralimbic** cortex. It is phylogenetically new and ascendent, covering most of the cerebral surface. Like mesocortex, it directs the vast majority of its efferent axons inward and receives its afferents from the deep white matter.

        c. The exuberant overgrowth of ectocortex accounts for the increasing brain size in higher animals. It is what fulfills the process of encephalization and leads to the need for the extensive sulcation and fissuration of the brain in higher animals.

D. **Six horizontal layers of the ectocortex**

    1. Nissl-stained sections disclose **six horizontal layers** of neuronal perikarya and also their tendency to align in vertical columns (Fig. 13-32 and Table 13-6; see Fig. 13-32A).

    2. Golgi-stained sections show the full branching patterns of the various types of cortical neurons (see Fig. 13-32B).

    3. Myelin-stained sections show a gridwork of entering and exiting nerve fibers, obviously designed for vertical **and** horizontal dispersion of nerve impulses (see Fig. 13-32C).

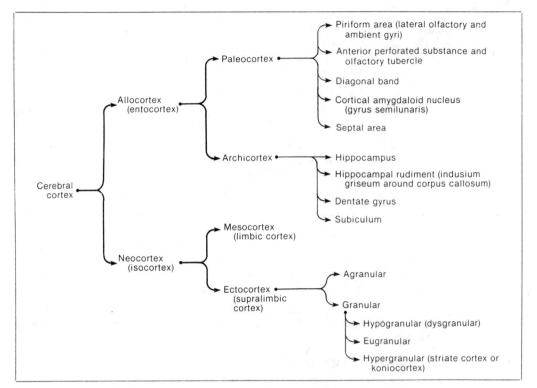

Figure 13-31. Dendrogram of phylogenetic terminology for the cerebral cortex.

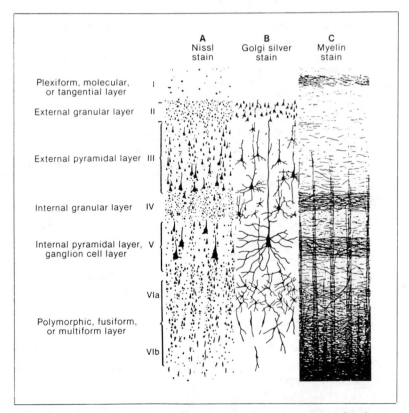

Figure 13-32. Histologic sections of the ectocortex. (*A*) Nissl stain. (*B*) Golgi silver impregnation. (*C*) Myelin stain. (Reprinted with permission from Brodal A: *Neurological Anatomy.* New York, Oxford University Press, 1981, p 63.)

Table 13-6. Horizontal Laminae of the Ectocortex As Seen in Nissl Stain*

Layer	Average Width (%)	Synonyms	Outstanding Cellular Characteristics
I	10	Plexiform, molecular, or tangential layer	Neuronal perikarya very sparse; contains axons and dendrites
II	10	External granular layer	Numerous small pyramidal and stellate neurons
III	30	External pyramidal layer	Numerous medium-sized pyramidal neurons, increasing in size from superficial to deep parts of the layer
IV	10	Internal granular layer	Numerous small stellate (granular) neurons
V	20	Internal pyramidal layer, ganglion cell layer	Medium to very large pyramidal neurons with small numbers of stellate neurons
VI	20	Polymorphic, fusiform, or multiform layer	Many fusiform or polymorphic perikarya; some pyramidal and stellate neurons

*Compare to Figure 13-32.

    a. The larger cortical dendrites, as well as the entering and exiting nerve fibers, run in vertical columns, perpendicular to the cortical surface.

    b. When the vertically oriented nerve fibers or dendrites branch, their collaterals tend to run perpendicular to the vertical columns, forming horizontal laminae (Table 13-7; see Fig. 13-32C).

    c. The horizontal laminae of myelinated fibers (lines of Baillarger) are readily visible as stripes in the sensory receptive areas of the cortex, whence the name **striate cortex** for these areas.

E. Vertical (radial) arrangement of cortical neurons

    1. The vertical fibers of the cortex create a matrix that separates countless vertical stacks of 100 to 300 synaptically connected neurons.

      a. These countless vertical stacks may constitute the "functional units" of the cortex, more so than its horizontal lamination.

      b. Both the laminar and cylindrical arrangement of cortical neurons occur throughout the mammalia.

    2. The cylinders may vary in diameter up to several hundred micra. For example, a thalamocortical relay axon ends in a cylindrical tuft with a longitudinal spread of around 300 μ.

      a. The size of a cylinder as defined by the spread of thalamic afferents may differ from the size defined by association fiber afferents.

      b. Dendrites and axonal collaterals may spread over radii of different lengths.

      c. These arrangements provide for varying degrees of "cross talk" between the neurons in a vertical cylinder and between vertical cylinders.

    3. A cylinder in the sensory receptive cortex might receive afferents from a restricted group of sensory neurons. The more specific the sensory topography, as in the tonotopic auditory cortex or retinotopic visual cortex, the more restricted the afferents to the cylinder.

Table 13-7. Horizontal Strata of Myelinated Fibers of the Ectocortex

Layer	Name of Stripe or Plexus	Source of Fibers
I	Tangential plexus of Retzius	Horizontal neurons of layer I
II	None present	
III	Outer main layer (line of Kaes-Bekhterev)	Terminal collaterals of cortical association and commissural fibers
IV	Outer line of Baillarger (line of Gennari or Vicq d'Azyr in visual cortex)	Terminal plexus of incoming thalamocortical fibers; sometimes crowds into layer IIIc
V	Inner main layer or inner line of Baillarger	Collaterals of fibers in transit to and from the cortex
VI	Indistinct	Collaterals of fibers in transit to and from the cortex

   4. Although cylinders are not as evident in the motor cortex, a vertical stack might activate only a tiny group of lower motoneurons (LMNs). However, the localization in either motor or sensory systems should not be regarded too rigidly.
      a. Destruction of one vertical zone in the motor cortex does not cause paralysis of one tiny group of LMNs. Some overlap exists, and each vertical zone might function as the maximum or modal point for a particular LMN pool rather than having the fatality of a telephone switchboard.
      b. This issue reflects an old controversy as to whether the motor cortex represents "muscles" or "movements."

F. Five anatomical types of cortical neurons

   1. The five types of cortical neurons differ in the size and shape of their perikarya, which in turn relate to the pattern of dendritic branching and to the size and length of their axons (Fig. 13-33).

   2. The three most common types of neurons have a **pyramidal, fusiform,** or **stellate** perikaryon. The less common types, the **neurons of Martinotti** and **horizontal neurons of Cajal,** have a polygonal or fusiform perikaryon, respectively.

   3. The **pyramidal neurons,** named for their pyramid-shaped perikaryon, vary in height from 10 to 100 μ.
      a. A long **apical dendrite** extends vertically from the apex of the pyramid.
      b. Basal dendrites extend laterally in horizontal and oblique planes from the base of the pyramid. The horizontal spread of the basal dendrites and the distal branches of the apical dendrite is 50 to 300 μ.
      c. From the base of the pyramid, an axon extends into the white matter (Golgi type I neuron).
         (1) Typically the axon collateralizes into branches that form association, commissural, or projection fibers.
         (2) The recurrent axonal collaterals of the association fibers may end on other pyramidal neurons or cortical interneurons.
      d. The pyramidal neurons of layer V, along with the fusiform neurons of layer VI, provide the major efferent axons of the cerebral cortex. Two specialized large pyramidal efferent neurons are those of Betz and Meynert.
         (1) The **Betz neurons** are located in layer V of the motor cortex (Fig. 13-34; see area 4, Fig. 13-34A). The largest neurons of the cortex measure up to 100 μ in height. They originate the large, myelinated axons of the pyramidal tract.
         (2) The **Meynert cells** are moderately large pyramidal neurons located in layer V of the visual receptive cortex in the occipital lobe (see area 17, Fig. 13-34D). They send axons to the brainstem, which mediate visually directed reflex eye movements.

   4. The **stellate,** or **granular, neurons** have a small, round, polygonal, or triangular perikaryon, 4 to 8 μ in diameter, which reflects a very busy, more random pattern of dendritic branching (see Fig. 13-33).
      a. The dendrites extend only a short distance from the perikaryon, and the axon runs only a short distance (Golgi type II neuron) to form intracortical connections.
      b. The various types of stellate neurons and the Cajal and Martinotti neurons are interneurons whose axons remain within the cerebral cortex.
         (1) Stellate neuronal subtypes are either excitatory or inhibitory.
         (2) Each subtype produces characteristic axodendritic and axoaxonic synapses.

   5. The **fusiform neurons** are most common in layer VI. They have an elongated perikaryon, which gives off a dendrite from each end (see Fig. 13-33). Their axons enter the deep white matter (Golgi type I neurons).

   6. The **Martinotti neurons** are present in all cortical layers except layer I. They have a polygonal perikaryon with short dendrites. Their axons, directed vertically toward the cortical surface, give off collaterals to the neuronal layers as they ascend (see Fig. 13-33).

   7. The **horizontal neurons of Cajal** are confined to layer I.
      a. The long axis of their fusiform perikaryon and their dendrites and axons run **horizontal** to the surface and remain in layer I (see Fig. 13-33).
      b. Since layer I has only Cajal neurons and they are infrequent, it has the fewest neurons of any of the cortical layers.

G. Connections and synaptic relationships of the cortical neurons

   1. The outer four cortical layers (layers I through IV) tend to be **receptive** and **interneuronal** in function.

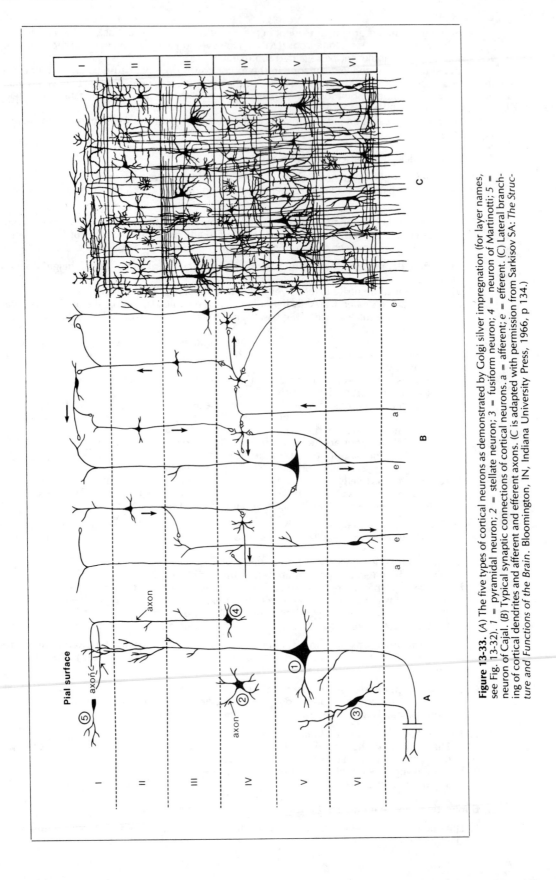

304 *Neuroanatomy*

Figure 13-33. (A) The five types of cortical neurons as demonstrated by Golgi silver impregnation (for layer names, see Fig. 13-32). *1* = pyramidal neuron; *2* = stellate neuron; *3* = fusiform neuron; *4* = neuron of Martinotti; *5* = neuron of Cajal. (B) Typical synaptic connections of cortical neurons. *a* = afferent; *e* = efferent. (C) Lateral branching of cortical dendrites and afferent and efferent axons. (C is adapted with permission from Sarkisov SA: *The Structure and Functions of the Brain.* Bloomington, IN, Indiana University Press, 1966, p 134.)

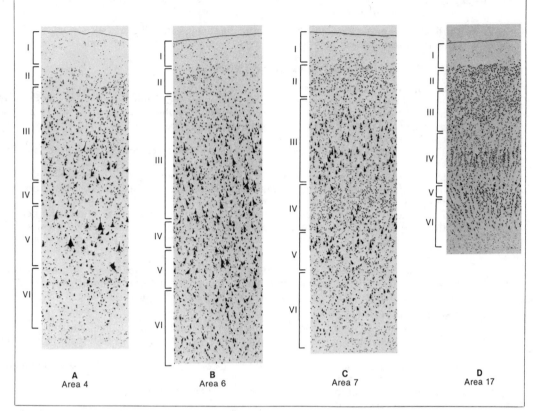

Figure 13-34. Nissl-stained sections of the cerebral cortex showing regional variations in its cytoarchitecture (for layer names, see Fig. 13-32). (A) Agranular, area 4. (B) Dysgranular, area 6. (C) Eugranular, area 7. (D) Hypergranular, area 17. (Adapted with permission from Campbell AW: *Histological Studies on the Localization of Cerebral Function*. Cambridge, University Press, 1905.)

2. The inner two layers (layers V and VI) tend to be **efferent**, but the dichotomy is by no means strict.

3. All layers contain intracortical interneurons, and all except layer I contribute some axons to the white matter.
   a. Cortical commissural and association axons arise mainly from neurons in layers II and III.
   b. Corticothalamic axons arise in layer VI and possibly layer V.
   c. Corticostriatal, corticorubral, corticotectal, corticoreticular, corticopontine, corticobulbar, and corticospinal axons arise mainly in layer V.

4. Sources of afferent fibers to the cortical neurons include:
   a. Corticocortical association and commissural axons (of the synapses on a cortical neuron, 95% or more come from other cortical neurons)
   b. Thalamic nuclei (the thalamic nuclei provide perhaps 1% of the cortical input)
   c. Nucleus locus ceruleus (noradrenergic) and ventral tegmental nucleus (dopaminergic)
   d. Nucleus basalis of Meynert (cholinergic)
   e. Nuclei of brainstem raphe (serotonergic)

5. Mode of termination of thalamic afferents
   a. The **specific thalamic afferent fibers** that carry topographic information generally ascend without branching to synapse in layer IV and the deeper part of layer III.
      (1) On reaching these layers, the fibers branch horizontally, forming a conspicuous outer stripe of Baillarger.
      (2) The axons end as tufts. They synapse on the pyramidal dendrites or granular neurons, which relay to the pyramidal neurons.
   b. Nonspecific thalamic afferents are thought to be collaterals of thalamostriatal fibers.
      (1) They terminate diffusely in all layers, spreading over a much greater diameter than the specific thalamic tufts.

(2) Their role would appear to be dispersion of ascending reticular activating system activity, rather than localization.

6. **Cortical interneurons** receive afferents from the same sources listed in section V G 4. The interneurons connect with the pyramidal neurons and neurons of Martinotti.

H. Areal subdivisions of the neocortex (cortical maps)

1. **Cytoarchitectural subdivisions**
   a. Nissl-stained sections from various cortical areas show differences in the size and shape of neuronal perikarya, their density in the various layers, the thickness of the layers, and the degree of radial striation. These characteristics are spoken of as the **cytoarchitecture** of the cortex (see Fig. 13-34).
   b. The underlying theory that cytoarchitectural differences correlate with functional differences is only partially true.
   c. Some cortical regions, such as the paracentral motor and sensory cortex, obviously differ in cytoarchitecture and function, but the functions overlap the cytoarchitectural boundaries even in these regions.
   d. Even when similar in cytoarchitecture, cortical regions may not function alike because their afferent and efferent connections differ. For example, the cerebellar cortex, with its monotonous, uniform cytoarchitecture, shows localization of function because of its differing connections.

2. **Brodmann's cytoarchitectural map (1904)**, the one most commonly used, divides the cerebral cortex into some 52 regions. Brodmann assigned the numbers arbitrarily and did not intend their sequence on the map to imply any cytoarchitectural kinship (Fig. 13-35).

3. **Von Bonin and Bailey's map (1951)**
   a. After Brodmann, some authors proposed as many as 200 cytoarchitectural areas, causing Von Bonin and Bailey in 1951 to suggest that these authors had over-read minor differences.
   b. Von Bonin and Bailey emphasized that most cortical areas look much alike and offered a simplified map of a dozen areas.
      (1) They used color to identify the areas and gradations of color to emphasize gradual transitions between areas.
      (2) They rejected Brodmann's system of numbers and stippling, contending that it failed to reflect the degree to which a given area resembled or differed from others and gave a false impression of the sharpness of areal boundaries.
   c. Today, authors use Brodmann's numbers in two ways:
      (1) In their original sense to designate cytoarchitectural areas as such
      (2) As a shorthand system to designate some region on the cerebral surface

4. **Granular layer as a cytoarchitectural criterion**
   a. A glance at various cortical sections (see Fig. 13-34) reveals great variation in the width of layer IV, which is packed with granular neurons and is receptive in function. Using this one layer allows the separation of four cortical variants:
      (1) Agranular: no distinct granular layer
      (2) Hypogranular (dysgranular): thin, discontinuous granular layer
      (3) Eugranular: average-width granular layer
      (4) Hypergranular (koniocortex or striate cortex): excessively wide granular layer
   b. The cortex in front of and behind the central sulcus aptly demonstrates the value of this criterion.
      (1) Commencing precentrally, **area 4** of Brodmann's map (see Fig. 13-35) is **agranular**.
      (2) Going forward into **area 6**, the granular layer appears sporadically, making this area **hypo- or dysgranular**.
      (3) Forward of area 6, the **prefrontal** cortex, and continuing through **area 10** of the frontal pole, the cortex is **eugranular**.
   c. Just posterior to the central sulcus and the agranular cortex of area 4 lie **areas 3, 1, and 2**. These areas have a very wide internal granular layer, making them **hypergranular** or **striate** cortex.

I. Cytoarchitectural areas of the frontal lobe neocortex

1. **Motor cortex, areas 4 and 6**
   a. Area 4 of the precentral gyrus is agranular, very thick, lacks distinct radial striations, and has huge pyramidal neurons of Betz in layer V (see Fig. 13-34A).
      (1) The Betz neurons, which originate large myelinated fibers for the pyramidal tract, are largest where area 4 extends onto the medial side of the hemisphere (see Fig. 13-35B).

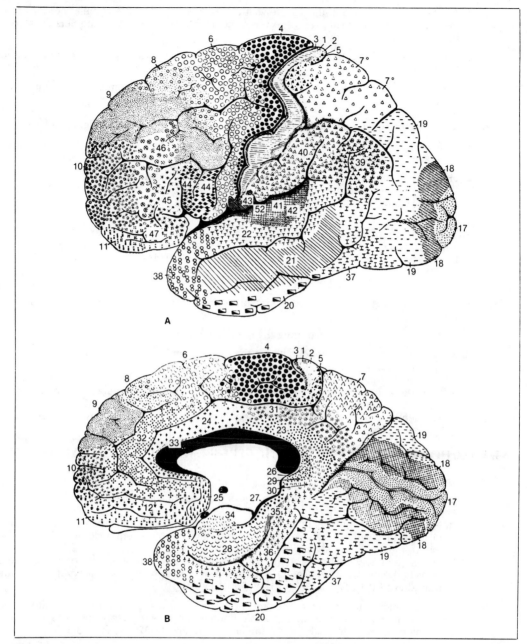

Figure 13-35. Brodmann's cytoarchitectural map of the cerebral cortex. (A) Lateral view of the cerebral hemisphere. (B) Medial view. (Reprinted with permission from Brodmann K: Physiologie des Gehirns, in Die Allgemeine Chirurgie der Gehirnkrankheiten. *Neue Deutsch Chirurgia*, vol 11. Stuttgart, Ferdinand Enke Verlag, 1914, p 1.)

    (2) Betz neurons gradually get smaller as they extend laterally over the superior hemispheric crest and ventrally down along the precentral gyrus in a triangular field (see Fig. 13-35A).

  b. Identification of area 4 as part of the motor cortex rests on functional evidence, not sheer anatomy.

    (1) Electrical stimulation of the region elicits movements of the contralateral extremities.

    (2) Destruction of the region results in contralateral "pyramidal tract" signs.

  c. The correlation between function and structure is imperfect even for such distinctive cytoarchitecture. Motor responses also occur following electrical stimulation of area 6 and the postcentral hypergranular sensory cortex.

2. **Area 6**, forward of area 4, thins somewhat and is hypogranular. The granular neurons commence to appear in small patches. A few large neurons reminiscent of the Betz cells occur here and there.

3. **Prefrontal cortex**, in front of area 6, is eugranular and shows a well-developed internal granular layer.

4. **Area 10**, the frontal pole cortex, gets thinner, as is typical of polar cortex, but it maintains the standard six layers.

J. Cytoarchitecture of the parietal, temporal, and occipital neocortex (see Fig. 13-34)

1. The hypergranular (striate) cortex (see Fig. 13-34*D*) of areas 3, 1, and 2 of the postcentral gyrus undergoes a gradual transition posteriorly to eugranular cortex (see Fig. 13-34*C*).

2. Striate cortex characterizes the primary sensory receptive cortex of:
   a. Areas 3, 1, and 2 (somesthetic) of the parietal lobe
   b. Areas 41 and 42 (auditory) of the temporal lobe
   c. Area 17 (visual) of the occipital lobe

3. The remainder of the parietal, temporal, and occipital lobes is eugranular and resembles the eugranular cortex of the prefrontal region. While variations do exist in the cytoarchitecture in these regions, they are not as striking as the differences in motor and sensory cortex.

K. Cytoarchitecture of the limbic lobe

1. In limbic cortex, the granular neurons occur less frequently in layers II and IV, with more neurons being pyramidal.

2. The radial striations are less distinct than in many other areas.

3. Specific thalamic afferents tend to end in the external lamina, layers I to III, and the efferents tend to arise from the internal lamina, layers IV to VI.
   a. Looked at in another way, the thalamic afferents tend to be offset a layer closer to the surface. This apparently reflects a more primitive phylogenetic feature because in the rodent, thalamic afferents extend to layer I.
   b. The dendrites of the neurons in layer II of limbic cortex extend into layer I to receive the synaptic contacts.

VI. FUNCTIONAL LOCALIZATION IN THE CEREBRUM AND CLINICAL SYNDROMES

A. Representation of movement

1. In the past, the criterion for **motor areas** was that electrical stimulation elicited movements and lesions caused paralysis.
   a. Now, new scanning techniques allow direct, noninvasive identification of the active neural tissue involved in cerebral events by radioactive measurement of neuronal metabolism [positron emission tomography (PET) scanning].
   b. The old and new methods confirm the existence of three more or less contiguous motor areas in the frontal lobes bilaterally: **classic motor area**, **supplementary motor area**, and **frontal eye fields** (Fig. 13-36).

2. The **classic motor area** occupies the precentral gyrus, areas 4 and 6, with some spillover into the postcentral gyrus. Stimulation causes a discrete, upside-down somatotopic activation of contralateral muscles through the pyramidal system (Fig. 13-37; see Fig. 13-37*B*).

3. The **supplementary motor area** occupies the medial hemispheric wall, in area 6, just anterior to the lumbosacral representation in area 4 of the classic motor area.
   a. Stimulation of the supplementary motor area produces postural movements, which are more complex and more bilateral than the discrete movements resulting from stimulation of the classic motor area.
   b. Unilateral destruction of this area causes no clear motor syndrome in man, but radioactive scanning suggests that it may be involved in motor planning. For example, when a person thinks about moving one hand, this area shows an increase in metabolism before the classic motor area shows activation.
   c. In some patients, infarction of the left supplementary area causes aphasia (see section VI G).

4. The **frontal eye field** is in the posterior part of the middle frontal gyrus, approximately the inferior part of area 8.
   a. Stimulation causes **contra**lateral conjugate deviation of the eyes. Destruction results in **ipsi**lateral conjugate deviation of both eyes.

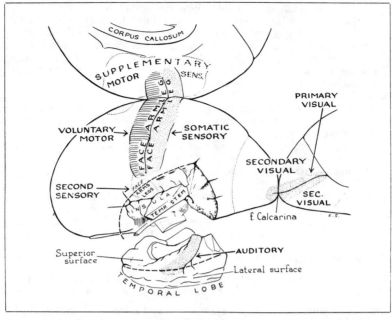

Figure 13-36. Map showing the location of the motor (*lined*) and sensory (*dotted*) areas of a cerebral hemisphere. (Reprinted with permission from Penfield W, Roberts L: *Speech and Brain Mechanisms*. Princeton, University Press, 1959, p 32.)

b. An **occipital eye field** is located on facies lateralis of the occipital lobe. It turns the eyes contralaterally.

5. Apraxia
   a. Definition. Apraxia is the inability of a previously normal person with an acquired cerebral lesion to execute a normal volitional act, even though the motor systems and mental status are relatively intact and the person is not paralyzed. The lesions affect cerebral areas around or distant from the primary motor area but do not involve it.

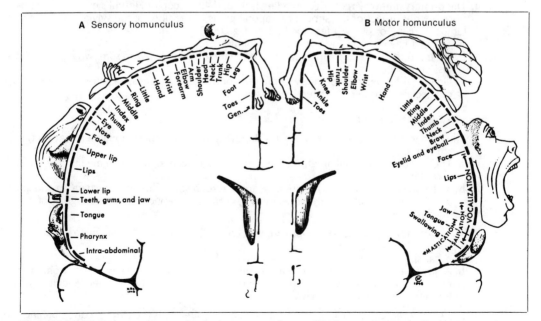

Figure 13-37. (*A*) Sensory representation in the postcentral gyrus. (*B*) Motor representation in the precentral gyrus. (Reprinted with permission from Penfield W, Rasmussen T: *The Cerebral Cortex of Man*. New York, Hafner Publishing, 1968, pp 44, 57.)

(1) The apraxias differ from the well-categorized LMN, pyramidal (see Table 7-3), cerebellar (see Fig. 9-13), and basal motor (see Table 11-2) syndromes. The patient behaves as if the motor engrams or templates for movements have been lost.

(2) As with the pyramidal tract, the discussion of apraxia is limited to the effects of postnatal lesions inflicted on previously normal brains. Transfer of the concepts and terminology of adult neurology to children with prenatal lesions and learning disabilities is fraught with scientific pitfalls.

b. Speech apraxia

(1) An area in the posterior end of the inferior frontal gyrus, approximately area 44, close to the primary motor cortex, controls the bulbar muscles to produce speech.

(2) After its destruction on the left side, the patient loses the ability to utter words, but the bulbar muscles are not paralyzed for other voluntary actions, such as biting, if the primary motor area is spared.

c. Writing apraxia (dysgraphia). Lesions of the left angular gyrus region may cause dysgraphia. The patient loses the ability to form letters, although the arm is not paralyzed.

d. In **dressing apraxia,** the patient cannot orient the clothes to place them on the body. Dressing apraxia usually results from a lesion in the posterior part of the right parietal lobe.

e. In **gait apraxia,** the patient becomes unable to stand and walk, although he is not paralyzed. Gait apraxia is usually associated with diffuse cerebral disease.

B. Representation of general and special somatic sensation

1. Primary sensory areas are the **somatosensory area** of the postcentral gyrus, the **visual area** along the calcarine sulcus, and the **auditory area** of the transverse temporal gyri.

2. The primary **somatosensory area** (areas 3, 1, and 2) has a somatotopy closely resembling that of the classic motor area (see Fig. 13-37A).

a. A secondary sensory area is located on the superior lip of the sylvian fissure, adjacent to the insula (see Fig. 13-36).

b. Both sensory areas receive relays from the nucleus ventralis posterior, but as with the classic and supplementary motor cortices, the secondary sensory area has a less discrete somatotopy.

c. No special clinical syndrome related to destruction of the secondary sensory area is known in man.

3. The **primary visual receptive area** (area 17) occupies the superior and inferior banks of the calcarine sulcus. It has a strict retinotopic representation of the macula and contralateral visual field (see Fig. 10-9).

4. The **primary auditory receptive area** (areas 41 and 42) occupies Heschl's gyrus on the posterior–superior aspect of the superior temporal gyrus in the floor of the sylvian fissure (supratemporal plane or planum temporale) [see Fig. 13-7].

a. The gyri have a strict tonotopic representation.

b. Destruction of one auditory area reduces hearing bilaterally, with somewhat more severe loss contralaterally.

c. Unilateral lesions do not cause complete contralateral deafness because of the bilateral connections through the lateral lemniscus.

C. Sensory association areas

1. The primary sensory receptive areas just described represent their modalities in a strict, keyboard topography.

a. The cerebrum must still interpret the symbolic significance or overall meaning of the sensory stimuli.

b. The cortex surrounding the primary areas rerepresents the sensory data to integrate, analyze, or **associate** it with the memories, current perceptions, and future goals of the individual.

2. The **visual association cortex,** approximately areas 18 and 19, gives meaning to visual stimuli, either words or objects.

a. A car speeding toward a person is a pattern of dots on area 17.

b. Areas 18 and 19 rerepresent the car's configuration and associate it with data from the rest of the brain. Thus, the brain recognizes the car, perceives its direction and velocity, and interprets it as a threat to survival.

3. The **somatosensory association area,** approximately area 7, is the strip of cortex behind the postcentral sulcus. It gives meaning or recognition to impulses from the skin afferents and proprioceptors.

4. The **auditory association area**, approximately area 22, gives meaning to sounds and, more importantly, to spoken words.

D. Contrasting effects of lesions of primary sensory and association areas

1. Destruction of primary sensory areas or of the pathways leading to them through receptors, nerves, the spinal cord, lemnisci, the thalamus, or thalamic peduncles causes defects that match the topography and modality of the pathway. The patient suffers numbness, hypesthesia or anesthesia, blindness, or deafness.

2. Irritative lesions of the respective sensory pathways or their primary sensory cortex cause tingling or paresthesias, flashes of light, or ringing, buzzing sounds.

3. Destructive lesions of association cortex rob the individual of the **meaning** or **symbolic significance** of the primary sensation. Such defects of perception are called **agnosias**.

E. Agnosias

1. **Definition**. Agnosia is the inability of a previously normal person who has an acquired cerebral lesion to recognize the symbolic significance or meaning of a sensory stimulus, even though the sensory pathway and primary sensory cortex are sufficiently intact to register the stimulus and the mental status is relatively intact.

2. **Common somatosensory agnosias due to lesions of the parietal lobe association area**
   a. **Astereognosis** (a means not; stereo means form; gnosis means knowing) is the inability to recognize the form of an object placed in the hand. For example, a patient cannot distinguish a paper clip from a safety pin by feeling the objects.
   b. **Astatognosia** (a means not; stat means station; gnosia means knowing) is the inability to recognize the position of the body parts.

3. **Common visual agnosias due to occipital lobe lesions**. Two important visual agnosias are for faces (prosopagnosia) and words (dyslexia).
   a. **Prosopagnosia** is the inability to recognize faces (face blindness) in the presence of intact visual pathways and primary visual cortex. The lesion responsible for prosopagnosia is in the association cortex of the temporo-occipital region on facies inferior (inferomedialis) of the hemisphere.
   b. **Dyslexia** is the inability to recognize written words or the meaning of words (word blindness) in the presence of intact visual pathways and primary visual cortex. The lesion responsible for word agnosia is in the association cortex of the left occipital lobe on facies lateralis.

4. The auditory agnosia for spoken words (word deafness) resulting from lesions of the auditory association area (area 22) of the temporal lobe compares with dyslexia (word blindness).

F. Anatomical connections of the primary cortical sensory areas and the association areas

1. The primary cortical sensory areas receive their thalamocortical afferents from the sensory relay nuclei. The association areas receive their thalamic afferents from the association (ectocortical) nuclei of the thalamus.

2. The primary sensory areas connect with their association areas by means of horizontal fibers in the laminae of the cortex and arcuate fibers.

3. The more generalized meanings may come from:
   a. Numerous progressive arcuate cascades (see Fig. 13-25), which extend the associations like a Huygens wave front
   b. Long association fibers
   c. Callosal connections

4. The **primary sensory areas** have few commissural connections through the corpus callosum. These areas are for discrete, topographic representations.

5. The **association areas** have rich callosal connections in keeping with their role to disperse their information to form the widest associations of the primary sensory data.

G. Representation of language: the aphasias

1. **We express language, or we receive it**. We express it through **speaking** or **writing** or receive it through **auditing** or **reading**. Thus, we **speak/listen** or **write/read**. Disorders in expressing or receiving words as symbols for communication are called **aphasia**.

2. Definition. Aphasia is the inability of a previously normal person with an acquired cerebral lesion to understand or express words as symbols for communication, even though the primary sensory systems, motor mechanisms of phonation, and mental state (sensorium) are relatively intact.

3. Anatomical basis for language reception and expression

    a. In most normal individuals, the critical region for receiving and expressing language is the left parasylvian area (Fig. 13-38) and its connections with itself by means of arcuate fasciculi and with the left thalamus through the thalamic peduncles.

    b. Anatomically, the left sylvian fissure is somewhat longer than the right, and the supratemporal plane is larger in area. A prominent **arcuate fasciculus** runs around the posterior ramus of the sylvian fissure into the posterior inferior frontal region, connecting the centers for receptive and expressive speech.

    c. Lesions of the left thalamus, which connects with the parasylvian area, give rise to syndromes of aphasia similar to those resulting from lesions of the cortex or intervening white matter of the thalamic peduncles.

    d. Speech is also represented to some extent in the left supplementary motor area, since its destruction may cause aphasia.

4. Types of aphasia and localizing significance. The types of expressive and receptive aphasia correlate fairly well with the location of the lesion within the aphasic zone (Table 13-8; see Fig. 13-38). Lesions in site 1 of Figure 13-38 cause mainly a nonfluent, expressive aphasia, with relative preservation of receptive language. In this nonfluent, or Broca's, aphasia, the patient produces few words. Lesions in sites 2–4 of Figure 13-38 tend to impair language reception. The patient produces many words and speech sounds, but they are garbled and incomprehensible, so-called Wernicke's fluent aphasia.

H. Gerstmann's syndrome: a left posterior parasylvian area syndrome

    1. Lesions of the left angular and supramarginal gyrus region tend to produce Gerstmann's syndrome, consisting of dysgraphia, dyscalculia, right–left disorientation, and finger agnosia (inability to recognize and name one's own or the examiner's fingers).

    2. Some degree of aphasia, including dyslexia, is also present. The aphasia and other components of the syndrome vary from patient to patient.

I. Left-sided hemineglect: a right posterior parasylvian area syndrome

    1. Right hemisphere lesions, almost mirroring in location those causing Gerstmann's syndrome, spare language, but cause a very different set of deficits. The patient:

        a. Lacks awareness of the left half of space—he or she ignores tactile, auditory, and visual stimuli from the left side and even ignores food on the left half of the plate

        b. Is unable to draw the left half of figures or designs and is unable to reproduce match-stick constructions (constructional apraxia)

        c. Is unable to orient clothes for dressing (dressing apraxia)

        d. Often does not appreciate the existence of neurologic defects, even when the lesion extends to the paracentral area, causing hemiplegia and hemianesthesia. Failure to recognize such defects is called **anosognosia** (a means not; noso means disease; gnosia means knowing).

    2. In summary, the patient shows left-sided inattention to sensory stimuli and unawareness of

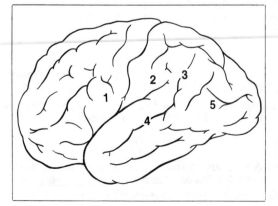

Figure 13-38. Lateral view of the left cerebral hemisphere, the one dominant for language. *1* = Posterior inferior frontal area of Broca. *2* = Inferior parietal lobule (parietal operculum). *3* = Angular gyrus. *4* = Posterior superior temporal gyrus area of Wernicke. *5* = Confluence of the parietal, occipital, and temporal lobes.

Table 13-8. Types of Aphasia As Related to the Site of the Lesion*

Type	Clinical Features	Lesion Site
Global aphasia	Inability to speak/audit or read/write	Entire left parasylvian area (sites 1–4 of Figure 13-38)
Motor aphasia (speech apraxia, Broca's aphasia, nonfluent aphasia)	Inability to utter words; comprehension of speech by auditing or reading remains relatively intact	Posterior part of inferior frontal gyrus (site 1 of Figure 13-38)
Agraphia (writing apraxia, without conspicuous speech apraxia)	Inability to write words, spell, or form letters correctly	Left angular-supramarginal gyrus area (site 3 of Figure 13-38); agraphia of another type may follow lesions of the posterior third of the middle frontal gyrus
"Pure" word deafness	Inability to understand spoken words	Posterior part of the superior temporal gyrus (site 4 of Figure 13-38)
"Pure" word blindness	Inability to understand written words	Anterior part of the occipital lobe at its junction with the temporal lobe (site 5 of Figure 13-38)
Wernicke's aphasia (fluent aphasia)	Inability to comprehend spoken or written language; the patient makes fluent vocalizations, which have the phrasing and rhythm of language but consist of parts of words mixed together—a "word salad," devoid of meaning; dyslexia may also be present	Inferior posterior part of the parietal lobe at its junctions with the temporal and occipital lobes (site 3 of Figure 13-38, extending toward sites 2 and 4)
Conduction aphasia	Similar to Wernicke's aphasia, but the patient retains understanding of written and spoken words while being unable to produce them	Interruption of the upper limb of the arcuate bundle (site 2 of Figure 13-38) resulting in disconnection of the auditory and visual receptive area from Broca's area

*Compare to Figure 13-38.

the left half of space (left-sided spatial agnosia), left-sided constructional apraxia, and dressing apraxia; the patient is often unaware of the deficits (anosognosia).

J. Syndromes of the right and left cerebral hemispheres are summarized in Figure 13-39.

K. Representation of recent memory

1. The discussion involves only recent memory, since we know much more about its anatomical substrate than about memory for remote events.

2. **Pure amnestic syndrome**
   a. This syndrome is characterized by temporal disorientation—the patient cannot remember the day, date, time, or current events but can remember previously learned information and skills. The memory is, as it were, frozen in time.
   b. Other mental functions, along with motor and sensory functions, remain relatively intact. The patient walks around, talks normally, reads, and can calculate. The patient shows no motor or sensory loss, apraxia, or agnosia, and may do well on IQ tests.

3. **Anatomical basis of the pure amnestic syndrome.** Lesions that cause pure amnesia involve one or more of the following structures, usually bilaterally (Fig. 13-40), the:
   a. Medial, inferior quadrant of the temporal lobe, including the hippocampal formation
   b. Stalk of white matter connecting it with the thalamus (inferior thalamic peduncle)
   c. Nucleus medialis dorsalis of the thalamus
   d. Fornix/mamillary bodies

4. Although the lesion frequently involves the hippocampus–fornix and mamillary body circuit,

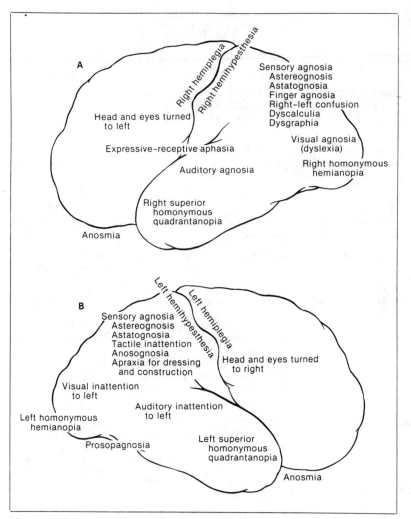

Figure 13-39. Summary of some of the outstanding neurologic signs and symptoms that occur with focal destructive lesions in the right or left cerebral hemisphere as detected upon neurologic examination. (*A*) Lateral view of the left cerebral hemisphere. (*B*) Lateral view of the right cerebral hemisphere. Notice that some signs and symptoms, such as hemiplegia, are common to both hemispheres.

particularly in Korsakoff's syndrome (see Chapter 12, section III E 7), the exact role of the individual parts of the circuit is unclear.

    a. Neurosurgical section of the anterior pillars of the fornix, as has been done in an attempt to treat epileptic seizures, does not cause amnesia, nor do pure lesions of the mamillary bodies.

    b. However, recent work suggests that a lesion of the fornix in its commissural region may cause loss of recent memory.

  5. Any diffuse cerebral disease, including the normal effects of aging, also selectively impairs recent memory before remote memory. However, as the disease advances, the patient shows global dementia rather than pure amnesia for recent memory.

L. Representation of ''higher'' mental functions

  1. To this point the text has described clinical deficits that correlate strongly with local lesions of the cerebrum.

  2. The cerebrum appears to represent many so-called higher mental functions generally or in several sites, rather than in specific centers. Focal brain lesions may impair but do not specifi-

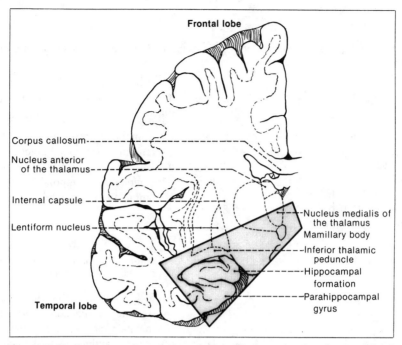

Figure 13-40. Coronal section of a cerebral hemisphere showing the "corridor," which, when damaged bilaterally, causes amnesia. (Adapted with permission from Horel JA: The neuroanatomy of memory. *Brain* 101: 403–445, 1978.)

cally abolish functions such as foresight, planning, socially appropriate behavior, conscience, and cognition. Lesions of limbic circuits may alter mood and affective responses. Limbic lesions may result in hypersexuality and murderous aggression or passivity and taming effects, but again correlation of these clinical disorders with lesion sites is imperfect.

VII. EPILOGUE. As humans, we all share an ultimate, common perception of life as a process, as a series of ongoing events, of **who** we and others are, **where** we are, **when** it is, and **what** is happening. Answering these adverbial questions of who, where, when, and what, we arrive at a common sense of **how** it is appropriate to behave. We come in out of the rain and do not try to walk through walls. We speak gently to the ill, the old, and the unfortunate, and we don't shout "Fire!" in a crowded theater. Our common sense warns us not to try to mount our neighbor's mate, even though our limbic system urges us on. This common sense, the **sensorium commune** of ancient philosophers, depends on reticular formation, thalamic, and cortical circuitry, but to try to specify which neurons and which circuits would require an idiot's audacity. Nevertheless, our mind has a structural basis. Lesions of this structure alter thought, will, and behavior. To understand the brain/thought/behavior triumvirate is the Holy Grail of neuroanatomy, as compelling to the researcher as a cyclonic vortex.

STUDY QUESTIONS

Directions: Each question below contains five suggested answers. Choose the **one best** response to each question.

1. The stem of the lateral (sylvian) fissure extends

(A) medially from the parahippocampal gyrus
(B) laterally from the vallecula (the anterior perforated space)
(C) from the anterior ascending ramus to the tip of the posterior ramus
(D) vertically through the inferior frontal gyrus
(E) none of the above

2. The main efferent layers of the cerebral cortex are

(A) layers IV and VI
(B) layers V and VI
(C) layers I and II
(D) layers III and IV
(E) none of the above

3. One of the great differences between archicortex and ectocortex (neocortex) is

(A) absence of lamination in archicortex
(B) lack of significant function of archicortex
(C) presence of a superficial layer of white matter in archicortex
(D) absence of pyramidal neurons in archicortex
(E) scarcity of pathways between archicortex and the limbic system

4. The inferior longitudinal fasciculus connects the

(A) frontal and occipital lobes
(B) temporal and frontal poles
(C) parietal lobe and frontal poles
(D) occipital and temporal lobes
(E) limbic and temporal lobes

5. After interruption of the corpus callosum the patient would be unable to

(A) feel sensation in the hands
(B) execute a verbal command with the left hand
(C) maintain bladder and bowel control
(D) perform arithmetical calculations
(E) maintain consciousness

6. Anosognosia is most characteristic of which of the following lesions?

(A) Diffuse cerebral disease
(B) Left posterior parasylvian area lesions
(C) Right posterior parasylvian area lesions
(D) Left temporal lobe lesions
(E) Right frontal lobe lesions

Directions: Each question below contains four suggested answers of which **one or more** is correct. Choose the answer

A if **1, 2, and 3** are correct
B if **1 and 3** are correct
C if **2 and 4** are correct
D if **4** is correct
E if **1, 2, 3, and 4** are correct

7. The body parts having a large relative representation in the sensorimotor cortex include the

(1) trunk
(2) thumb and little finger
(3) neck
(4) tongue

8. The cerebellar cortex differs from the cerebral cortex in having

(1) a surface layer of white matter
(2) indistinct lamination of its layers
(3) only two types of neurons
(4) only one neuronal type that originates corticofugal axons

9. Correct statements about the corpus callosum include which of the following?

A

(1) It is the largest bundle of fibers that crosses the midline of the CNS
(2) Its splenium connects cortex of the posterior parts of the cerebral hemispheres
(3) The fornix and fornix commissure attach to its ventral surface
(4) It conveys most of the projection fibers from the two cerebral hemispheres to lower centers

10. Characteristic features of the cerebral cortex include which of the following?

(1) Radial or columnar arrangement of neurons
(2) Laminar arrangement of neurons
(3) Grossly visible stripes of myelinated fibers
E (4) Numerous pyramidal neurons

without dementia & paralysis, inability to dress up & draw.

11. Correct statements about apraxia include which of the following?

B

(1) Bilateral pyramidal tract interruption would preclude testing a patient for apraxia
(2) Language apraxia implies a right hemisphere lesion
(3) Apraxia can result from lesions of the cortex and the thalamocortical circuits as well
(4) Dyslexia is a form of aphasic apraxia

PIPC

12. The ring of limbic cortex includes which of the following structures?

(1) Parahippocampal gyrus
(2) Cingulate gyrus
(3) Posterior orbital cortex of frontal lobes
E (4) Insular cortex

FM

13. Pathways in the classic Papez (visceral brain) circuit include the

(1) occipitofrontal fasciculus
(2) fornix
(3) ansa lenticularis
(4) mamillothalamic tract

14. Fissures differ from sulci because they

A

(1) form earlier
(2) are longer
(3) are deeper
(4) are more numerous

FM

15. The Papez circuit, which Papez proposed as the anatomical substrate of emotional experience and expression, consists of the

(1) hippocampus/fornix
(2) mamillothalamic tract
(3) cingulum
(4) fasciculus lenticularis

16. True statements about the surface contours of the brain include which of the following?

A

(1) The medial face is the flattest surface
(2) The lateral face is strongly convex
(3) The orbital surface is faintly concave
(4) The temporo-occipital region of the inferomedial face is concave

Directions: The groups of questions below consist of lettered choices followed by several numbered items. For each numbered item select the **one** lettered choice with which it is **most** closely associated. Each lettered choice may be used once, more than once, or not at all.

Questions 17–21

Match the cortical areas with their identifying anatomical characteristics.

(A) Has a conspicuous internal granular layer and an outer line of Baillarger
(B) Has very large pyramidal neurons in layer V
(C) Has three layers of neurons
(D) In general is the thinnest cortex
(E) Has no striking features

17. Precentral gyrus (area 4)
18. Calcarine cortex
19. Association cortex
20. Polar cortex
21. Postcentral gyrus (areas 3, 1, and 2)

Questions 22–26

Match the clinical deficit with the expected lesion site.

(A) Left posterior parasylvian area
(B) Right posterior parasylvian area
(C) Either parietal lobe, behind areas 3, 1, and 2
(D) Inferior medial quadrants of temporal lobes
(E) Medial inferior temporo-occipital region

22. Expressive (fluent) aphasia
23. Loss of recent memory
24. Dyscalculia, dysgraphia, right–left disorientation, and finger agnosia
25. Prosopagnosia
26. Astereognosis

Questions 27–31

Match the cortical cell type with the usual orientation of its axon.

(A) Directed toward the white matter
(B) Directed toward the cortical surface
(C) Directed tangential to the cortical surface
(D) More or less randomly directed on leaving the perikaryon
(E) None listed

27. Pyramidal neurons
28. Stellate neurons
29. Martinotti neurons
30. Fusiform neurons of layer VI
31. Horizontal neurons of Cajal

Questions 32–36

Match each description below with the relevant fissure or space.

(A) Choroid fissure
(B) Cavum veli interpositi
(C) Sylvian fissure
(D) Cavum septi pellicidi
(E) Transverse cerebral fissure

32. Forms by invagination of the medial wall of the cerebral hemispheres
33. Located between the fornices and the anterior part of the corpus callosum
34. Formed when the corpus callosum enlarges posteriorly from the commissural plate
35. The roof of the third ventricle forms its floor
36. The hippocampal formation forms its floor

ANSWERS AND EXPLANATIONS

1. The answer is B. [*I E 1 (a) (1); Figure 13-9*] The stem of the lateral fissure commences at the anterior perforated substance in a little depression called the vallecula and extends laterally from that region, separating the temporal pole from the overlying posterior inferior aspect of the frontal lobe.

2. The answer is B. (*V G 2*) The cortical layers can be divided according to whether they are mainly receptive or efferent in nature. The superficial layers from IV up tend to be receptive, and the deeper layers, including V and VI, tend to be efferent; however, this is by no means a dichotomous classification.

3. The answer is C. (*V C 2 a*) Archicortex and neocortex are both distinctly laminated. Both types of cortex contain pyramidal neurons, and both have numerous connections with the limbic system. One major difference is that archicortex has a distinct superficial layer of nerve fibers or white matter in comparison to ectocortex or neocortex, which has its white matter on its inner surface and forms the deep white matter of the cerebral wall.

4. The answer is D. (*IV D 2 b*) The inferior longitudinal fasciculus is one of the many bundles that connects different regions of the cerebral cortex. Although it is generally depicted as a single bundle of long axons, recent studies suggest that it consists of a series of arcuate cascades rather than a single pathway composed of long fibers.

5. The answer is B. (*IV F 4*) The corpus callosum connects the two hemispheres and functions for the interhemispheric transfer of information. After interruption of the corpus callosum, the patient cannot execute a command with his left hand but will do so readily with the right. The left hemisphere understands the command and can direct the right extremities by means of the pyramidal tract to execute the command. The right hemisphere does not understand the command because it lacks a language center. After interruption of the corpus callosum, the left hemisphere cannot inform the right hemisphere of the command.

6. The answer is C. (*VI I 1 d*) Functional localization in the two hemispheres differs even though anatomically the hemispheres appear to be mirror images of each other. A large acute destructive lesion of the right hemisphere, extending from the motor area into the posterior parietal or posterior parasylvian area, will result in left-sided hemiparesis and left-sided inattention, with the patient often being unaware of these defects. The condition of unawareness of a bodily defect is called anosognosia. A lesion of the corresponding region of the left hemisphere causes aphasia, not anosognosia.

7. The answer is C (2, 4). (*Figure 13-37*) Several of the body parts have a larger area of cortex devoted to their motor and sensory representation than other parts. The largest representations involve the tongue, the thumb and little finger, and the corresponding digits of the foot, as well as the hands and feet in general. Apparently the complexity of motor actions and sensory contacts of these regions requires a larger cortical circuitry than the simpler movements and sensations mediated by the trunk.

8. The answer is D (4). (*V D, F, G*) The cerebellar cortex differs from the cerebral cortex in having only three layers; the cerebral cortex typically has six. It has five types of neurons but only one type, the Purkinje cell, originates corticofugal axons.

9. The answer is A (1, 2, 3). [*IV F 1 b, c (1); Figure 13-28*] The corpus callosum is the largest bundle of commissural fibers in the CNS. It connects mirror image points of the two cerebral hemispheres. Anteriorly it has a rostrum, genu, and body and posteriorly a splenium, which connects the cortex of the posterior parts of the cerebral hemispheres.

10. The answer is E (all). (*V D 1, 3 c, E 1, F 3*) The cerebral cortex in general is characterized by a laminar arrangement of neurons, which also form radial or columnar groupings. It contains numerous pyramidal neurons, which have their axons directed toward the white matter and which constitute most of the commissural, projection, and association fibers of the cerebrum. Several sections of the cortex contain grossly visible stripes of myelinated fibers. These are most conspicuous in the sensory receptive areas.

11. The answer is B (1, 3). [*VI A 5 a, b (1), c (2)*] Apraxia is the inability of a patient who is not paralyzed and who does not have dementia to perform a normal volitional act. Examples would be dressing apraxia (inability to orient the clothes to put them on) or construction apraxia (inability to copy or draw geometric figures). The expressive forms of aphasia, involving spoken or written language, can be thought of as language apraxia.

12. The answer is E (all). (*I G; Table 13-1; Figure 13-11*) The so-called limbic lobe forms a ring of structures around the hemispheric hilus. It is bordered internally by the rhinencephalon and externally by ectocortex. The cortical surface of the ring consists of the cingulate gyrus and its isthmus to the parahippocampal gyrus, the uncus and insula, the posterior orbital cortex, and the parolfactory and subcallosal gyri. The latter gyri lead back to the cingulate gyrus to complete the ring.

13. The answer is C (2, 4). (*II D 1, 2; Figure 13-16*) The classic Papez circuit includes the hippocampus, fornix, mamillary bodies, mamillothalamic tract, and the thalamocortical projection from the nucleus anterior to the cingulate gyrus and then through the cingulum back to the temporal lobe and hippocampus. This pathway mediates emotional experience and its expression through visceral activities.

14. The answer is A (1, 2, 3). (*I D*) The surface of the cerebrum shows furrows of two types, fissures and sulci. Fissures form earlier than sulci and are longer and deeper. In general, they result from evagination of the cerebral hemispheres from the forebrain and from evagination of the temporal lobes from the hemispheres themselves. After the process of evagination has created the fissures, numerous smaller crevices called sulci commence to appear on the cerebral surface at about the twentieth week of gestation.

15. The answer is A (1, 2, 3). (*II D 1; Figure 13-16*) James Papez proposed that a circuit linking limbic structures was essential for the experience and behavioral expression of emotion and certain instinctive behaviors. The various pathways of the basal motor nuclei and thalamus, related to somatomotor control and feeding back mainly through the pyramidal tract, are not part of this circuit.

16. The answer is A (1, 2, 3). (*I B 1*) The medial face is flat where the cerebral hemispheres abut on the cerebral falx. At the superior margin of the hemispheres, the lateral face is distinctly convex, reflecting the contours of the calvaria. The temporo-occipital region inferomedially is convex, reflecting the contour of the tentorium cerebelli, upon which this part of the cerebrum rests. The orbital surface of the frontal lobe is made concave by the bulging orbital roof upon which it rests.

17–21. The answers are: 17-B, 18-A, 19-E, 20-D, 21-A. (*V H 4 c, I 1 a, 4, J 3*) Some regions of neocortex or ectocortex have specific structural features, whereas the majority of the cortex, generally called association areas, looks much the same, lacking conspicuous regional differences or unique characteristics.

The motor and sensory cortices have the most striking regional variations. The precentral gyrus is thick and has the largest cortical neurons, the neurons of Betz, in layer V. It has no distinct internal granular layer.

Sensory cortex (somatosensory, visual, and auditory) has a thick, distinct layer IV (internal granular layer) and a distinct outer stripe of Baillarger. This stripe represents the incoming thalamic afferents from the sensory relay nuclei of the thalamus. They penetrate the deeper layers of the cortex at right angles to the cortical surface and then branch horizontally to run parallel to the cortical surface as stripes of Baillarger.

Even the cortical areas lacking these conspicuous features show minor variations from site to site in the thickness of the individual layers and in the density and size of neurons in the layers. On the crests of the gyri, the cortex is thicker than where it bends around the depths of the sulci.

The cortex of the poles in general is the thinnest and has the least number of neurons per unit of volume. The first and, to a lesser extent, second cortical layers show the least regional variations from site to site.

22–26. The answers are: 22-A, 23-D, 24-A, 25-E, 26-C. (*VI E 2 a, 3 a, G 3 a, H 1, K 3 a*) Lesions of some areas of the cerebrum cause definite clinical syndromes with specific defects, whereas lesions of the parts of the cortex known as association areas may cause some personality and behavioral changes without having specific features. For example, lesions of the frontal poles do not cause any evident hemiplegia, sensory loss, or disturbance of language, but will reduce the general drive of the individual and may cause subtle changes in the personality.

Lesions of the left posterior parasylvian area, if located more toward the occipital lobe, tend to cause a syndrome of dyscalculia, dysgraphia, right–left disorientation, and finger agnosia. These features tend to merge with some degree of receptive aphasia. The receptive aphasia would be more obvious with lesions of the posterior parasylvian area, which involve the inferior part of the parietal lobe and extend around into the posterior superior part of the temporal lobe.

Loss of recent memory will result from lesions of the medial quadrant of the temporal lobe. Such individuals again will have no obvious motor, sensory, or language deficits. They tend to retain their remote memory.

Lesions that affect the inferior part of the temporo-occipital region tend to cause a peculiar agnosia for faces, a defect known as prosopagnosia. These patients cannot recognize a person's face either with the person present or in the form of a photograph. In prosopagnosia, there may be some encroachment on the geniculocalcarine pathway if the lesion is large, but the visual field defect does not cause the agnosia for faces.

Lesions of the parietal lobe behind the postcentral gyrus will cause astereognosis or stereoagnosia, in which the patient fails to recognize the form of objects felt with the fingers but not looked at. This will usually be combined with other forms of agnosia, such as the inability to recognize numbers written on the skin of the palm or fingers. If the lesion is anterior in the parietal lobes, affecting the postcentral gyrus and its sensory receptive area, the patient may not recognize the form of the object. If the primary cortex were interrupted, the condition would be called stereoanesthesia rather than stereoagnosia. In agnosia, the sensory pathway to the cortex and the primary receptive cortex have to be intact. The lesion causing agnosia involves the so-called association areas adjacent to the primary sensory areas. The association areas of the cortex give meaning and recognition to the primary sensory stimuli.

27–31. The answers are: 27-A, 28-D, 29-B, 30-A, 31-C. (*V F 3 c, 4 a, 5, 6, 7 a*) Although the cerebral cortex consists of neurons that vary greatly in size and type, they can be classified into five fundamental groups.

Pyramidal neurons are found throughout the first three layers of the cortex; they increase in size toward the depth of the cortex and encroach into layer IV.

Layer V in particular and, to a lesser degree, layer VI have large numbers of pyramidal neurons and fusiform neurons. Both types of neurons have their axons directed toward the white matter and give rise to cortical efferent pathways. The pyramidal neurons have the greatest variation in the size of the perikaryon, dendritic branching, and axon diameter. The large Betz cells with their myelin sheaths may be upward of 20 μ in diameter. Although providing perhaps only 25,000 of the 1,200,000 axons of the pyramidal tract, they are the fastest conducting axons.

The stellate or granular neurons are concentrated in layer IV, a very thick layer in the sensory receptive cortex; they have a more random orientation of both axons and dendrites. These are mainly intracortical association neurons or cortical interneurons.

Similarly, Martinotti neurons and the horizontal neurons of Cajal are cortical interneurons. Their circuits modify the afferent input into the cortex and integrate it to affect ultimately the efferent neurons of the cortex. The Martinotti neurons have their axons directed toward the surface of the cortex. The horizontal neurons of Cajal are confined to the first layer of the cortex. They are the only neuronal type in that layer, which has the fewest neurons of any of the six standard cortical layers.

32–36. The answers are: 32-E, 33-D, 34-B, 35-B, 36-A. (*I D 2 c, d; II C 1; III C 2 b, 3; Figure 13-19*) The midline anatomy of the cerebrum can only be understood by reference to its embryology (ontogeny). The roof plate of the prosencephalon is a membrane that covers the lateral and third ventricles (see Fig. 13-19). Invagination of the medial hemispheric wall with rolling in of the hippocampal formation creates the transverse cerebral fissure. As the hippocampus migrates posteriorly and inferiorly with the evagination of the temporal lobe, the transverse cerebral fissure is continued as the choroid fissure, with the hippocampal formation forming its floor in the temporal lobe.

As the corpus callosum enlarges posteriorly, it covers the fornix and fornix commissure, which constitute the immediate roof of the cavum veli interpositi. The roof of the third ventricle is the floor of the cavum. In agenesis of the corpus callosum, no cavum veli interpositi is present.

The cavum septi pellucidi has as its floor the anterior pillars of the fornices and as its roof the undersurface of the corpus callosum. Its lateral walls are the septum pellucidum, one leaf of which extends to the corpus callosum from each fornix.

14
Chemical Neuroanatomy

I. SPECIFICATION OF NEURONS AND TRACTS BY NEUROTRANSMITTER CHEMISTRY

A. Discovery of the chemical transmission of the nerve impulse

1. The theory that electrical messages crossed synapses began to topple in the 1920s and 1930s when neuroscientists discovered that peripheral nerves, when stimulated, released chemical substances at their endings. The chemical substances, catecholamines and acetylcholine, reproduced the effects of nerve stimulation when applied directly to the postsynaptic neuron or effector.

2. Beginning in the mid-1950s, new techniques confirmed the presence of peripheral nervous system (PNS) neurotransmitters in the central nervous system (CNS) and disclosed many new neurotransmitters.
   a. The new techniques include analytic chemistry, enzyme histochemistry, immunocytochemistry, radioactive labeling of metabolites, and the use of fluorescence microscopy for demonstration of catecholamines in situ in CNS neurons.
   b. Many catecholaminergic tracts, now readily demonstrated by fluorescence microscopy, eluded the classic methods of tract demonstration because they consist of fine axons that lack myelin sheaths and do not readily accept silver impregnation.

B. According to their neurotransmitters, tracts are classified into one of four types:

1. **Monoaminergic**
   a. **Catecholaminergic**
      (1) **Adrenergic**
      (2) **Noradrenergic**
      (3) **Dopaminergic**
   b. **Serotonergic**

2. **Cholinergic**

3. **Gabergic**

4. **Peptidergic**

II. CATECHOLAMINERGIC NEURONS AND THEIR PATHWAYS IN THE CNS

A. General location of catecholaminergic perikarya

1. Catecholaminergic perikarya are found in the following locations:
   a. **Brainstem tegmentum**. Dopaminergic perikarya are most numerous in the midbrain, noradrenergic in the pons, and adrenergic in the medulla, but considerable overlap occurs.
   b. **Subthalamus, hypothalamus**, and **retina** of the diencephalon
   c. **Olfactory bulb** and **septal region** of the telencephalon

2. Catecholaminergic perikarya do **not** occur in the following structures:
   a. Spinal cord gray matter
   b. Motor and sensory nuclei of the cranial nerves
   c. Cerebellar and cerebral cortices
   d. Thalamic nuclei

B. Dopaminergic pathways

1. **Dopaminergic perikarya** occur predominantly in the midbrain tegmentum.

   a. Caudally, they dwindle quickly in the transition from the midbrain tegmentum to the pontine tegmentum.
   b. Rostrally, they extend as scattered groups through the zona incerta and hypothalamus and into the retina. The olfactory bulbs contain the only dopaminergic perikarya of the telencephalon.

2. The **substantia nigra** and **ventral paramedian tegmental nucleus** are the two largest dopaminergic nuclei of the midbrain.
   a. The **substantia nigra**, pars compacta and pars reticulata, occupies a grossly visible, darkly pigmented zone covering the midbrain basis (see Fig. 8-36).
   b. The **ventral paramedian tegmental nucleus** is mediodorsal to the medial part of the substantia nigra.

3. Distribution of dopaminergic axons. The dopaminergic perikarya can be classified by the **length** and **extent** of their axons, beginning with the shortest.
   a. Dopaminergic neurons of the **retina** and **olfactory bulb** have no axons at all. They function as amacrine interneurons by means of dendrodendritic contacts on adjacent neurons (see Fig. 10-4).
   b. The **diencephalic** dopaminergic perikarya of the zona incerta and hypothalamus project short axons, mainly to the hypothalamus itself. Within the hypothalamus, a short tuberoinfundibular tract runs from the arcuate and periventricular nuclei to the median eminence and infundibulum. It controls hormone release.
   c. The **substantia nigra**, mainly pars compacta, sends nigrostriatal and nigrodiencephalic tracts of moderate length.
      (1) The **nigrostriatal tract** projects to the striatum (Fig. 14-1A).
         (a) The nigrostriatal tract turns medially from its origin to enter field H_2 of Forel, ventral to the zona incerta. At the level of the subthalamic nucleus, the axons veer into the internal capsule and fan out as they ascend to innervate all parts of the striatum.
         (b) In reaching the head of the caudate nucleus, many fibers run just dorsal to or in the medial forebrain bundle.
      (2) The **nigrodiencephalic tract** runs to the ventral thalamic motor nuclei, hypothalamus, and basal forebrain.
   d. The **ventral paramedian tegmental dopaminergic pathway** is extensive, reaching from the spinal cord to the cerebral cortex (see Fig. 14-1B).
      (1) Caudally projecting axons from dopaminergic perikarya of the ventral paramedian nuclei of the midbrain and from some dopaminergic perikarya in the hypothalamus run to the spinal cord.
      (2) Rostrally projecting axons run ventromedial to and in close association with the nigrostriatal pathway and then enter the medial forebrain bundle.
         (a) At the retrochiasmatic level, some of these dopaminergic axons veer laterally into the ansa peduncularis to reach the amygdala, piriform cortex, and entorhinal area (area 28) of the limbic mesocortex (see Fig. 14-1B).
         (b) Axons proceeding rostrally enter the nucleus accumbens (ventromedial part of the caudate nucleus) and the anterior perforated substance.
            (i) Some extend forward to the olfactory bulb.
            (ii) Others run through and around the head of the caudate nucleus to reach the septal region, cingulate gyrus, and general frontal cortex.
   e. Some authors, to give uniform names to the dopaminergic pathways, refer to them as **mesostriatal, mesolimbic, mesocortical**, and **mesospinal**, to indicate the predominantly **mesencephalic** location of their perikarya.

C. Noradrenergic pathways

1. Location of noradrenergic perikarya
   a. Noradrenergic perikarya commence in the medulla and extend through the brainstem and ventral diencephalon to the olfactory bulb and septal area.
   b. The noradrenergic perikarya in the pons form two groups: the **nucleus locus ceruleus** and **several additional nuclei.**

2. The **nucleus locus ceruleus** is a grossly visible, darkly pigmented area in the dorsal pontine tegmentum, lateroventral to the aqueduct and fourth ventricle.
   a. Afferents to the nucleus locus ceruleus come from:
      (1) Cerebral and cerebellar cortices
      (2) Hypothalamus
      (3) Reticular formation, particularly the dorsal raphe nucleus of the midbrain, which is the largest serotonergic nucleus and the largest single source of afferents to the nucleus locus ceruleus.

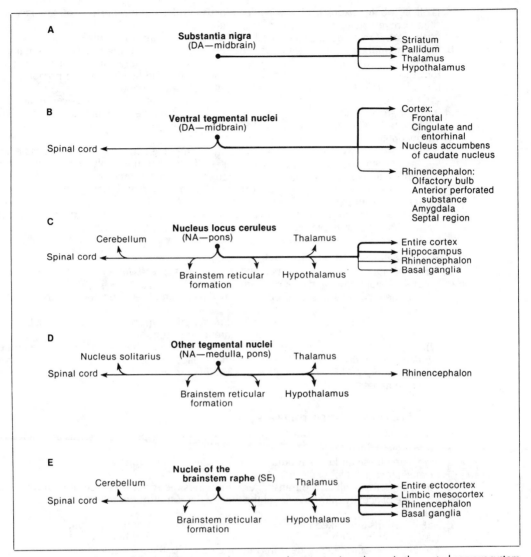

Figure 14-1. Distribution of dopaminergic, noradrenergic, and serotonergic pathways in the central nervous system (CNS). *DA* = dopaminergic; *NA* = noradrenergic; *SE* = serotonergic.

    b. Efferents from the nucleus locus ceruleus disperse more widely than those of any other known nucleus (see Fig. 14-1C).

      (1) In keeping with efferent reticular formation neurons, the axons undergo a T-like bifurcation into ascending and descending branches (see Fig. 8-39).

      (2) The individual axons from the nucleus locus ceruleus collateralize locally and then sprout hundreds of thousands of axonal endings that extend into all major subdivisions of the neuraxis: cerebral cortex, diencephalon, brainstem, cerebellum, and spinal cord.

  3. Other noradrenergic perikarya of the pontine tegmentum, apart from the nucleus locus ceruleus, distribute their axons in a similar but less extensive manner (see Fig. 14-1D).

    a. Rostrally, the axons probably do not extend past the olfactory bulb and septum.

    b. Scattered noradrenergic neurons in the medulla send axons to the spinal cord and to the nucleus solitarius.

  4. Course of rostrally running noradrenergic pathways. Noradrenergic axons from the pons are distributed by periventricular and tegmental pathways.

    a. The **periventricular pathway** extends in the periaqueductal gray matter from the medulla to the periventricular region of the thalamus and hypothalamus.

(1) It distributes axons from the nucleus locus ceruleus, the other pontomedullary noradrenergic nuclei, and serotonergic nuclei.

(2) In part, it may include the dorsal longitudinal fasciculus of Schütz.

b. The **tegmental pathway** runs through the region designated as the central tegmental tract (see Figs. 8-28 through 8-34). The noradrenergic axons concentrate in the dorsomedial sector of the tract as the **dorsal tegmental bundle**. This bundle splits as the noradrenergic fibers fan out in the midbrain into dorsal and ventral components.

(1) The **dorsal bundle**, mostly from the nucleus locus ceruleus, ascends ventrolateral to the periaqueductal gray matter, en route to midbrain, diencephalic, and telencephalic targets. Traversing the diencephalon in the medial forebrain bundle, it reaches the telencephalon by two routes.

(a) The majority of the fibers veer dorsally to enter the cingulum, internal capsule, and adjacent deep white matter to disperse diffusely and uniformly to the entire cortex.

(b) Other fibers veer ventrolaterally through the ansa peduncularis and inferior thalamic peduncle to reach the piriform cortex, amygdala, and hippocampus.

(c) Hippocampal fibers travel with the cingulum.

(2) The **ventral bundle**, mostly from the noradrenergic perikarya outside the nucleus locus ceruleus, ascends through the central tegmental tract, en route to its midbrain and forebrain targets. In the forebrain, it roughly follows the medial forebrain bundle.

5. Cortical distribution of noradrenergic terminals

a. Noradrenergic axons from the nucleus locus ceruleus spread uniformly and diffusely to the entire cerebral cortex and hippocampus.

b. Noradrenergic axons to the cerebral cortex differ from other subcortical afferents in two respects.

(1) They run directly to the cortex without undergoing synaptic interruption in a thalamic relay nucleus (although they may collateralize to the thalamus).

(2) The noradrenergic terminals end in close proximity to the membranes of the cortical neurons but do not form distinct terminal synaptic bars. In this respect, they resemble the endings of the serotonergic axons but differ from the dopaminergic endings, which are synapses.

D. Function of catecholaminergic pathways

1. Facile generalizations about the function of the chemically specified systems are difficult to make for several reasons.

a. Many are diffuse and have modulating influences on many functions rather than initiating or mediating specific functions.

b. The receptor as well as the transmitter determines the effect on different neurons.

c. The state of activity of the system at the time of neurotransmitter release may alter the outcome.

d. Some systems are linked in loops of alternating excitation and inhibition.

(1) Stimulation of inhibitory neurons may reduce a specified behavior.

(2) Inhibition of inhibitory neurons may increase a particular behavior.

(3) Stimulation or inhibition of excitatory neurons produces converse effects.

2. The amacrine dopaminergic neurons of the olfactory bulb and retina may function to inhibit the lateral transfer of excitatory activity, thus increasing the signal-to-noise ratio in these systems.

3. The effect of catecholamine neurotransmitters on motor function is complex, depending on the amount of the neurotransmitter and the degree of sensitivity of the receptors.

a. An excess of dopamine causes involuntary movements or rigidity.

b. A decrease in dopamine causes hypokinesia and rigidity of the muscles (parkinsonism); affected patients, in spite of their hypokinesia and difficulty in initiating movements, also display a necessity to move, called **akathisia**.

4. In schizophrenia, the limbic dopaminergic system is thought to be overactive because drugs that block the action of dopamine improve the condition. Most of the effective medications also cause extrapyramidal syndromes such as parkinsonism or other involuntary movements because they also block dopaminergic activity in the basal motor nuclei. Chronically treated patients may show a variety of involuntary movements called **tardive dyskinesia**. Long-term blockade is thought to cause the dopaminergic receptors in the basal motor nuclei to become hypersensitive to dopamine, resulting in the tardive dyskinesia.

5. In Alzheimer's disease and parkinsonism, the neurons of the nucleus locus ceruleus degenerate, as do those of the nucleus basalis and the substantia nigra.

6. The response of noradrenergic neurons to injury differs strikingly from that of other CNS neurons because, at least in lower animals, their axons tend to regenerate following interruption, whereas the other tracts of classic neuroanatomy do not regenerate.

III. SEROTONERGIC PATHWAYS

A. Location and morphology of serotonergic perikarya

1. Serotonergic neurons tend to be large and isodendritic in character (see Fig. 8-39).

    a. The dendrites from the serotonergic perikarya may intertwine in bundles with the dendrites of other reticular formation neurons and the shafts of glial cells (tanycytes) in the floor of the fourth ventricle of the medulla.

    b. These bundles run as vertically oriented shafts that extend in the median plane from the floor of the fourth ventricle to the ventral margin of the medullary tegmentum.

    c. Blood vessels frequently abut on these bundles.

2. The main groups of serotonergic perikarya extend from the caudal medulla to the rostral end of the midbrain. They make up varying proportions of the raphe and medial nuclei, the more definite nuclei of the reticular formation (see Fig. 8-40).

    a. The midbrain contains two large serotonergic nuclei in the raphe and paramedian zone, the **dorsal raphe nucleus** and the **median raphe nucleus** (see Fig. 8-40).

    b. The decussation of the brachium conjunctivum separates the two nuclei.

3. The hypothalamus contains scattered serotonergic neurons, but few or none extend rostral to this level.

B. Afferents to the serotonergic nuclei

1. Sensorimotor cortex

2. Limbic periventricular and habenular systems

3. Reticular formation

4. Fastigial nucleus of the cerebellum

5. Spinal cord

C. Efferents from the serotonergic nuclei

1. The serotonergic distribution resembles the noradrenergic, although ectocortex is less extensively innervated.

2. The axons divide into ascending and descending branches, which reach all major divisions of the CNS (see Fig. 14-1E).

3. The **caudal serotonergic nuclei**, in the medulla, tend to project caudally, forming a bulbospinal tract.

4. The **intermediate nuclei**, in the pons, project caudally to the medulla and spinal cord; rostrally to the midbrain, diencephalon, and cerebrum; and dorsally into the cerebellum.

5. The **rostral serotonergic nuclei**, in the midbrain, project rostrally to the forebrain.

6. The serotonergic neurons of each brainstem segment project strongly to surrounding reticular formation.

7. The serotonergic axons project to the nonspecific thalamic nuclei (i.e., those not relaying specific pathways from basal motor nuclei, the cerebellum, and the senses).

8. The majority of serotonergic axons ascending to the forebrain reach the striatum, rhinencephalon, and limbic system through the medial forebrain bundle.

D. Functions of the serotonergic system

1. The widespread connections of the serotonergic system in general suggest that it plays an augmenting or modulating role rather than initiating specific behaviors or mediating highly focal, point-to-point functions like those of the visual system. The general action of serotonin appears to be inhibitory.

2. The serotonergic neurons of the raphe make an inhibitory monosynaptic connection with sympathetic neurons of the spinal cord, establishing a link in a pathway for the control of cardiovascular responses.

3. The bulbospinal serotonergic pathway also reaches the substantia gelatinosa and may play a role in pain modulation.
   a. Electrical stimulation of the raphe, which causes serotonin release at axonal endings, produces analgesia in animals by increasing the pain threshold.
   b. Serotonin depletion decreases the pain threshold.

4. Destruction of the raphe serotonergic nuclei or pharmacologic inhibition of serotonin synthesis causes insomnia, suggesting a sleep-initiating role for the serotonergic system.

5. Some serotonergic axons terminate on CNS blood vessels and ventricular surfaces as do some noradrenergic axons. Their function is unclear.

6. The anatomical arrangement of the medullary dendritic bundles suggests a route by which cerebrospinal fluid (CSF) and blood-borne chemical substances might directly influence reticular formation neurons.

7. In summary, stimulation or destruction of the serotonergic system alters the following visceral and behavioral functions:
   a. Homeostatic functions, such as water balance, blood flow, temperature regulation, and sleep
   b. Activity level and aggression
   c. Self-stimulation and the learning of avoidance behavior
   d. Sexual behavior
   e. Pain responses

IV. CHOLINERGIC PATHWAYS

A. Identification of cholinergic neurons

1. Current techniques do not directly localize acetylcholine itself in the CNS. The inference that a neuron acts by cholinergic transmission rests largely on histochemical demonstration of the degradative enzyme, acetylcholinesterase, or in some cases on the presence of the synthesizing enzyme, choline acetyltransferase.

2. Unfortunately, the presence of these enzymes does not establish acetylcholine as a transmitter because it may have metabolic roles other than neurotransmission. Also, it is not always clear whether the enzymes act pre- or postsynaptically.

3. The highest concentrations of these enzymes occur in the central segments of the dorsal roots (but not the peripheral segments), the interpeduncular region, the striatum, and the retina.

4. In the monkey cerebral cortex, which receives its cholinergic innervation from nucleus basalis and adjacent nuclei, the association areas show the lowest (but still significant) activity, the sensorimotor regions show intermediate activity, and the limbic mesocortex area, except for the cingulate gyrus, shows the greatest activity. In addition, enzyme activity is strong in the hippocampus and amygdala.

B. Probable and possible cholinergic perikarya and pathways are listed in Table 14-1.

C. Function of the cholinergic system

1. Acetylcholine generally functions as an excitatory transmitter.

2. Acetylcholine is the probable transmitter in many pathways that have clearly recognized functions, such as those of autonomic and somatic motoneurons and perhaps the pyramidal tract, and in those sensory systems with point-to-point representation, such as the visual system.
   a. This pattern contrasts with the monoaminergic pathways that tend to have more generalized modulating functions.
   b. Nucleus basalis, however, is a cholinergic pathway with a generalized distribution, whereas the dopaminergic pathway from the substantia nigra to the striatum is topographically organized.

3. Midbrain–forebrain cholinergic pathway
   a. The interpeduncular region has the highest concentration of acetylcholine enzymes of any area of the CNS. This region and the overlying reticular formation, the region called nucleus cuneiformis, may originate a series of cholinergic cascades, which play upon the thalamus, hypothalamus, striatum, rhinencephalon and adjacent limbic structures, and ultimately the cortex in general.

Table 14-1. Cholinergic Pathways of the Central Nervous System

Probable cholinergic pathways

Primary afferents for vision and hearing

Ascending reticular activating system

Septohippocampal tract

Habenulointerpeduncular tract

Recurrent collaterals to Renshaw neurons

Nucleus basalis of Meynert

Possible cholinergic pathways

Caudate efferents

Efferents of ventral and posteromedial thalamic nuclei

Lateral geniculate and cochlear nuclei; hence, secondary (as well as primary) neurons of visual and auditory pathways

Supraoptic pathway

Hippocampus

Pyramidal neurons of the cerebral cortex

b. This system could be the anatomical substrate of the ascending reticular activating system, which is necessary for consciousness.

V. GABERGIC PATHWAYS [gamma-aminobutyric acid (GABA) pathways]

A. Location of gabergic perikarya

1. Technically, it is easy to identify GABA-positive axonal terminals but difficult to identify the perikarya of origin. The description of the gabergic system is offered tentatively, based on the concentrations of GABA and gamma-aminodecarboxylase (GAD). The concentration of GAD is preferred as a criterion because glial cells also take up GABA.

2. GABA is mainly found in short interneuronal circuits, rather than in the long tracts. Gabergic interneurons with short axons (Golgi type II) are probably present in all parts of the CNS, although in differing numbers. GABA is present in a few tracts of intermediate length, such as the striatonigral and Purkinje projections.

3. Concentrations of GABA and GAD are highest in the dorsal horns, cerebellum, collicular plate, substantia nigra, hypothalamus, pallidum, and anterior perforated substance (substantia innominata).

4. In the **spinal cord**, GABA and GAD concentrations are highest in the substantia gelatinosa, nucleus dorsalis of Clarke, and nuclei gracilis and cuneatus. The remainder of the dorsal horns and the ventral horns also contain gabergic interneurons.

5. In the **cerebellum**, Purkinje neurons are the best-characterized gabergic system.
   a. The entire output of the Purkinje neurons to the deep cerebellar nuclei and the vestibular nuclei is inhibitory.
   b. The other inhibitory intrinsic cerebellar neurons are thought to be gabergic. The one excitatory intrinsic cerebellar neuron, the granule cell, is glutaminergic.

6. The **striatum** sends a gabergic pathway to the pallidum and substantia nigra and many of its interneurons are gabergic.

7. In the **telencephalon**, the **rhinencephalon** contains gabergic interneurons in the olfactory bulb, substantia innominata, septal region, and medial amygdalar region. The **cortex** contains only average amounts of gabergic interneurons, but they appear to be evenly distributed. The **hippocampus** has gabergic interneurons that synapse upon its granular and pyramidal neurons.

B. Function of the gabergic system

1. GABA and glycine are regarded as inhibitory transmitters.

2. In Huntington's chorea, the amount of GABA in the striatum is very small; this correlates with the predominant loss of the small interneurons seen histologically and the choreiform movements seen clinically.

VI. NEUROPEPTIDE PATHWAYS

A. Definition of peptides. Peptides are compounds that consist of 2–40 amino acids linked to each other.

B. Discovery of peptides as messengers and neurotransmitters

1. About 50 years ago scientists discovered that substance P, a peptide found in the gut and brain, serves as a chemical messenger to act on smooth muscle and glands. In recent decades, peptides were discovered in the brainstem, pituitary gland, and hypothalamus, and the hypothalamus was found to use peptide messengers to cause the release of pituitary hormones (see Fig. 12-16A). The first hypothalamic–hypophyseal releasing peptide discovered was thyrotropin releasing factor (TRF).

2. Neuropeptides of the CNS are generally concentrated in axonal terminals. Calcium-dependent mechanisms release them, as with other transmitters.

3. A veritable explosion of interest in the neuropeptides followed the discovery in the mid-1970s that opiates (e.g., morphine) localize in regions of the brain known to be involved in affective experiences and pain perception.
    a. Later, two naturally occurring endogenous neuropeptides called **enkephalins** were found to bind to the opioid receptors of neurons and to reproduce the action of morphine. Naloxone blocks the action of these peptides and of morphine.
    b. Now, the term **endorphins** (from "endogenous" and "morphine") is used generically for a whole class of endogenous neurotransmitter or neuromodulator peptides having opioid activity.
    c. Thus, peptides are now known to act as neurotransmitters or neuromodulators, as releasing factors for adenohypophyseal hormones and as hormones themselves. The same peptide may serve one or more of these functions.

C. Neuroactive peptides fall into three classes (selected examples are included below).

1. **Neurohypophyseal neuropeptides** are the actual hormones released from the neurohypophysis (see Fig. 12-16B) and include oxytocin and vasopressin.

2. **Adenohypophyseal releasing neuropeptides** are manufactured in the hypothalamus and act on adenohypophyseal cells to release or inhibit the release of their hormones. They include:
    a. TRF
    b. Gonadotropin releasing factor (GRF)
    c. Corticotropin releasing factor (CRF)
    d. Somatotropin (growth hormone) inhibiting factor or somatostatin (SST)

3. **Neurotransmitter neuropeptides** include the following:
    a. Opioid neuropeptides
        (1) Opiocortins
            (a) Adrenocorticotropic hormone (ACTH; corticotropin)
            (b) β-endorphin
            (c) Melanocyte stimulating hormone (MSH)
        (2) Enkephalins
        (3) Dynorphin
    b. Substance P and vasoactive intestinal peptides (found in the gut and CNS)

D. Opiocortin neuropeptides: location of perikarya and distribution of axons

1. **Hypothalamic nuclear groups**
    a. **Arcuate** and **paramedian nuclei** distribute their axons widely to reticular formation (including monoaminergic groups), periaqueductal gray matter, the hypothalamus–pituitary gland, the thalamus, and rhinencephalic–limbic forebrain structures.
    b. **Laterodorsal hypothalamic neurons** distribute axons to forebrain structures: the olfactory bulb, hippocampal formation, and ectocortex.

2. Medullary group
 a. The perikarya are located in the commissural division of nucleus tractus solitarii and extend ventrolaterally through nucleus reticularis of the medulla into the catecholaminergic region, medial to nucleus ambiguus.
 b. Axons are distributed to the reticular formation of the medulla and to the central gray matter of the spinal cord at all levels.

3. Medullary and arcuate opiocortin axonal terminals strongly overlap the perikarya containing CRF, giving them a unique codistribution.
 a. CRF perikarya are scattered from the rostral level of the spinal cord to the septal region.
 b. The codistribution is strong in the periventricular region of the hypothalamus and in the paraventricular nucleus, which has about the greatest concentration of CRF perikarya in the CNS.

4. Function
 a. The medullary corticotropin system is in a prime location to mediate cardiovascular, respiratory, and gastrointestinal reflexes of CN IX and CN X.
 b. The hypothalamic and paraventricular nuclear connections provide a pathway for regulating the release of vasopressin (antidiuretic hormone) or oxytocin by the paraventricular nucleus.

E. Substance P

1. Substance P, a peptide originally isolated from the gastrointestinal tract and CNS, was found to cause contraction of intestinal muscle and dilation of blood vessels. It has a particularly high concentration in the following areas:
 a. Small dorsal root axons and axonal terminals ending on the substantia gelatinosa of the spinal cord and on the spinal nucleus of CN V. It is also found in dental pulp nerves and in about 20% of the dorsal root ganglion perikarya.
 b. Periaqueductal gray matter, substantia nigra, and interpeduncular region of the brainstem
 c. Medial preoptic area and habenula of the diencephalon
 d. Striatum and medial amygdaloid nucleus of the telencephalon

2. Substance P is regarded as the primary neurotransmitter for pain, although it may not function as a pain mediator in the striatum.
 a. Figure 14-2 illustrates one theory of the mechanism of pain control by interactions of several transmitter systems.
 b. The primary sensory neuron releases substance P to excite the neurons in the substantia gelatinosa or other secondary neurons of the spinothalamic pain pathway.

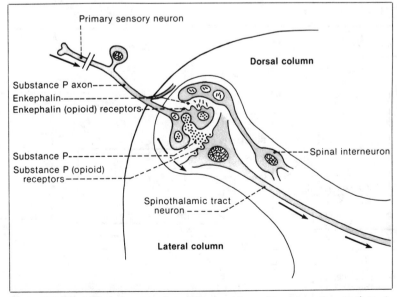

Figure 14-2. Simplified diagram of possible neurotransmitter interactions in the pain pathway in the dorsal quadrant of the spinal cord. *Arrows* indicate the direction of flow of pain impulses. See text for further explanation.

c. Certain spinal interneurons, if activated, release enkephalin, which attaches to the enkephalin (opioid) receptors on the terminals of substance P axons. Opiate drugs such as morphine may also attach to these receptors. Activation of these receptors by enkephalin or opiate drugs blocks the release of substance P into the synaptic cleft and hence transmission of pain impulses through the spinothalamic tract. Such an action is called **presynaptic inhibition**.

d. The exact way in which serotonergic bulbospinal axons inhibit pain transmission is uncertain.

F. Model of excitatory and inhibitory neurotransmitter interactions

1. The basal motor nuclei, which are rich in many known neurotransmitters, illustrate the complex interaction of excitatory and inhibitory neurons in circuits (Fig. 14-3).

2. Figure 14-3 also serves as a model to explain the action of two different medications, levodopa and atropine, used to treat Parkinson's disease. This disease results from degeneration of dopaminergic neurons of the substantia nigra.

   a. Dopamine, conveyed from the substantia nigra to the striatum by the nigrostriatal pathway, inhibits the intrinsic small cholinergic neurons of the striatum. These small cholinergic neurons in turn excite the large neurons, which project to the globus pallidus. According to this theory, overaction of the large striatal neurons (see Figs. 11-7 and 11-8) results in the tremor, rigidity, and bradykinesia that characterize Parkinson's disease.

   b. The drug, levodopa, given by mouth, passes the blood–brain barrier to be converted to dopamine in the striatum, tending to restore the normal excitatory–inhibitory balance that regulates the excitation of the large striatal neurons by the small ones.

   c. On the other hand, atropine-like drugs block the cholinergic excitation of the large neurons by the small neurons, and thus counter the loss of inhibition produced by dopamine deficiency. It is also quite possible that the two drugs act at other sites in the circuit.

   d. High doses of the drugs used to treat schizophrenia cause parkinsonism by blocking dopaminergic inhibition of the small striatal neurons. Atropine-like drugs then enable the patient to continue to take the high doses of medication required to alleviate the symptoms of schizophrenia.

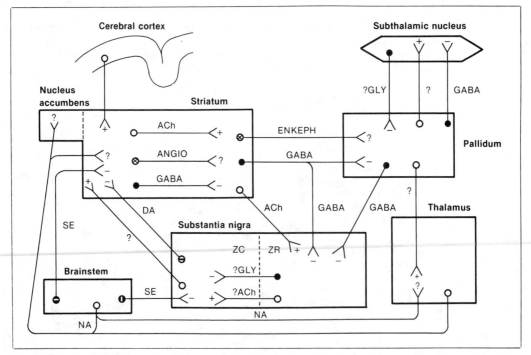

Figure 14-3. Simplified diagram for the conceptual understanding of the interaction of numerous neurotransmitter pathways in the motor circuitry. *ACh* = acetylcholine; *ANGIO* = angiotensin; *DA* = dopaminergic pathway; *ENKEPH* = enkephalin; *GABA* = gamma-aminobutyric acid; *GLY* = glycine; *NA* = noradrenergic pathway; *SE* = serotonergic pathway; *ZC* = zona compacta; *ZR* = zona reticularis; + = excitatory; − = inhibitory.

substance P isolated is a peptide in CNS from GI of muscle — contracts GI muscle blood vessels — dilates

STUDY QUESTIONS

Directions: Each question below contains four suggested answers of which **one or more** is correct. Choose the answer

A if **1, 2, and 3** are correct
B if **1 and 3** are correct
C if **2 and 4** are correct
D if **4** is correct
E if **1, 2, 3, and 4** are correct

1. Statements that characterize serotonergic neurons include which of the following? *pathways*

(1) Perikarya are concentrated in the median raphe region
(2) Perikarya extend through the entire brainstem
(3) Neurons are large and of the isodendritic type
(4) Electrical stimulation of serotonergic nuclei produces analgesia

2. Correct statements about cholinergic pathways include which of the following?

(1) The axons of the nucleus basalis have the widest distribution of any of the cholinergic nuclei
(2) The ventral motoneurons of the brainstem and spinal cord are cholinergic
(3) Very high concentrations of acetylcholine enzymes occur in the interpeduncular region of the midbrain and may be part of the anatomical substrate of the ascending reticular activating system
(4) Cholinergic pathways in general tend to be inhibitory

3. Statements that characterize the dopaminergic neurons of the midbrain include which of the following?

(1) They have small, obscure perikarya that are difficult to distinguish from glia
(2) They send their main axonal connections to structures rostral to the location of their perikarya
(3) They lack conformity with any previously known cytoarchitectural subdivisions of the brainstem
(4) Their perikarya are concentrated in the ventral part of the midbrain tegmentum

4. Correct statements about peptides include which of the following?

(1) The gut, pituitary gland, and hypothalamus release similar peptides
(2) Hypothalamic nerve endings release neuropeptides, which release growth hormone from the pituitary gland
(3) Periaqueductal gray matter receives large numbers of peptidergic nerve endings from the hypothalamus
(4) The cerebral cortex receives no peptidergic nerve endings

5. Gabergic neurons are thought to be which of the following? *inhibitory neurons*

(1) Purkinje neurons
(2) Granule neurons of the cerebellum
(3) Interneurons of the caudate nucleus
(4) Ganglion layer of the retina

6. Correct statements concerning the perikarya of the noradrenergic neurons include which of the following?

(1) They were discovered only after the development of fluorescence microscopy
(2) They are concentrated in largest numbers in the pontomedullary tegmentum
(3) They produce small, unmyelinated axons with tremendous numbers of collaterals
(4) They do not all group neatly into the known cytoarchitectural subdivisions of the reticular formation

ANSWERS AND EXPLANATIONS

1. The answer is E (all). (*III A 1, 2 a, D 3 a*) Serotonergic neurons are concentrated in the median raphe and extend throughout the entire brainstem; but they are present in largest numbers in the dorsal raphe nucleus and median raphe of the caudal midbrain tegmentum, extending into the rostral pons. Electrical stimulation reduces the response to pain. Destruction of the raphe nuclei or pharmacologic blockade of serotonin action causes insomnia, suggesting a sleep-initiating role for the serotonergic system.

2. The answer is A (1, 2, 3). (*IV C 1, 2 b, 3*) The cholinergic pathways in general tend to be excitatory. The ventral motoneurons are almost certainly cholinergic as are many of the axon terminals in the midbrain and basal ganglia. The nucleus basalis of Meynert has the widest distribution of any of the cholinergic neurons.

3. The answer is C (2, 4). [*II B 1, 3 d (2)*] The dopaminergic perikarya have a much more restricted location in the brainstem than the noradrenergic perikarya. The perikarya are concentrated in the midbrain, where they form two well-delineated and well-recognized nuclei: the substantia nigra and the ventral paramedian tegmental nucleus. These nuclei contain large cells, the former being strongly pigmented. In general, they project to structures rostral to the location of their perikarya rather than having the widespread distribution of the catecholaminergic axons, which typically produce ascending and descending branches.

4. The answer is A (1, 2, 3). (*VI B 1, D 1 a*) Neuropeptides act as transmitters and releasing factors throughout the CNS, including the cortex. Some opiocorticoid and neuropeptide perikarya in the hypothalamus project widely to the forebrain. Others, in the medulla, project widely to the reticular formation and the catecholaminergic nuclei of the brainstem. They also have strong connections with the periaqueductal and periventricular gray matter, including the central gray matter of the spinal cord.

5. The answer is B (1, 3). (*V A 5; Figure 14-3*) A number of inhibitory interneurons scattered throughout the nervous system, including those in the caudate nucleus, are thought to be gabergic. The Purkinje cells and the other inhibitory neurons of the cerebellar cortex are all thought to be gabergic. The granule neurons, which are excitatory, are glutaminergic.

6. The answer is E (all). [*I A 2 b; II C 1, 2 b (2)*] Some noradrenergic perikarya form discrete nuclei, such as the nucleus locus ceruleus, but others are quite scattered and do not conform to specific known nuclear configurations of the reticular formation. The axons from these neurons have the widest distribution of any axonal system in the nervous system. Each axon typically bifurcates numerous times to produce hundreds of thousands of synapses and distributes them to virtually every region of the nervous system. In spite of their wide distribution, the axons, being small and unmyelinated, were not discovered until the advent of fluorescence microscopy.

15
Blood Supply of the Central Nervous System

I. EMBRYOGENESIS OF CENTRAL NERVOUS SYSTEM VESSELS

A. Surface origin of vessels

1. The vessels of the central nervous system (CNS) originate as coalescing channels in the mesenchyme, which coats the surface of the neural tube and also produces its meninges.

2. From the initial, almost random, network of anastomoses, particular channels enlarge while others atrophy and disappear (Fig. 15-1).

3. One product of coalescence—essentially a single **ventral median artery**—extends along the entire neuraxis, although it splits and reunites rostrally (see Fig. 15-1C).

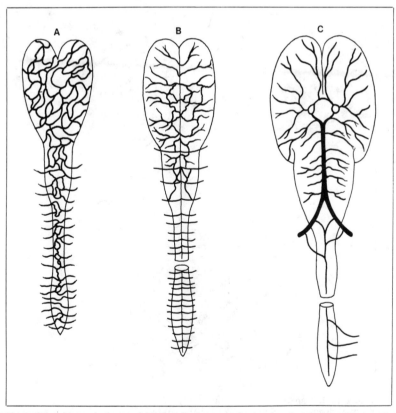

Figure 15-1. Ventral aspect of the developing neural tube showing the arterial pattern. (A) Early stage of random vascularization. (B) Theoretical stage of single ventral artery with segmental feeders. Branchial-arch vessels are not shown. (C) Final plan of arterial vessels. A few channels enlarge while others diminish or atrophy entirely.

B. Basic pattern of cerebral arteries

1. The ventral median artery receives its blood from somite arteries, which branch off at regular intervals from the aorta, or from branchial-arch arteries (see Fig. 15-1C).

2. After receiving its blood from extracranial sources, the ventral arterial channel distributes the blood through **paramedian** and **circumferential** arteries, which then perforate the wall of the neuraxis (Fig. 15-2).

   a. The **paramedian arteries** branch off at right angles to the longitudinal ventral trunk and perforate the neural tube wall just dorsal to their origin (see Fig. 15-2B).

   b. The **circumferential arteries** circumnavigate the neuraxis, sending perforating branches into it. The circumferential arteries form two groups: short and long.

      (1) The **short** circumferential arteries reach only around the circumference of the spinal cord or brainstem.

      (2) The **long** circumferential arteries extend around the brainstem and around the circumference of the cerebellar and cerebral hemispheres. They form on the hemispheric surface before the completion of fissuration and before sulcation commences. Then they fold into these crevices (Fig. 15-3).

II. BLOOD SUPPLY OF THE SPINAL CORD

A. Spinal arteries

1. A spinal artery enters the intervertebral foramina with each spinal nerve and travels to the cord along each dorsal and ventral root.

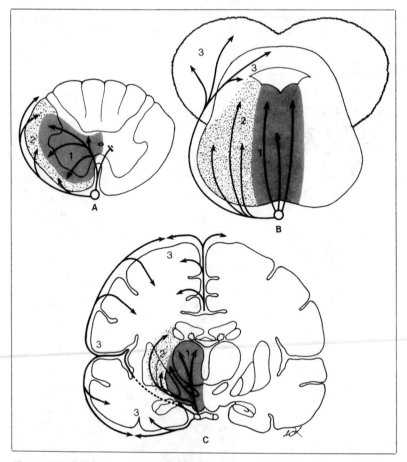

Figure 15-2. Transverse sections of the (*A*) spinal cord, (*B*) brainstem, and (*C*) cerebrum, showing how a ventral arterial channel provides paramedian branches and short and long circumferential branches that then perforate the wall of the neural tube. *Shaded area* (1) indicates median–paramedian vessels; *dotted area* (2) indicates short circumferential vessels; *white area* (3) indicates long circumferential vessels.

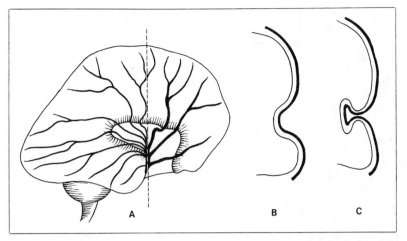

Figure 15-3. (A) Lateral view of the right cerebral hemisphere. The cerebral vessels form on the surface of the cerebrum and are then infolded into the sulci and fissures, in this case the insular region of the sylvian fissure. (B) Coronal section at the level indicated by the *interrupted line* in (A). (C) Coronal section at the same level at a later stage, showing further infolding of the cerebral arteries as the opercula grow over the sylvian fissure.

    a. Although each radicular artery remains, only a few develop into major feeders for the ventral spinal artery.
    b. The largest feeder is the artery of Adamkiewicz (Fig. 15-4).

  2. Paramedian branches of the ventral spinal artery enter the cord via the ventral median sulcus. **Circumferential branches** send short perforating arteries into the peripheral part of the ventral and lateral white columns (Fig.15-5).

  3. The dorsal root arteries coalesce into paired longitudinal **dorsal spinal arteries**.
    a. These dorsal arteries take a wavy, irregular course along the line of attachment of the dorsal roots, rather than running straight like the ventral spinal artery, and are of lesser importance.
    b. The dorsal arteries form many circumferential anastomoses with each other and circumferential branches of the ventral spinal artery (see Fig. 15-5).

  4. All in all, the ventral spinal artery irrigates about the ventral two-thirds of the cord; the dorsal spinal arteries irrigate about the dorsal one-third (see Fig. 15-5).
    a. Figure 7-24C shows the classic area of spinal cord infarction resulting from occlusion of the ventral spinal artery.
    b. Because the ventral spinal artery is the main source of arterial blood, occlusion of it or of one of its major feeders may infarct the whole diameter of the cord.

B. Spinal veins

  1. The blood from the spinal cord drains into three longitudinal systems, which anastomose extensively: the **spinal cord plexus** itself, the **epidural**, or **internal vertebral**, **plexus**, and the **external vertebral plexus**.
    a. The **spinal cord plexus** occupies the subarachnoid space. It communicates freely with the internal vertebral plexus.
    b. The **internal vertebral**, or **epidural**, **plexus** extends the length of the vertebral column in the epidural space. This space ends at the foramen magnum, where the dura mater becomes tightly adherent to the skull, forming its inner periosteum.
    c. The internal vertebral plexus communicates freely through the intervertebral foramina with the **external vertebral plexus**, which runs along the outside of the vertebral column.

  2. Since these venous systems lack valves, blood readily refluxes from one compartment to the other.
    a. Infected emboli or cancer cells may disseminate through and lodge in the plexuses.
    b. The resultant abscess or enlarging tumor in the epidural space then compresses the spinal cord or roots.
    c. Emboli in the external vertebral plexus may result in a retroperitoneal mass.

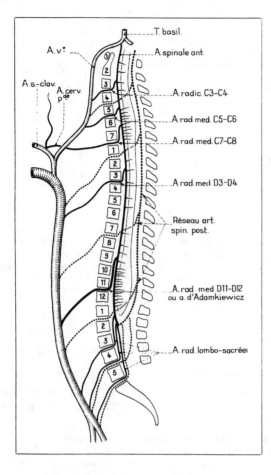

Figure 15-4. Lateral view of the arterial blood supply of the spinal cord. Most of the blood is supplied by means of enlargement of only a few of the original 31 pairs of somite arteries from the aorta. *A. cerv.* = cervical artery; *A. radic.* or *A. rad. med.* = radiculomedullary artery; *A. rad. lombo-sacrées* = lumbosacral radiculomedullary artery; *A. s.-clav.* = subclavian artery; *A. spinale ant.* = ventral spinal artery; *A. v.* = vertebral artery; *Réseau art. spin. post.* = network of posterior spinal arteries; *T. basil.* = trunk of basilar artery. (Reprinted with permission from Djindjian R: *Angiography of the Spinal Cord.* Baltimore, University Park Press, 1970, p 16.)

III. ARTERIAL BLOOD SUPPLY OF THE BRAIN

A. Metabolic requirements of the brain

1. The brain must receive oxygen and glucose continuously to survive. Neurons commence to die within 5 minutes of complete cardiac arrest, which deprives the brain of both substrates.

2. The brain comprises only about 2% of the body weight; however, it utilizes about 20% of the inspired oxygen and receives about 20% of the cardiac output. Cerebral blood flow is 50 ml/100 g of brain tissue/min.

3. Figure 15-6 shows the tremendous volume of the CNS occupied by the arteries.

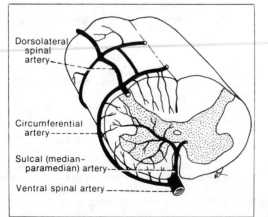

Figure 15-5. Segment of the spinal cord showing the arterial irrigation pattern.

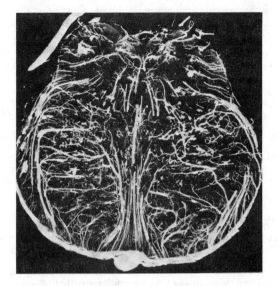

Figure 15-6. Transverse section of the pons with the arteries injected to show the volume of neural tissue occupied by arteries alone. (Reprinted with permission from Hassler O: Arterial pattern of human brainstem. *Neurology* 17:368–375, 1967.)

B. Four major arterial feeders for the brain

1. The brain receives its blood from two pairs of arteries: two **vertebral arteries** (VAs) and two **internal carotid arteries** (ICAs).

2. These four arteries penetrate foramina at the base of the skull to approach the brain ventrally, where they coalesce incompletely into a ventral median trunk (Fig. 15-7).

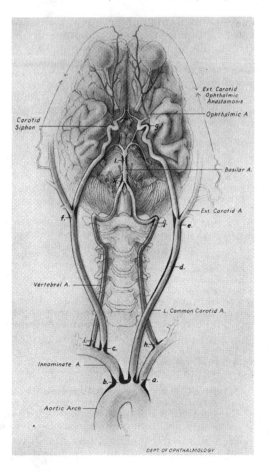

Figure 15-7. The four major arteries that supply the brain: two carotid arteries and two vertebral arteries. All of these approach the brain ventrally. The letters a–g indicate common sites for arteriosclerotic plaques, which may lead to insufficiency of arterial blood flow or actual arterial occlusions. (Reprinted with permission from Hoyt WF: Some neuro-ophthalmologic considerations in cerebral vascular insufficiency. *Arch Ophthalmol* 62:260–274, 1959.)

3. The **ICAs** run through the neck to enter the carotid canal at the skull base. They enter the intracranial space through the foramen lacerum, located just posterolateral to the sella turcica.

4. The **VAs** run through the transverse processes of the cervical vertebrae. They enter the skull through the foramen magnum, where they pierce the dura mater. Then they course rostrally through the subarachnoid space ventral to the medulla to unite into the **basilar artery** (BA).

C. Arterial patterns at the base of the brain

1. The branches of the four major arteries at the base of the brain and those of the coronary arteries are the two most important vascular patterns in the body. Study the progressogram in Figure 15-8 in relation to Figure 15-9.

2. **Anterior anastomotic circle (of Willis).** A bug commencing at the BA bifurcation may crawl through the right or left posterior communicating artery (PComA), cross the ICA lumen, enter the anterior cerebral artery (ACA), cross the anterior communicating artery (AComA), and return through the opposite vessels to the BA bifurcation, having negotiated the **circle of Willis** (see Fig. 15-9).

3. **Posterior anastomotic circle.** A bug commencing in the ventral spinal artery can reach the VA by its right or left posterior communicating branch, circle the apex of the posterior diamond-shaped circuit, and return unimpeded to its starting point (see Fig. 15-9).

4. The lumen size of the vessels of the anastomotic circles varies considerably.
   a. The PComA on one side may be small or absent; or the VAs may differ greatly in diameter, and one may be missing.
   b. These anatomical variations determine the site and extent of infarction in cerebrovascular disease.

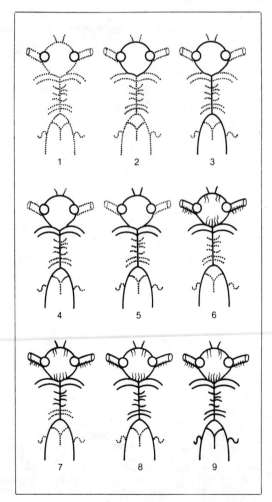

Figure 15-8. Progressogram of an insect figurine representing the arterial pattern at the base of the brain. To learn it, make your own drawing as follows:
1. Draw a pair of eyes: ICAs (Fig. 15-9 has the key to the arterial abbreviations).
2. Draw in the facial outline, completing the anterior anastomotic circle (of Willis): ICA, ACA, AComA, PComA, and PCA.
3. Add a trunk and a pair of hind legs: BA and VAs.
4. Draw four forelegs (all insects have six legs): SCA and extension of PCA.
5. Add antennae (feelers): extension of ACA.
6. Put a tube in each ear and striate it with hair: the lenticulostriate arteries or lateral striate arteries, LSAs; add hair: MSAs; and a beard: PSAs (Fig. 15-17).
7. Create a few irregular ribs: unnamed paramedian arteries.
8. Add a belt: IAAs and AICAs.
9. Attach some feelers to the hind legs: PICAs; add a penis, completing the posterior anastomotic circle: VSA.
10. Label the arteries on part 9 from Fig. 15-9.
11. Transpose the arteries onto the ventral aspect of the brain, and relate them to the cranial nerves (Fig. 15-9).
12. Mentally connect the two ICAs and two VAs of Fig. 15-8 with those of 15-7.

(Reprinted with permission from DeMyer W: *Technique of the Neurologic Examination: A Programmed Text*, 3rd ed. New York, McGraw-Hill, 1980, p 92.)

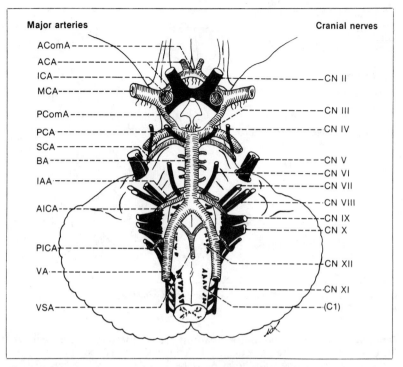

Figure 15-9. Ventral aspect of the brainstem and cerebrum with the arteries in place. *ACA* = anterior cerebral artery; *AICA* = anterior inferior cerebellar artery; *AComA* = anterior communicating artery; *BA* = basilar artery; *IAA* = internal auditory artery; *ICA* = internal carotid artery; *MCA* = middle cerebral artery; *PCA* = posterior cerebral artery; *PICA* = posterior inferior cerebellar artery; *PComA* = posterior communicating artery; *SCA* = superior cerebellar artery; *VA* = vertebral artery; *VSA* = ventral spinal artery.

D. Distribution of the vertebrobasilar system (posterior circulation) [Fig. 15-10]

   1. The **VA** on each side gives off the following vessels:
   a. Many small, unnamed paramedian perforating arteries to the medulla oblongata
   b. A posterior communicating branch to the anterior spinal artery
   c. One long circumferential branch, the posterior inferior cerebellar artery (PICA)

   2. The **BA** commences at the pontomedullary junction where the VAs unite. It extends the length of the pons to reach the interpeduncular fossa. The BA gives off the following vessels:
   a. Numerous unnamed paramedian perforating arteries to the pons
   b. One short circumferential artery, the internal auditory artery (IAA)
   c. Three named long circumferential arteries:
      (1) Anterior inferior cerebellar artery (AICA)
      (2) Superior cerebellar artery (SCA)
      (3) Posterior cerebral artery (PCA)

   3. Embryologically, the PCA arises from the PComA. Thus, the segment between the BA and PCA is the true "communicating" branch. Some authors call this segment the **basilar communicating artery** or **mesencephalic artery** to acknowledge this fact.

   4. Superficial and deep distributions of the vertebrobasilar system are illustrated in Figures 15-10, 15-11, and 15-12.

E. External and surface distribution of the internal carotid system (anterior circulation)

   1. Cavernous and parasellar segment of the ICA. After penetrating the foramen lacerum, the ICA pierces the dural layer that forms one wall of the cavernous sinus.
   a. Traversing the split in the dura, which is the cavernous sinus, the ICA folds itself into an S-shaped **carotid siphon.**
   b. The ICA then pierces the other dural leaf of the sinus to emerge into the vallecular region of the subarachnoid space, where it gives off several important branches (Fig. 15-13).

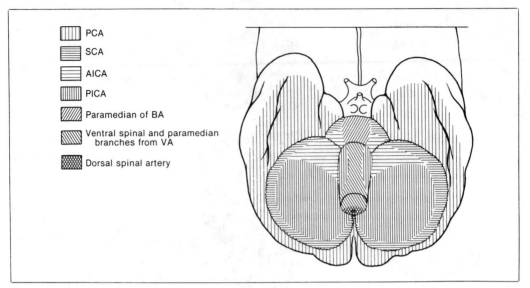

Figure 15-10. Ventral view of the brainstem and cerebellum showing the surface distribution of the vertebrobasilar arteries (posterior circulation).

2. **Terminal branches of the internal carotid artery: the middle cerebral artery (MCA) and ACA.** After ending at the vallecula, the ICA divides into two major terminal arteries, the MCA and ACA, which, along with the PCA, irrigate the cerebrum (see Fig. 15-10). Thus, both the cerebrum and cerebellum receive three large, long circumferential arteries—the ACA, MCA, and PCA for the cerebrum and the SCA, AICA, and PICA for the cerebellum.

3. **Surface distribution of the ACA, MCA, and PCA** (Fig. 15-14)
   a. To remember the distribution of the three cerebral arteries, you need learn only one—the MCA. Clasp your head between your hands with your fingers pointing backward: your hand exactly covers the distribution of the MCA. Notice that the curve of your thenar eminence covers the temporal pole (Fig. 15-15).
   b. The three poles of the cerebrum receive blood from one of the three cerebral arteries—the **frontal (anterior) pole** from the **ACA,** the **occipital (posterior) pole** from the **PCA,** and the **temporal (middle) pole** from the **MCA.**
   c. Notice that **medially** the ACA and PCA meet slightly anterior to the parieto-occipital sulcus (see Figs. 15-14B and 15-15B).
   d. Notice that **laterally** the junction of the ACA and MCA delineates a "basket handle" arc (see Figs. 15-14A and 15-15A).

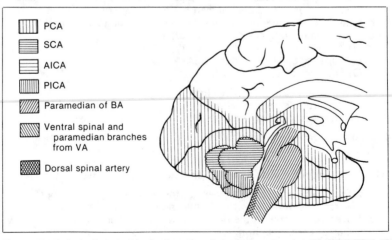

Figure 15-11. Sagittal view of the brainstem and cerebellum showing the distribution of the vertebrobasilar arteries (posterior circulation).

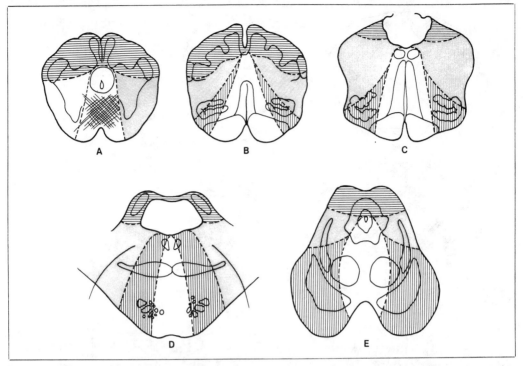

Figure 15-12. Transverse sections of the brainstem showing the arterial distributions. See also Figure 15-2A and B. (A) Medullocervical junction. (B) Medulla oblongata, caudal level. (C) Medulla oblongata, middle level. (D) Pons. (E) Midbrain. *White area* indicates paramedian vessels; *vertical lines* indicate short circumferential vessels, intermediate group; *shaded area* indicates short circumferential vessels, lateral group; *horizontal lines* indicate long circumferential vessels or, in the caudal part of the medulla, dorsal spinal arteries.

F. Internal distribution of the cerebral arteries (Fig. 15-16)

1. Paramedian and striate arteries

   a. From the anterior spinal and vertebral arteries up through the ACAs to their AComA, the ventral arterial trunk gives off numerous small, unnamed penetrating vessels to the paramedian zone of neural tissue.

   b. In three regions—**medial**, **lateral**, and **posterior**—these paramedian vessels form tufts or leashes of numerous fine branches, called **striate arteries**, from their resemblance to the striations of a comb.

   c. The **medial striate arteries** arise from the ACA and perforate the medial part of the basal forebrain. The more medial striate artery, often the largest, is called the **recurrent artery of**

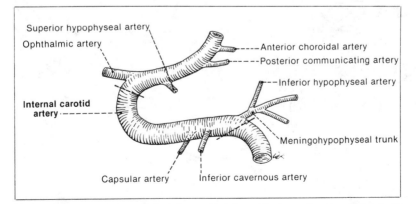

Figure 15-13. Lateral view of the left carotid siphon. The *lower interrupted line* indicates where the carotid artery enters the cavernous sinus and the *upper interrupted line* where it exits.

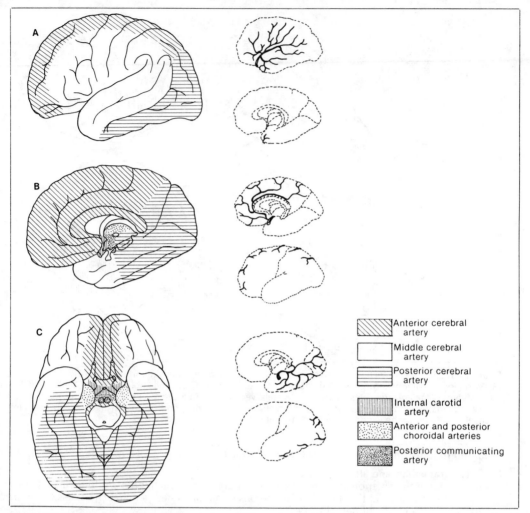

Figure 15-14. Surface distribution of the anterior, middle, and posterior cerebral arteries. (*A*) Lateral view of the left cerebral hemisphere. (*B*) Medial view of the left cerebral hemisphere. (*C*) Ventral view of the cerebrum. The figures to the right show the branches of the arteries.

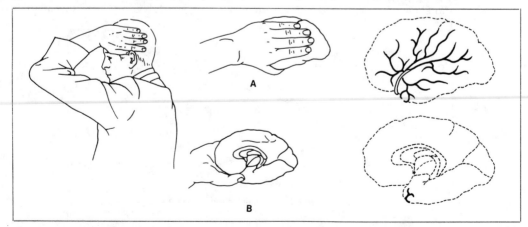

Figure 15-15. A handy method is shown for remembering the surface distribution of the middle cerebral artery, and, therefore, all three major cerebral arteries (i.e., place your palms on the sides of your head with your fingers and thumbs in a horizontal position). (*A*) Lateral aspect of the left cerebral hemisphere. (*B*) Medial aspect of the right cerebral hemisphere. The figures to the right show the branches of the middle cerebral artery.

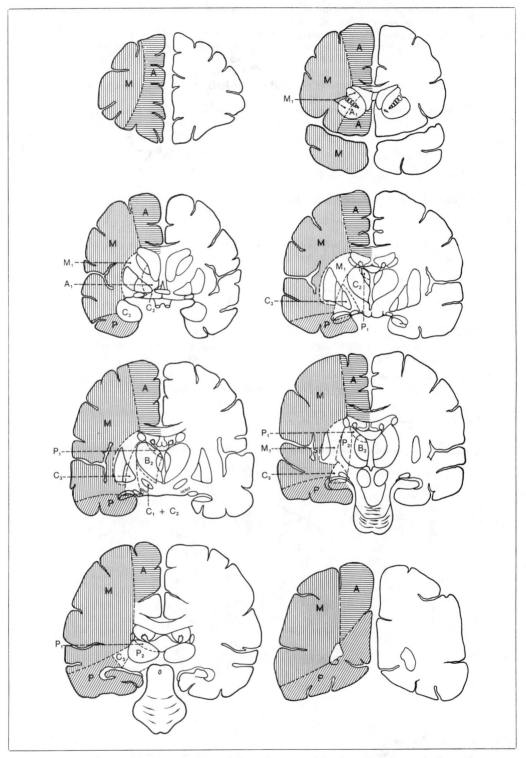

Figure 15-16. Coronal sections of the cerebrum showing the internal distributions of the cerebral arteries. A = anterior cerebral artery; A_1 = medial striate arteries; B = basilar communicating artery (mesencephalic artery); B_1 = paramedian arteries; B_2 = thalamoperforate artery; C = internal carotid artery; C_1 = paramedian perforating arteries to the wall of the third ventricle, hypothalamus, and subthalamus (ventral diencephalon); C_2 = posterior communicating artery, including the thalamotuberal artery; C_3 = anterior choroidal artery; M = middle cerebral artery; M_1 = lateral striate arteries (lenticulostriate arteries); P = posterior cerebral artery (proper); P_1 = posterior choroidal artery; P_2 = thalamogeniculate artery.

Heubner, which irrigates the basal third of the caudate nucleus and may reach the anterior limb or genu of the internal capsule (Fig. 15-17).

d. The **lateral striate arteries** arise from the MCA.

(1) They enter the basal forebrain by perforating the **anterior perforated substance**, which is the roof of the vallecula. They irrigate the basal ganglia and arch over them to reach the superior parts of the internal capsule.

(2) Because they irrigate the lentiform nucleus, they are often called **lenticulostriate arteries** (Fig. 15-18; see Fig. 15-18A).

e. The **posterior striate arteries** arise from the PCA and the basilar communicating artery. They enter the midbrain–diencephalic junction through the posterior perforated substance, which is the roof of the interpeduncular fossa (see Fig. 15-17).

2. The arterial supply of the internal capsule is illustrated in Figure 15-18.

3. The arterial supply of the thalamus is illustrated in Figure 15-19.

IV. VENOUS DRAINAGE OF THE BRAIN

A. Basic plan

1. The veins of the brain, unlike those of other organs, run their courses independent of the arteries. In contrast to the arteries, they anastomose freely.

2. There are four venous systems: the **intraparenchymal**, **superficial**, and **deep venous systems** and a system of **intradural sinuses**. It is convenient to describe the sinuses first since the veins drain into them.

B. Intradural venous sinuses

1. The layers of the dura split to create endothelium-lined venous channels called sinuses (Table 15-1; Figs. 15-20 and 15-21).

2. The venous sinuses empty into extracranial veins by means of several emissary veins that exit through foramina in the calvaria or the base of the skull.

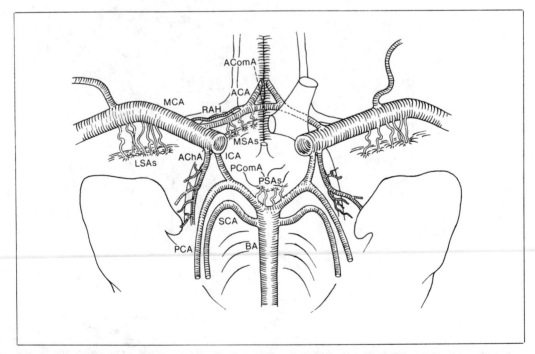

Figure 15-17. Ventral view of the circle of Willis showing the medial, lateral, and posterior perforating groups of arteries. *ACA* = anterior cerebral arteries; *AChA* = anterior choroidal artery; *AComA* = anterior communicating artery; *BA* = basilar artery; *ICA* = internal cartoid artery; *LSAs* = lateral striate arteries; *MCA* = middle cerebral artery; *MSAs* = medial striate arteries; *PCA* = posterior cerebral artery; *PComA* = posterior communicating artery; *PSAs* = posterior striate arteries; *RAH* = recurrent artery of the Heubner; *SCA* = superior cerebellar artery.

3. The most important and the largest such vein, the **jugular vein**, exits through the jugular foramen as a continuation of the **sigmoid sinus**. The jugular vein travels through the neck in a
sheath with the ICA and the vagus nerve.

C. Superficial cerebral veins (Table 15-2; see Fig. 15-20)

1. The lateral and medial superior superficial veins drain into the superior sagittal sinus, which
drains mainly into the right transverse dural sinus.

2. The inferior lateral superficial veins drain into the superior petrosal and transverse sinuses,
which ultimately drain into the jugular vein.

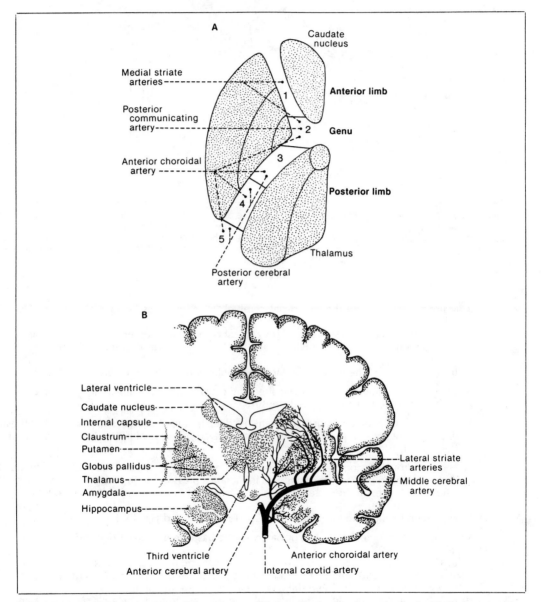

Figure 15-18. Arterial irrigation areas of the superior and inferior levels of the internal capsule. (A) Horizontal section
of the inferior level of the internal capsule showing the areas irrigated by different arteries. *1* = anterior limb; *2* = genu;
3 = anterior part of posterior limb; *4* = posterior part of posterior limb; *5* = retrolenticular part. (B) Coronal section
of the internal capsule through the genu. The superior part of the entire capsule receives blood only from the ar-
cades of lateral striate (lenticulostriate) arteries. At the coronal level shown, the anterior choroidal artery supplies
the inferior part of the internal capsule and the medial part of the globus pallidus. It may also send a small branch
into the ventrolateral aspect of the thalamus, but the lateral striate arteries do not supply the thalamus.

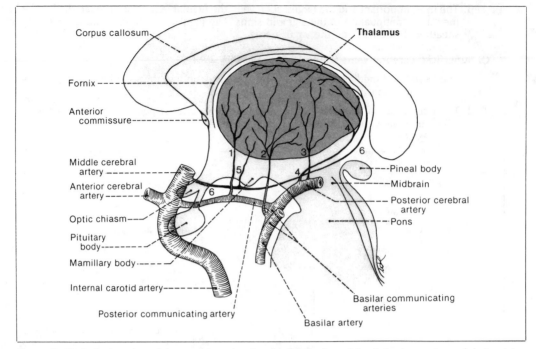

Figure 15-19. Sagittal section of the cerebrum showing the distribution of the thalamic arteries and their origins from the internal carotid, posterior communicating, and posterior cerebral arteries. *1* = thalamotuberal (premamillary) artery; *2* = thalamoperforant (postmamillary) artery; *3* = thalamogeniculate artery; *4* = posterior choroidal artery; *5* = lateroventral artery; *6* = anterior choroidal artery. (Adapted from Plets C, et al: The vascularization of the human thalamus. *Acta Neurol Belg* 70:687–770, 1970.)

3. Major anastomoses of the superficial cerebral veins on facies lateralis of a cerebral hemisphere include:
  a. Anastomosis of the veins of Trolard and Labbé with each other (the vein of Trolard then empties into the superior sagittal sinus, and the vein of Labbé empties into the transverse sinus)
  b. Anastomosis of the veins of Trolard and Labbé with the middle cerebral (sylvian) veins

4. The superficial middle cerebral veins reach the cavernous sinuses via the sphenoparietal sinuses or via the superior petrosal sinuses.

5. The superficial middle cerebral vein joins the deep middle cerebral vein, which drains the insular and opercular regions. It joins the basal vein of Rosenthal of the deep venous system (see section IV D).

6. The numerous anastomoses of the superficial and deep systems and the sinuses allow quick shifts of blood in response to changes in intracranial pressure; such changes may be related to intrathoracic pressure reflected via the jugular system or to intrinsic intracranial lesions.

D. Deep cerebral veins: the galenic system (see Table 15-2 and Fig. 15-21)

1. The major tributaries of the vein of Galen are the **basal vein of Rosenthal** and the **internal cerebral vein**.
  a. The **basal vein** commences at the vallecula with the union of the anterior internal frontal vein, striate veins, and deep middle cerebral vein. After collecting blood from the insular region and basal forebrain, the basal vein circles the midbrain.
  b. The basal vein then joins the **internal cerebral vein** to form the **great vein of Galen**.

2. The resultant galenic vein then enters the **straight sinus**, which mainly empties into the left transverse sinus (see Fig. 15-20).

3. Lower animals have a large confluent sinus (torcular Herophili), where the superior and straight sinuses meet to form the two transverse sinuses, but usually in humans only a modest-sized anastomosis exists (see Fig. 15-20).

Table 15-1. Intradural Venous Sinuses

Sinus	Location	Receives	Empties Into
Superior longitudinal (sagittal) sinus	Falx, attached margin	Superior superficial cerebral veins from upper part of facies medialis and facies lateralis	Transverse sinus, mainly the right
Inferior longitudinal (sagittal) sinus	Falx, free margin	Superficial cerebral veins from inferior part of facies medialis (excepting inferior frontal lobe) and from corpus callosum	Sinus rectus
Straight sinus (sinus rectus)	Junction of falx with tentorium	Inferior longitudinal sinus and great vein of Galen	Transverse sinus, mainly the left
Transverse sinus	Margin of tentorium attached to occipital bone	Superior longitudinal sinus, straight sinus, superior petrosal sinus	Sigmoid sinus
Sigmoid sinus	Between transverse sinus and jugular vein	Transverse sinus and inferior petrosal sinus	Jugular bulb and vein
Cavernous sinus	Parasellar area	Ophthalmic vein and sphenoparietal sinus	Superior and inferior petrosal sinuses and numerous emissary veins into nasopharynx; circular (intercavernous) sinuses connect the two cavernous sinuses
Superior petrosal sinus	Margin of tentorium attached to petrous ridge of temporal bone	Cavernous sinus, superficial middle cerebral vein, adjacent temporal lobe, superior cerebellar veins	Transverse sinus
Inferior petrosal sinus	Line of petro-occipital suture	Inferior cerebellar veins, medulla, pons, middle ear	Jugular bulb

V. CLINICAL CORRELATIONS WITH VASCULAR ANATOMY. Major forms of cerebrovascular disease are infarction and hemorrhage.

A. Infarction

1. Occlusion, or narrowing, of arteries leads to infarction of the territory supplied by the artery. The arterial territories are relatively constant, and the arteries act as end-arteries, with relatively little anastomosis between territories. Thus, the clinical syndromes of infarction are fairly reproducible.

2. Infarction in the **MCA distribution** leads to contralateral hemiplegia and hemisensory loss, with aphasia if it affects the left hemisphere, or loss of left-side spatial awareness if it affects the similar region of the right hemisphere.

3. Infarction in the **ACA territory** may cause contralateral crural (leg) monoplegia because the ACA irrigates the "leg area" on the medial hemispheric wall (see Figs. 13-36 and 13-37).

4. Infarction in the **internal capsule** may cause pure contralateral motor or sensory loss, or both (see Fig. 15-18).

5. Infarction in the **vertebrobasilar distributions** in the brainstem leads to alternating signs.

6. "Watershed" infarcts occur along the junction zones of major vessels if the systemic blood pressure drops or if the patient suffers anoxia.
   a. These watershed zones are farthest from the origins of the vessels and have the most precarious lifeline of blood.
   b. A common site of watershed infarction is the "basket handle" arc at the junction of the ACA and MCA.

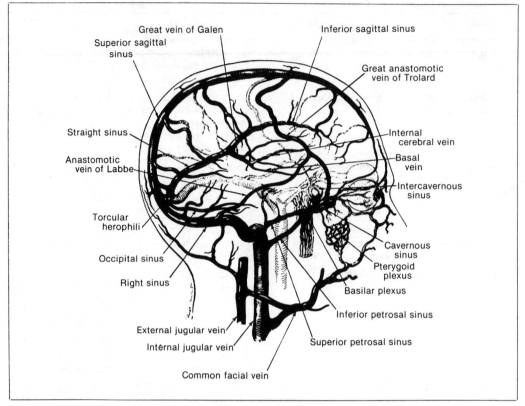

Figure 15-20. Lateral perspective view of the dural sinuses. (Reprinted with permission from Shenkin HA: Dynamic anatomy of cerebral circulation. *Arch Neur Psychiatry* 60:245, 1948. Original drawing by Ralph Sweet.)

7. Transient ischemic attacks may affect any of the distributional areas of the posterior or anterior circulation, giving rise to transient signs of dysfunction of the affected neural tissue. Transient ischemic attacks in the BA distribution cause cranial nerve and long tract signs often accompanied by transient vertigo, diplopia, and loss of consciousness.

B. Intracranial hemorrhage (subarachnoid or intracerebral)

1. Intracranial hemorrhage results from rupture of any artery, vein, or aneurysm.

2. Intracerebral hemorrhage
   a. Although any cerebral vessel may bleed, the lenticulostriate arteries have the most marked predilection for hypertensive intracerebral hemorrhage.
   b. The blood may dissect through the basal ganglia to enter the ventricles. Massive intraventricular hemorrhage of any origin is usually fatal.

3. Arterial aneurysms
   a. Aneurysms occur most frequently where the major arteries of the circle of Willis branch.
   b. The aneurysm may act as a mass, compressing cranial nerves, brain tissue, the optic chiasm, or the pituitary gland. Commonly, an aneurysm of the ICA causes palsy of CN III.
   c. If the aneurysm bursts, it causes subarachnoid hemorrhage or, less frequently, intracerebral or intraventricular hemorrhage.

4. Arteriovenous malformations
   a. Errors in the development of the vascular channels may leave abnormal tangles of vessels in various regions of the brain.
   b. In the cerebrum, such lesions frequently cause seizures. They may act as arteriovenous shunts that rob the normal vessels of blood, causing ischemia of the rest of the brain.
   c. Arteriovenous malformations that empty into the galenic system may cause an aneurysmal dilation of the vein of Galen. Such a dilation may cause an output type of cardiac failure in an infant due to the large amount of blood shunted into the dilated vein.

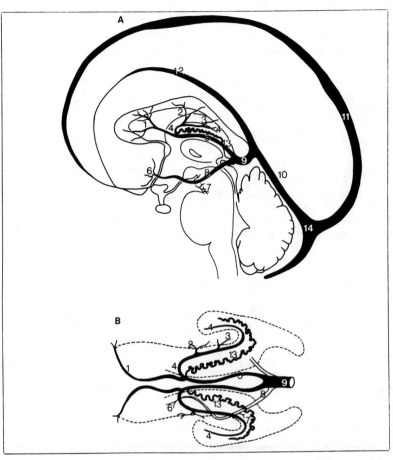

Figure 15-21. Deep cerebral venous system. (A) Sagittal section, medial aspect of the right cerebral hemisphere, showing the deep cerebral venous system. (B) Dorsal perspective view of the deep venous system, in relation to the cerebral ventricles (*interrupted lines*). *1* = septal vein; *2, 3* = thalamostriate branches; *4* = terminal vein; *5* = internal cerebral vein; *6* = anterior perforating veins; *7* = posterior perforating veins; *8* = basal vein of Rosenthal; *9* = vein of Galen; *10* = straight sinus; *11* = superior sagittal sinus; *12* = inferior sagittal sinus; *13* = choroid vein; *14* = confluent sinus.

Table 15-2. Drainage of Cerebral Veins

Brain Region Drained	Sinus Outlet
Superficial cerebral veins	
Superior	
Upper part of facies medialis and facies lateralis	Superior longitudinal sinus
Inferior	
Facies inferior and lower part of facies lateralis and facies medialis	Superior petrosal and transverse sinuses; some superficial posterior cerebral veins enter the vein of Galen
Deep cerebral veins	
Galenic system	
Corpus striatum, dorsal thalamus, periventricular white matter, choroid plexus	Sinus rectus
Miscellaneous basal veins	
Ventral thalamus, midbrain, pons, medulla	Through galenic system to sinus rectus or basal channels

STUDY QUESTIONS

Directions: Each question below contains five suggested answers. Choose the **one best** response to each question.

1. Which one of the following statements concerning the cerebral blood supply is correct?

(A) The blood vessels penetrate the CNS from the pial surface
(B) The terminal arterial distributions tend to have irregular, overlapping margins
(C) The longest brain arteries irrigate the paramedian zone of the brain
(D) The branching pattern of the major veins closely matches the branching pattern of the major arteries
(E) The blood from the right and left half of the brain intermingles freely at the torcular Herophili and the circle of Willis

2. All of the following statements about the basilar artery are correct EXCEPT

(A) it is formed by the union of the vertebral arteries
(B) it commences at the level of the pontomedullary junction
(C) it extends along the ventral aspect of the brainstem to the optic chiasm
(D) it terminates by bifurcating into the posterior cerebral arteries
(E) it sends numerous paramedian branches into the brainstem

3. All of the branches or connections listed for the following major vessels are correct EXCEPT

(A) anterior cerebral artery/Heubner's artery
(B) middle cerebral artery/lateral striate arteries
(C) Galenic vein/inferior longitudinal (sagittal) sinus
(D) Basilar artery/posterior inferior cerebellar artery
(E) Carotid artery/middle cerebral artery

4. All of the following vessels are part of the circle of Willis EXCEPT

(A) the anterior communicating artery
(B) the posterior communicating artery
(C) the connection of the posterior cerebral arteries with the basilar artery
(D) the anterior cerebral artery
(E) the lateral striate arteries

Directions: The group of questions below consists of lettered choices followed by several numbered items. For each numbered item select the **one** lettered choice with which it is **most** closely associated. Each lettered choice may be used once, more than once, or not at all.

Questions 5–10

Match each clinical deficit that is typically caused by arterial occlusion with the responsible artery.

(A) Paramedian branch of basilar artery
(B) Posterior cerebral artery
(C) Lateral striate arteries
(D) Posterior inferior cerebellar artery
(E) Anterior cerebral artery

5. Contralateral monoplegia of the leg
6. Contralateral hemiplegia and hemisensory loss
7. Contralateral hemianopia
8. Contralateral loss of pain and temperature and ipsilateral ataxia and Horner's syndrome
9. Medial longitudinal fasciculus syndrome
10. Ipsilateral palsy of CN VI and contralateral hemiplegia

ANSWERS AND EXPLANATIONS

1. The answer is A. (*I A 1; V A 1*) The cerebral blood vessels penetrate the CNS from the pial surface. The terminal distributions are regular in most patients, and infarcts due to occlusion of the major vessels have predictable distributions. The longest brain arteries are the long circumferential vessels.

2. The answer is C. (*III D 2*) The basilar artery commences with the union of the vertebral arteries at the pontomedullary junction, and it extends essentially the length of the pons, bifurcating into the posterior cerebral arteries at the interpeduncular fossa. Thus, it stops short of the full length of the midbrain and does not extend to the optic chiasm.

3. The answer is D. [*III D 2 c (1)*] The basilar artery gives rise to the posterior cerebral arteries, the superior cerebellar arteries, and the anterior inferior cerebellar arteries. The posterior inferior cerebellar arteries are usually branches of the vertebral artery. These are all long circumferential arteries.

4. The answer is E. (*III C 2*) The circle of Willis is an anastomotic circle connecting the large arteries at the base of the forebrain and midbrain. The circle is comprised of the bifurcation of the internal carotid arteries into two middle cerebral and two anterior cerebral arteries; the anterior communicating artery, two posterior communicating arteries, and two posterior cerebral arteries. These arteries connect the internal carotid arteries with the terminal end of the basilar artery. The lateral striate arteries, which come from the middle cerebral arteries, are distal to the circle of Willis and are not part of it.

5–10. The answers are 5-E, 6-C, 7-B, 8-D, 9-A, 10-A. (*V A*) Infarctions in the distributions of the major cerebral arteries produce characteristic clinical syndromes. Occlusion of the anterior cerebral artery may cause a contralateral monoplegia of the leg because it supplies the medial hemispheric wall. The "leg area" of the motor strip is represented over the crest of the hemisphere and down into the cortex of the interhemispheric fissure of the medial hemispheric wall.

Occlusion of the middle cerebral or lateral striate arteries generally gives rise to contralateral hemiplegia and hemisensory loss, due to involvement of the pre- and postcentral gyri or the internal capsule. Extensive infarcts of the middle cerebral artery distribution in the left hemisphere will also cause aphasia. When infarcts affect the right cerebral hemisphere, they may cause disturbances in the awareness of the left half of space.

Occlusion of the posterior inferior cerebellar artery typically gives rise to ipsilateral ataxia and contralateral loss of pain and temperature. Ataxia is a result of infarction of the cerebellar hemisphere. Horner's syndrome is the result of interruption of descending sympathetic fibers in the dorsolateral part of the medulla, which is supplied by the posterior inferior cerebellar artery. The artery also supplies the lateral medullary region dorsal to the inferior olivary nucleus, which conveys the pain and temperature fibers from the contralateral side of the body. Because of involvement of the descending root of CN V, the patient may also lose the corneal reflex and pain and temperature sensations over the ipsilateral side of the face. Involvement of the nucleus ambiguus or its fibers, which enter CNs IX and X, may cause some degree of paralysis of the pharyngeal and laryngeal muscles.

Occlusion of the basilar artery itself generally causes quadriplegia and loss of consciousness, due to involvement of the basis of the brainstem and the tegmentum of the midbrain or rostral pons. A more restricted infarct in the basilar artery distribution in the basis pontis interrupts the pyramidal tracts bilaterally and causes the locked-in syndrome. If the lesion affects one pyramidal tract at the caudal end of the pons, it may also involve the CN VI fibers that run through the paramedian pontine region at that level. The patient then has an ipsilateral CN VI palsy and contralateral hemiplegia.

Another characteristic syndrome related to restricted occlusion of the paramedian branches of the basilar artery is the syndrome of contralateral hemiplegia with ipsilateral CN III involvement, when the lesion affects the midbrain level, or the medial longitudinal fasciculus syndrome, when the infarct affects the pontine tegmentum. Occlusion of one posterior cerebral artery results in occipital lobe infarction, causing contralateral hemianopia or complete blindness (double hemianopia) if both occipital lobes undergo infarction.

Appendix:
Basic Clinical
Neurologic Examination

I. DETECTING THE MANIFESTATIONS OF NEUROLOGIC DISEASE

A. Neurologic disease can cause changes in the mental, motor, and sensory function of the patient.

B. The clinical neurologic examination consists of a series of observations, questions, commands, and maneuvers designed to detect mental, motor, and sensory dysfunction.

C. The clinician should execute each observation, question, command, and maneuver according to a strict protocol of correct technique and judge the results with knowledge of the limits of normality.

D. The clinician should use prescribed equipment in conducting the clinical neurologic examination (Table A-1).

E. The examination is divided into several areas of investigation, which are outlined in this appendix.

II. HISTORY TAKING. Much of the neurologic examination can be completed as the history is being taken.

A. Inspect the patient's facial features, movement patterns, and posture, and assess the content and production of speech.

B. The history and preliminary observations can determine the examination plan and the areas to be emphasized.

C. The history may suggest additional tests that can be given, tailored to a patient's particular problems.

D. The conditions that the patient thinks precipitate or aggravate his or her condition should be reproduced during the history taking and preliminary examination, such as:

1. Weakness in climbing stairs: The clinician should watch the patient climb stairs.

2. Dizziness when standing up: The clinician should check for orthostatic hypotension.

III. MENTAL STATUS

A. General behavior and appearance. Describe the patient's behavior as normal, hypoactive, or hyperactive, and note the mode and appropriateness of his or her clothing.

B. Flow of speech. Describe the patient's conversation as normal, too slow, too rapid or insistent, as well as the degree of spontaneity, discursiveness, and ability to follow the line of the conversation.

C. Mood and affective responses. Is the patient emotionally labile, agitated, inappropriately gay or euphoric, giggling, silent, weeping, or angry? Does the patient's mood match the subject matter of the conversation?

The appendix has been adapted with permission from the "Summarized Neurologic Examination" that appears in *Technique of the Neurologic Examination, A Programmed Text,* 3rd ed. by William DeMyer, New York, McGraw-Hill, 1980.

Table A-1. Equipment Required for the Neurologic Examination

Article	Use
1. Flexible steel measuring tape	Measuring occipitofrontal and other body circumferences, size of skin lesions, length of extremities, etc.
2. Flashlight with rubber adapter	Checking pupillary reflexes; inspection of pharynx, and transillumination of the head
3. Transparent mm ruler	Measuring pupillary size, diameter of skin lesions, and distances on radiographic films
4. Ophthalmoscope	Funduscopy; examination of ocular media and skin surface for beads of sweat
5. Tongue blades (three per patient)	One for depressing tongue, one for eliciting gag reflex, and one (broken) for eliciting abdominal and plantar reflexes
6. Opaque vial of coffee	Testing sense of smell
7. Opaque vials of salt and sugar	Testing sense of taste
8. Tuning fork	Testing vibratory sensation and hearing (256 cps recommended)
9. Otoscope	Examination of auditory canal and drum
10. 10 cc syringe	Caloric irrigation of the ear
11. Cotton wisp	One end rolled for eliciting corneal reflex; the other loose for testing light touch
12. Reflex hammer	Eliciting muscle stretch reflexes
13. Two stoppered tubes	Testing hot and cold discrimination
14. Disposable straight pins	Testing pain sensation
15. Penny, nickel, dime, paper clip, and key	Testing stereognosis
16. Page of stimulus figures (Halstead-Reitan screening test) and table of examiner's instructions and patient's tasks	Screening cerebral and intellectual functions

D. **Content of thought.** Does the patient have illusions, hallucinations, or delusions? Does the patient display phobias or preoccupation with bodily functions?

E. **Intellectual capacity.** Estimate if the patient is bright, average, dull, mentally retarded, or obviously demented.

F. **Sensorium.** Assess the following:

1. Consciousness

2. Attention span

3. Orientation for time, place, and person

4. Memory, recent and remote, as disclosed during the history taking

5. Fund of information

6. Insight, judgment, and planning capabilities

7. Calculation ability

IV. **SPEECH.** Does the patient display any of the following impairments of speech?

A. **Dysphonia,** difficulty in producing the voice sound

B. **Dysarthria,** difficulty in articulating the individual sounds or the units (phonemes) of speech;

that is, f's, r's, g's, vowels, consonants, the labials (CN VII), gutturals (CN X), and linguals (CN XII)

C. Dysprosody, difficulty with the stress of syllables, inflections, pitch of voice, and the rhythm of words

D. Dysphasia, difficulty in expressing or understanding words as symbols of communication

V. HEAD AND FACE

A. Inspection

1. Record the general impression of the patient's face. Does it show normal motility and emotional expression, or is it a diagnostic facial gestalt?

2. Inspect the eyes for ptosis, the width of the palpebral fissures, the relation of iris to lid, pupillary size, and interorbital distance.

3. Inspect the contours of the nose, mouth, chin, and ears.

4. Inspect the hair of the scalp, eyebrows, and beard.

5. Inspect the head for abnormalities in shape and symmetry.

B. Palpate the skull for lumps, depressions or tenderness, and asymmetries. Measure and record the occipitofrontal circumference, and palpate the skull sutures and fontanelles of all infants.

C. Auscultate for bruits over the great vessels, eyes, temples, and mastoid processes.

D. Percuss sinuses and mastoid processes for tenderness if the patient has headaches.

E. Transilluminate the sinuses if the patient has headaches. Attempt to transilluminate the skull of every infant.

VI. CRANIAL NERVES

A. Optic group (II, III, IV, and VI)

1. Inspect the width of the palpebral fissures, the relation of limbus to lid margins, and the interorbital distance, and check for en- or exophthalmos.

2. **Visual functions.** Test acuity of central fields with newsprint (each eye separately) and peripheral fields by confrontation. Test for inattention to simultaneous stimuli if a cerebral lesion is suspected.

3. **Ocular motility.** Test the range of ocular movements by having the patient's eyes follow your finger through all fields of gaze. During convergence, check for miosis. Record nystagmus and any effects of eye movements on it.

B. Branchiomotor group and tongue (V, VII, IX and X, XII, and XI)

1. **CN V.** Inspect masseter and temporalis muscle bulk, and palpate the masseter when the patient bites.

2. **CN VII.** Check forehead wrinkling, eyelid closure, mouth retraction, and labial articulation; have patient whistle or puff out the cheeks and wrinkle the skin over the neck to check the platysma muscle. Check for Chvostek's sign in selected cases.

3. **CNs IX and X.** Assess swallowing, gag reflex, and palatal elevation, and assess phonation and nasality of articulation.

4. **CN XII.** Assess lingual articulations and midline and lateral tongue protrusion, and inspect the tongue for atrophy and fasciculations.

5. **CN XI.** Inspect sternocleidomastoid and trapezius contours, and test the strength of head movements and shoulder shrugging.

C. Special sensory group (I, VII, VIII)

1. **Olfaction (CN I).** Use an aromatic, nonirritating substance and test each nostril separately.

2. **Taste (CN VII).** Use salt or sugar. Check particularly if a CN VII lesion is suspected.

3. **Hearing** (CN VIII)
   a. Do an otoscopy.
   b. Assess **threshold and acuity** by testing the patient's ability to hear conversational speech, a tuning fork, a watch tick, and rustling of fingers.
   c. If the history or preceding tests suggest a deficit, do the air–bone conduction test of Rinne and the vertex lateralizing test of Weber.
   d. If the history suggests a cerebral lesion, test for auditory inattention to bilateral simultaneous stimuli, using finger rustling.

4. **Vestibular function** (CN VIII). Do caloric irrigation in selected patients, and test for positional nystagmus.

D. **Somatic sensation of the face (CN V)**

   1. Assess the corneal reflex (CNs V–VII arc).

   2. Check light touch over the three divisions of CN V.

   3. Check pain perception over the three divisions of CN V.

   4. Assess temperature discrimination.

   5. Test the buccal mucosa sensation in selected cases.

VII. SOMATIC MOTOR SYSTEM

A. **Inspection**

   1. Inspect the patient's somatotype, posture, general activity level, and look for tremors or involuntary movements.

   2. Search the entire skin surface for lesions, particularly neurocutaneous stigmata, such as café au lait spots.

   3. Observe the size and contour of the muscles; look for atrophy, hypertrophy, body asymmetry, joint malalignments, fasciculations, tremors, and involuntary movements.

   4. Assess the patient's gait by observing free walking, toe and heel walking, tandem walking, and deep knee bends. Have children hop on each foot and run.

B. **Palpation.** Palpate muscles if they seem atrophic or hypertrophic or if the history suggests that they may be tender or in spasm.

C. **Strength testing**

   1. **Shoulder girdle.** Try to press the patient's arms down after he or she abducts them to shoulder height. Look for scapular winging.

   2. **Upper extremities.** Test biceps, triceps, wrist dorsiflexors, and grip. Test the strength of finger abduction and extension.

   3. **Abdominal muscles.** Have the patient do a sit-up; watch for umbilical migration.

   4. **Lower extremities.** Test hip flexors, abductors and adductors, knee flexors, foot dorsiflexors, invertors, and evertors. (The knee extensors were tested by the deep knee bends at section VII A 4.)

   5. Grade the patient's strength on a scale of 0 to 5, or describe the patient as having paralysis; severe, moderate, or minimal weakness; or normal strength. Observe if any weakness follows a distributional pattern, such as proximal–distal, right–left, or upper extremity–lower extremity.

D. **Percussion.** Percuss the thenar eminence for myotonia, and test myotonic grip if the patient has generalized muscular weakness.

E. **Muscle tone assessment.** Make passive movements of the joints to test for spasticity, clonus, or rigidity.

F. **Muscle stretch (deep) reflex testing.** Grade on a scale of 0 to 4+, and observe whether they are clonic (Fig. A-1).

   1. Jaw jerk (CN V afferent, CN V efferent)

   2. Biceps reflex (C5–C6)

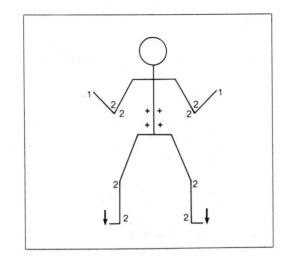

Figure A-1. Figure for recording the results of a reflex examination. The numbers represent a normal reflex pattern.

3. Triceps reflex (C7–C8)

4. Finger flexion reflex (C7–T1)

5. Quadriceps reflex (L2–L4)

6. Hamstrings reflex (L5–S1–S2)

7. Triceps surae reflex or ankle jerk (L5–S1–S3)

8. Toe flexion reflex (S1–S2)

G. Skin–muscle (superficial) reflex testing

1. Abdominal skin–muscle reflexes (upper quadrants T8–T9). Do an umbilical migration test for Beevor's sign, if a thoracic cord lesion is suspected.

2. Cremasteric reflex (afferent L1–efferent L2)

3. Anal pucker (S4–S5) and bulbocavernosus reflexes in patients suspected of having sacral or cauda equina lesions

H. Cerebellar system testing. (Also see gait testing in section VII A 4 of this appendix.)

1. Request the finger-to-nose and heel-to-knee maneuvers for dystaxia (incoordination) of voluntary movements.

2. Request rapid alternating hand movements to test for incoordination (dysdiadochokinesia).

I. Nerve root stretch testing. (Do in selected cases.)

1. If meningitis is suspected, test for nuchal rigidity and concomitant leg flexion (Brudzinski's sign) and do leg raising tests.

2. If disk or low-back disease is suspected, do leg raising tests: straight-knee leg raising test (Lasègue's sign) and bent-knee leg raising test (Kernig's sign).

VIII. SOMATIC SENSORY SYSTEM

A. Superficial sensory modality testing

1. Light touch perception over hands, trunk, and feet (use cotton wisp)

2. Pain perception over hands, trunk, and feet

3. Temperature discrimination

B. Deep sensory modality testing

1. Vibration perception at knuckles, fingernails, and malleoli of the ankles

2. Position sense of fingers and toes (fourth digits)

3. Romberg (swaying) test

4. Stereognosis

C. Determination of the distributional pattern of any sensory loss: dermatomal, peripheral nerves, central pathway, or nonorganic

IX. CEREBRAL FUNCTIONS

A. When the history or preliminary examination suggests a cerebral lesion, test for agraphognosia, finger agnosia, poor two-point discrimination, right–left disorientation, atopognosia, and tactile, auditory, and visual inattention to bilateral simultaneous stimuli. Test for tactile inattention to simultaneous ipsilateral stimulation of face–hand and foot–hand.

B. Have the patient do the cognitive, constructional, and performance tasks of the Halstead-Reitan cerebral function screening test (Fig. A-2; Table A-2). The figure and table are used simultaneously by the examiner during the screening.

X. CASE SUMMARY. The examiner should prepare a summary of the pertinent positive and negative findings, a clinical diagnosis, a differential diagnosis, and a sequential plan of management.

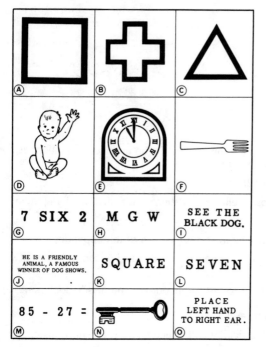

Figure A-2. Stimulus figures for the Halstead-Reitan cerebral function screening test.

Table A-2. Halstead-Reitan Cerebral Function Screening Test

Patient's Task	Examiner's Instructions to the Patient
1. Copy *square* (A)	First, draw this on your paper. (Point to square, item A.) I want you to do it without lifting your pencil from the paper. Make it about the same size.
2. Name *square*	What is that shape called?
3. Spell *square*	Would you spell that word for me?
4. Copy *cross* (B)	Draw this on your paper. (Point to the cross, item B.) Go around the outside like this until you get back to where you started. Make it about the same size.
5. Name *cross*	What is that shape called?
6. Spell *cross*	Would you spell that word for me?

Table A-2. Continued

Patient's Task	Examiner's Instructions to the Patient
7. Copy *triangle* (C)	Draw this on your paper. (Point to the triangle, item C.) Do it without lifting your pencil from the paper, and make it about the same size.
8. Name *triangle*	What is that shape called?
9. Spell *triangle*	Would you spell that word for me?
10. Name *baby* (D)	What is this? (Show baby, item D.)
11. Write *clock* (E)	Now, I am going to show you another picture, but do not tell me the name of it. I don't want you to say anything out loud. Just write the name of the picture on your paper. (Show clock, item E.)
12. Name *fork* (F)	What is this? (Show fork, item F.)
13. Read *7 six 2* (G)	I want you to read this. (Show item G.)
14. Read *M G W* (H)	Read this. (Show item H.)
15. Read item I	Now, I what you to read this. (Show item I.)
16. Read item J	Can you read this? (Show item J.)
17. Repeat *triangle*	Now, I am going to say some words. I want you to listen carefully and say them after me as well as you can. Say this word: *triangle*.
18. Repeat *Massachusetts*	The next one is a little harder, but do your best. Say this word: *Massachusetts*.
19. Repeat *Methodist Episcopal*	Now, repeat this phrase: *Methodist Episcopal*.
20. Write *square* (K)	Don't say this word out loud; just write it on your paper. (Point to item K.)
21. Read *seven* (L)	Can you read this word out loud? (Show item L.)
22. Repeat *seven*	Now, I want you to repeat this after me: *seven*.
23. Repeat and explain *He shouted the warning*	I am going to say something that I want you to say after me. So listen carefully: *He shouted the warning*. Now, you say it. Would you explain what that means?
24. Write *He shouted the warning*	Now, I want you to write that sentence on the paper.
25. Compute *85 − 27* (M)	Here is an arithmetic problem. Copy it on your paper in any way you like and try to work it out. (Show item M.)
26. Compute *17 × 3*	Now, do this one in your head: *17 × 3 = ?*
27. Name *key* (N)	What is this? (Show item N.)
28. Demonstrate the use of a *key*	If you had one of these in your hand, show me how you would use it. (Show item N.)
29. Draw *key*	Now, I want you to draw a picture that looks just like this. Try to make your key look enough like this one so that I will know it is the same key from your drawing. (Point to key, item N.)
30. Read item O	Would you read this? (Show item O.)
31. *Place left hand to right ear*	Now, would you do what it says?
32. Place left hand to left elbow	Now, I want you to place your left hand to your left elbow. (The patient should quickly realize the impossibility of the task.)

Post-test

QUESTIONS

Directions: Each question below contains five suggested answers. Choose the **one best** response to each question.

1. The original somite–spinal nerve relationship is best shown at which level of the neuraxis?

(A) Cervical
(B) Thoracic
(C) Lumbar
(D) Sacral
(E) Coccygeal

2. The "jelly roll" hypothesis of myelination in peripheral nerves is based on which one of the following?

(A) The fact that a Schwann cell can accommodate only one myelinated fiber
(B) Embedding of small axons in the surface cytoplasm of the Schwann cell
(C) Encircling of large axons by a lip of Schwann cell cytoplasm
(D) Enfolding of several Schwann cells by one axon
(E) None of the above

3. The tentorium cerebelli can be most accurately described as

(A) a fold of arachnoid between the cerebellar hemispheres
(B) separating the cerebellum from the occipital lobe
(C) the membranous roof between the cerebellum and the fourth ventricle
(D) covering the ventral surface of the cerebellum
(E) none of the above

4. The correct dorsoventral order of tracts along the paramedian plane of the medulla is

(A) medial longitudinal fasciculus, tectospinal tract, medial lemniscus, and pyramidal tract
(B) tectospinal tract, medial lemniscus, pyramidal tract, and medial longitudinal fasciculus
(C) medial lemniscus, medial longitudinal fasciculus, tectospinal tract, pyramidal tract
(D) pyramidal tract, medial lemniscus, tectospinal tract, and medial longitudinal fasciculus
(E) none of the above

5. All of the following associations of a nerve and its distribution or function are correct EXCEPT

(A) median nerve/flexion of the wrist and distal interphalangeal joints
(B) ulnar nerve/abduction of the little finger
(C) obturator nerve/thigh adduction
(D) musculocutaneous nerve/biceps muscle
(E) common peroneal nerve/extension and flexion of the ankle

6. Use of horseradish peroxidase as a technique for identifying neuroanatomical pathways depends on

(A) transport along axons
(B) destruction of myelin sheaths
(C) wallerian degeneration
(D) inhibition of oxidative metabolism
(E) inhibition of protein synthesis

7. The two cranial nerves that differ radically in histology from that typical of peripheral nerves are

(A) CN I and CN II
(B) CN III and CN IV
(C) CN V and CN VI
(D) CN VII and CN VIII
(E) CN IX and CN XII

8. The tentorial notch provides an opening between

(A) the anterior fossa and the middle fossa
(B) the right supratentorial space and the left
(C) the supratentorial space and the infratentorial space
(D) the posterior fossa and the foramen magnum
(E) none of the above

9. All of the following structures derive in general from the neural crest EXCEPT

(A) neuronal perikarya in the PNS
(B) axons of ventral roots
(C) axons of dorsal roots
(D) autonomic ganglia
(E) adrenal medulla

10. All of the following statements about spinal nerves are true EXCEPT

(A) each spinal nerve innervates one somite
(B) the nerve trunk is formed by the union of dorsal and ventral roots
(C) each spinal nerve typically has one dorsal root ganglion
(D) most spinal nerves contain parasympathetic efferent axons
(E) all spinal nerves convey axons to skeletal muscles

11. According to the theory of nerve components, the white sympathetic rami contain

(A) general somatic efferent (GSE) axons
(B) GSE and general visceral afferent (GVA) axons
(C) GVA and general somatic afferent (GSA) axons
(D) general visceral efferent (GVE) axons
(E) GVE, GVA, and GSA axons

12. The spinal cord reflects the law of Bell and Magendie since

(A) the dorsal horn is sensory and the ventral horn is motor
(B) the spinal cord develops an intermediolateral cell column
(C) the corticospinal tracts run in the lateral columns
(D) the ventral horn contains no interneurons
(E) the ventral columns contain only sensory axons

13. The rostral-most somite receives innervation from which level of the CNS?

(A) Diencephalon
(B) Midbrain
(C) Pons
(D) Medulla
(E) C1 level

14. The sublenticular and retrolenticular parts of the internal capsule convey

(A) thalamoparietal and thalamocingulate radiations
(B) thalamoparietal and geniculocalcarine radiations only
(C) thalamofrontal and thalamoparietal radiations
(D) geniculocalcarine, temporal, and occipital radiations
(E) none of the above

15. A lesion that destroys the decussation of the brachium conjunctivum and surrounding tissue would also be likely to encroach on

(A) serotonergic nuclei
(B) dopaminergic nuclei
(C) the lateral lemniscus
(D) the CN IV nucleus
(E) the pretectal region

16. The subdivision of the CNS that lacks direct sensory connections with the external environment is the

(A) telencephalon
(B) diencephalon
(C) midbrain
(D) pons
(E) medulla oblongata

17. The nucleus ambiguus supplies axons to cranial nerves

(A) IX, X, XI, and XII
(B) VII, IX, X, and XI
(C) IX, X
(D) VII, XI, XII
(E) VIII, IX, X, XI

18. An example of a nerve cell process that is axonal in structure and dendritic in function is

(A) the distal process of a dorsal root ganglion neuron
(B) basal dendrites
(C) the proximal process of a bipolar ganglion neuron
(D) the distal process of a motoneuron axon
(E) none of the above

19. The pyramidal tract can be best described as

(A) arising only from area 4 (area gigantopyramidalis)
(B) synapsing almost exclusively directly on ventral horn cells
(C) having only small axons (less than 10 μ in diameter)
(D) having a somatotopic organization of its fibers at its origin
(E) conveying many axons from the rhinencephalon

20. Which of the following forms of aphasia would most likely be associated with a right-sided upper motor neuron (UMN) facial palsy?

(A) Dyslexia
(B) Auditory word agnosia
(C) Dyslexia plus dysgraphia
(D) Auditory word aphasia plus dyslexia (fluent aphasia)
(E) Expressive aphasia, nonfluent type

21. Which one of the following operations would denude the cerebellar vermis of spinal afferents?

(A) Section of the dorsal columns of the spinal cord
(B) Section of the middle cerebellar peduncle
(C) Section of the rostral (superior) cerebellar peduncle and the restiform body
(D) Section of the middle cerebellar peduncle and the ventral columns of the spinal cord
(E) None of the above

22. A lesion that would most effectively disconnect the frontal and temporal lobes would interrupt the

(A) uncinate fasciculus
(B) inferior longitudinal fasciculus
(C) central tegmental tract
(D) fornix
(E) frontal thalamic radiation

23. General characteristics of the dopaminergic neurons include all of the following EXCEPT

(A) they are concentrated in the midbrain tegmentum
(B) they send their main axonal connections rostrally, in contrast to the norepinephrinergic neurons
(C) they conform to well-delineated nuclear groups
(D) they consist mainly of small poorly branched neurons
(E) they receive strong connections from the basal ganglia and diencephalon

24. The one correct statement about the internal capsule is that it

(A) forms a large sheet between the thalamus and the tail of the caudate nucleus
(B) conveys the connections between the nucleus medialis dorsalis and the cingulate cortex
(C) conveys the somatosensory fibers between the thalamus and the postcentral gyrus
(D) receives its blood supply from the anterior communicating artery
(E) conveys few or no myelinated fibers

Directions: Each question below contains four suggested answers of which **one or more** is correct. Choose the answer

A   if **1, 2, and 3** are correct
B   if **1 and 3** are correct
C   if **2 and 4** are correct
D   if **4** is correct
E   if **1, 2, 3, and 4** are correct

25. Reduction in pain responses can be produced by which of the following procedures?

(1) Stimulation of the periaqueductal gray matter
(2) Anterolateral cordotomy
(3) Section of the lateral division of the dorsal roots
(4) Cingulotomy

26. Anatomical characteristics of the reticular formation include which of the following?

(1) Wide dispersion of axonal connections
(2) Sharply separated, discrete clumps of nuclei
(3) Heterogenous, multiple-afferent connections
(4) Output through a few discrete myelinated tracts

27. Section of both optic nerves in a young animal would ultimately have which of the following effects on the calcarine cortex?

(1) Decrease in capillarity
(2) Loss of the outer stripe of Baillarger
(3) Degeneration of cortical neurons
(4) Compensatory overgrowth of oligodendroglia

28. Neuronal perikarya assume which of the following patterns of organization?

(1) Laminations
(2) Nuclear masses
(3) Reticular formation
(4) Ganglia

29. Correct statements about substance P include which of the following?

(1) It is found in large concentration in the substantia gelatinosa and periaqueductal gray matter
(2) It combines with opioid receptors in the brainstem basis
(3) It is found in the smaller dorsal root ganglion neurons
(4) It is thought to inhibit pain transmission

30. A node of Ranvier has which of the following characteristics?

(1) It marks the site of discontinuity of the myelin sheath cells
(2) The theory of saltatory conduction presumes it to be the site of ionic flux
(3) It is visible in both electron and light microscopy
(4) The distance between two nodes is the length of a Schwann cell

31. The cavity of the CNS correctly matches the segment that contains it in which of the following pairs?

(1) Cerebrum/lateral ventricle
(2) Diencephalon/third ventricle
(3) Midbrain/aqueduct
(4) Pons–medulla/fourth ventricle

32. Dermatomal levels correctly matched with an area of the body include which of the following?

(1) C7/middle finger, index finger, or both
(2) T8/nipple line
(3) T10/umbilicus
(4) S1/perianal region

33. The thalamic fasciculus conveys which of the following pathways?

(1) Medial lemniscus
(2) Dentatothalamic tract
(3) Pallidothalamic tract
(4) Thalamofrontal radiation

34. Upon entering the spinal cord, dorsal root axons of the spinal nerves synapse on

(1) motoneurons
(2) sensory neurons
(3) interneurons
(4) isodendritic neurons

35. Major sites of neuroblast proliferation in the CNS include which of the following?

(1) Roof plate
(2) Marginal zone of the spinal cord
(3) White matter of the cerebrum
(4) Periventricular zone

36. Major sites at which large numbers of neurons lodge or accumulate after migration include the

(1) basis pontis
(2) cerebellar cortex
(3) olivary nuclei
(4) neurohypophysis

37. The epidural space of the cranium differs from the spinal epidural space in which of the following ways?

(1) It contains a plexus of blood vessels
(2) It is potential rather than actual space
(3) It does not distend with blood or pus
(4) It contains no fat cells

38. The pia mater can be described as being

(1) the outermost of the three meninges
(2) part of the leptomeninges
(3) in immediate contact with the arachnoid membrane
(4) enfolded into the crevices of the brain and spinal cord

39. Anatomical components of the blood–brain barrier include

(1) astrocytic end feet
(2) the arachnoid membrane
(3) capillary endothelium
(4) Nissl bodies

40. Fiber pathways through the anterior commissure include which of the following?

(1) Corticocortical connections of the parietal lobe
(2) Amygdalo–amygdalar connections
(3) Pallido–pallidal connections
(4) Habenulo–habenular connections

Directions: The groups of questions below consist of lettered choices followed by several numbered items. For each numbered item select the **one** lettered choice with which it is **most** closely associated. Each lettered choice may be used once, more than once, or not at all.

Questions 41–45

Match each procedure or operation with the neurotransmitter that it would deplete.

(A) Serotonin and catecholamines in the cerebral cortex
(B) Gamma-aminobutyric acid (GABA) and glycine in the spinal cord
(C) Substance P in the dorsal horns
(D) Acetylcholine in cerebral cortex
(E) Serotonin in the spinal cord

41. Destruction of spinal interneurons (by controlled hypoxia)

42. Section of dorsal roots

43. Section of the medial forebrain bundle

44. Destruction of the anterior perforated substance

45. Destruction of the medullary raphe

Questions 46–50

Match the cortical connections or projections listed below with the most closely related thalamic nucleus.

(A) Nucleus ventralis lateralis
(B) Nucleus pulvinaris
(C) Nucleus anterior and lateralis dorsalis
(D) Nucleus medialis dorsalis
(E) Lateral geniculate body

46. Projects visual impulses to the calcarine cortex

47. Connects with the frontal lobe anterior to the motor cortex (prefrontal area)

48. Projects to the nonstriate areas (eulaminate isocortex) of the parieto–occipito–temporal lobes

49. Projects to the motor cortex

50. Connects with the limbic cortex of the cingulate gyrus

Questions 51–55

Match the clinical deficit with the lesion site that would produce it.

(A) Precentral gyrus
(B) Postcentral gyrus
(C) Occipital lobe
(D) Left parasylvian region
(E) Medial temporal lobe/hippocampus

51. Aphasia
52. Hypesthesia
53. Hemiplegia
54. Hemianopia
55. Loss of recent memory

Questions 56–60

Match the characteristic properties of glial cells with each type of glial cell listed below.

(A) Medulloblast
(B) Oligodendrocyte
(C) Microglial cell
(D) Ependymal cell
(E) Fibrous astrocyte

56. Has numerous large branches that attach to the pial surface and blood vessel walls

57. Lines the cerebral aqueduct

58. Provides support and cohesion for the CNS

59. Has few processes, some of which may end on the neuronal surface, and its nuclei line up in rows in the white matter

60. Was once thought to produce macrophages in response to injury

ANSWERS AND EXPLANATIONS

1. The answer is B. (*Chapter 3 VII C*) Each somite of the body receives a single spinal nerve. In the arm and leg regions, the somites intermingle to form bones and muscles but they retain their original nerve supply. In the thoracic region, the somites remain in their original serial order and the spinal nerves run directly into the somite derivatives rather than going through plexuses.

2. The answer is C. (*Chapter 3 VIII A*) The "jelly roll" hypothesis of myelination assumes that the myelin sheath forms by a lip of Schwann cell encircling the individual axons. A single Schwann cell can myelinate more than one axon because its cytoplasm can encircle an axon wherever the axon contacts it.

3. The answer is B. (*Chapter 2 VI F*) The tentorium cerebelli is a fold of dura mater inserted between the occipital lobes and the posterior part of the temporal lobes and the cerebellum. Along its midline, the tentorium attaches to the cerebral falx, and along its posterior lateral margins, it attaches to the skull, where it splits to form the transverse sinuses.

4. The answer is A. (*Chapter 8 Figure 8-27*) The tracts along the paramedian plane of the medulla in dorsoventral order consist of the medial longitudinal fasciculus, tectospinal tract, medial lemniscus, and pyramidal tract. The tracts commence with the medial longitudinal fasciculus, which is a ground bundle of the somite nuclei of the brainstem, and then the other tracts laminate in an orderly manner, with the pyramidal tracts being most superficial. The pyramidal tracts are the longest and the latest to appear phylogenetically and, therefore, have the most superficial position, in contrast to the medial longitudinal fasciculus, which is a primitive tract and runs directly along the margin of the gray matter.

5. The answer is E. (*Chapter 5 Table 5-4*) The sciatic nerve divides at the popliteal space to form the common peroneal nerve and the tibial nerve. The common peroneal nerve is the extensor nerve of the foot and ankle, whereas the tibial is the flexor nerve of the foot and ankle. Both the median and ulnar nerves innervate muscles that flex the wrist.

6. The answer is A. (*Chapter 4 IV F*) The horseradish peroxidase technique for identifying pathways depends upon transport of the substance along axons. The material can be injected into the nervous tissue, where it will be incorporated into the nerve cell through the cell membrane and then distributed in either an anterograde or retrograde direction by internal transport mechanisms of the cell. The presence of the peroxidase is then demonstrated by exposing the tissue to a substrate that forms a reaction product that can be seen by microscopy. Other proteins as well as dyes can be used in a similar manner to outline cell processes and perikarya.

7. The answer is A. (*Chapter 3 II D 5; Chapter 8 VI A 1*) The histology of cranial nerves I and II differs radically from the typical histology of peripheral nerves. CN I consists of axonal filaments that perforate the cribriform plate, running from the olfactory mucosa to the olfactory bulb. CN II is actually a tract of central axons that extends from the retina to the diencephalon.

8. The answer is C. (*Chapter 2 VI F*) The opening in the tentorium cerebelli is called the tentorial notch. It separates the supratentorial space from the infratentorial space or, more particularly, the posterior fossa from the middle fossa. The part of the brain that runs from the middle to the posterior fossa through the tentorial notch is the midbrain. The rostral part of the vermis of the cerebellum extends slightly above the plane of the tentorial notch just dorsal to the quadrigeminal plate.

9. The answer is B. (*Chapter 3 IV D, E*) Much of the PNS derives from the neural crest. The crest derivatives include the dorsal root ganglia and their proximal and distal sensory processes, the sympathetic and parasympathetic ganglia, and the adrenal medulla. The axons of the ventral roots arise from the ventral motor neurons of the gray matter of the brainstem and spinal cord.

10. The answer is D. (*Chapter 3 V; VI*) The spinal nerves typically contain four components: visceral and somatic afferents and visceral and somatic efferents. For most spinal nerves, the visceral efferent axon derives from the sympathetic nervous system. Only sacral nerves 2, 3, and 4 carry large numbers of parasympathetic efferent axons.

11. The answer is D. (*Chapter 3 VI C*) The white sympathetic rami run from a nerve trunk to a sympathetic ganglion. These general visceral efferent (GVE) axons are preganglionic fibers, arising in the intermediolateral cell column of the thoracic and upper lumbar cord. The ramus is white because of the greater degree of myelination in the preganglionic fibers, as contrasted to the gray ramus, which conveys mainly unmyelinated postganglionic fibers. The color differences in the rami, however, are not striking.

12. The answer is A. (*Chapter 3 VI A 2, 3*) The law of Bell and Magendie states that the dorsal roots are afferent and the ventral roots are efferent. The internal structure of the spinal cord reflects this functional division since the dorsal horns are sensory and the ventral horns are motor.

13. The answer is B. (*Chapter 8 III D 1, 2*) The rostral-most somites give rise to the muscles that rotate the eyeballs. These muscles develop from somites that originally are opposite the midbrain and receive their innervation from CN III.

14. The answer is D. (*Chapter 12 Table 12-4; Figures 12-5 and 12-8*) The sublenticular and retrolenticular parts of the internal capsule are named for their relationship to the lentiform nucleus. The fibers that run from the thalamus under this nucleus connect the thalamus with the temporal and occipital cortices and convey, among important tracts, the geniculocalcarine tract and the auditory radiations to the temporal lobe.

15. The answer is A. (*Chapter 14 III A 2 a, b*) A lesion that would destroy the decussation of the brachium conjunctivum would affect the midline tegmentum of the caudal part of the midbrain. This region has a large concentration of serotonergic perikarya, located mainly in the dorsal median and raphe nuclei.

16. The answer is C. (*Chapter 8 XI B*) Of all the major subdivisions of the CNS, only the midbrain lacks direct primary afferent connections with the external environment. The olfactory nerve enters the telencephalon. The optic nerve enters the diencephalon. The pons has the huge gasserian ganglion of CN V, and the medulla receives direct afferents from CN IX and CN X. The third nerve of the midbrain may convey proprioceptive fibers, but these presumably go through the gasserian ganglion. The mesencephalic root of the trigeminal nerve serves proprioception rather than exteroception.

17. The answer is C. [*Chapter 8 VI C 3 f (1) (a)*] The nucleus ambiguus is a special visceral efferent nucleus located in the ventrolateral part of the medullary tegmentum. It supplies motor axons to skeletal muscle that derives from branchial arches and is innervated by CN IX and CN X.

18. The answer is A. (*Chapter 2 II C 3–5*) Classically, axons are distinguished from dendrites in being elongated processes that receive few or no synapses. Dendrites, on the other hand, tend to be short, stubby processes that receive numerous synapses. Axons conduct away from the perikaryon and dendrites toward it. The distal process of a dorsal root ganglion neuron is anomalous in having an axonal structure but conducting impulses toward the perikaryon and, therefore, being dendritic in function.

19. The answer is D. (*Chapter 13 VI A 2*) The pyramidal tract arises from areas 4 and 6 as well as from the anterior part of the parietal lobe. It consists of a mixture of axons ranging in size from small ones to very large. These fibers have a somatotopic organization as they originate from the motor cortex and, to a degree, maintain that organization as they descend through the brainstem and spinal cord.

20. The answer is E. (*Chapter 13 VI G 4*) In the parasylvian region, those lesions that are more anterior in the zone, in the posterior part of the inferior frontal gyrus, cause a nonfluent type of expressive aphasia. Since this region is adjacent to the motor cortex that supplies the upper motor neuron (UMN) fibers for the contralateral facial nucleus, a patient with expressive aphasia would be more likely to have a right-sided UMN facial palsy than a patient with a more posterior lesion and a more fluent type of receptive aphasia.

21. The answer is C. (*Chapter 9 IV B 1*) To denude the cerebellar vermis of spinal afferents would involve cutting the dorsal and ventral spinocerebellar tracts in the cord or section of the caudal and rostral cerebellar peduncles through which these tracts turn dorsally from the pons into the cerebellum. The middle peduncle conveys no spinocerebellar afferents.

22. The answer is A. (*Chapter 13 II D 1 c; Figure 13-25*) A large fiber tract, the uncinate fasciculus, bends around the stem of the sylvian fissure to connect the frontal and temporal lobes. This bundle is one of the U-fiber systems that typically skirt the depth of the cerebral crevices to connect adjacent gyri.

23. The answer is D. (*Chapter 14 II B 1–3*) Dopaminergic neurons concentrate in the midbrain in well-delineated masses, in the substantia nigra, and in the interpeduncular region. The neurons of the substantia nigra, in particular, are large and well-branched.

24. The answer is C. (*Chapter 12 II L 1–4*) The internal capsule separates the lentiform nucleus from the caudate and thalamus, forming a "V" around the apex of the globus pallidus of the lentiform nucleus. It consists of large numbers of myelinated, as well as some unmyelinated, fibers. The somatosensory, auditory, and visual pathways all run through some portion of the internal capsule.

25. The answer is E (all). (*Chapter 7 III B 3*) A number of surgical procedures may reduce pain, either by reducing the pain input or by reducing the patient's reaction to the pain input. Direct section of the ventrolateral quadrants of the spinal cord or of the lateral divisions of the dorsal roots will block the afferent pain impulses. Operations on the thalamus, the thalamofrontal connections, or the cingulum do not reduce the delivery of pain impulses but tend to reduce the patient's reaction or response to the pain.

26. The answer is B (1, 3). (*Chapter 8 XIII A, F*) The anatomical characteristics of the reticular formation include a diverse afferent input and a diverse efferent output. The perikarya that comprise the reticular formation generally do not form discrete nuclear clumps, although the regions of the reticular formation vary considerably in this regard. The reticular formation, with its diffuse nature and its intimate role in the control of visceral reactions, stands in direct contrast to the somatic systems, with their topographic point-to-point connections.

27. The answer is A (1, 2, 3). (*Chapter 2 III B 2*) Transection of the optic nerves in the young animal will cause transsynaptic degeneration of the geniculate bodies and the geniculocalcarine tract. Degeneration of this tract would deprive the calcarine cortex of its thalamic afferents and cause the outer line of Baillarger to disappear since it consists of myelinated fibers of thalamic origin. The deafferentation of the cortex would result in transsynaptic atrophy and degeneration of many of the cortical neurons. Because of the loss of neurons, the capillarity of the cortex decreases.

28. The answer is E (all). (*Chapter 3 III D 1*) Neuronal perikarya arrange themselves in basically four patterns: laminae, nuclear masses, reticular formation, and ganglia. Each of these arrangements may show a wide variety of neuronal types and a variety of degrees of concentration into nuclei or segregation into laminae.

29. The answer is B (1, 3). (*Chapter 14 VI E 3*) Substance P is found in high concentration in several of the sites of the nervous system concerned with pain transmission, particularly the substantia gelatinosa and periaqueductal gray matter. Enkephalins and morphine are thought to inhibit release of substance P by combining with opioid receptors and, therefore, to reduce pain sensations.

30. The answer is E (all). (*Chapter 5 I B*) A node of Ranvier marks the zone of apposition of two adjacent Schwann cells or oligodendroglial cells. The endoneurium continues across the node rather than dipping down in between the Schwann cell membranes to contact the axon. At this site, the axon surface would appear to be free to exchange the sodium and potassium ions that are involved in the depolarization of the axon that accompanies the nerve impulse.

31. The answer is E (all). (*Chapter 1 II D 4*) Each segment of the CNS has its own cavity, which continues with the adjacent cavities and represents the lumen of the original neural tube. The lateral ventricles occupy the cerebrum; the third ventricle, the diencephalon; the aqueduct, the midbrain; the fourth ventricle is present in both the pons and medulla; and the central canal occupies the spinal cord.

32. The answer is B (1, 3). (*Chapter 5 VI B 3 a, b; Figure 5-13*) While it is unnecessary to memorize dermatomal maps, it is clinically helpful to know the level of a few of the dermatomal boundaries. C7 innervates the index and middle fingers. T4 innervates the nipple line, and T10 innervates the level of the umbilicus. L5 innervates the big toe, and S1 innervates the little toe. S5 innervates the perianal region.

33. The answer is A (1, 2, 3). [*Chapter 11 II A 3 b (1)*] Field H_1, or the thalamic fasciculus, conveys the medial lemniscus, the dentatothalamic tract, and the pallidothalamic tract. It separates the ventral surface of the thalamus from the dorsal surface of the zona incerta.

34. The answer is A (1, 2, 3). (*Chapter 7 III B 1*) When dorsal roots enter the spinal cord, they separate into medial and lateral divisions and then synapse on sensory neurons of the dorsal horn, interneurons in both dorsal and ventral horns, and motoneurons in the ventral horns. Dorsal root axons of the spinal nerves do not synapse on the isodendritic neurons of the reticular formation.

35. The answer is D (4). (*Chapter 3 III A 1*) Major sites of proliferation of neuroblasts in the developing nervous system are the periventricular zone and, after migration, the subpial zone, where they form cortex. In general, neuroblasts do not invade the roof plate per se, except in the midbrain, where they form the quadrigeminal plate. The marginal zone of the spinal cord conveys only nerve fibers. It contains no neurons.

36. The answer is A (1, 2, 3). (*Chapter 3 II F 1–4*) Neuroblasts that remain in the periventricular zone form the gray matter that surrounds the cavities of the CNS, namely the nuclei of the spinal cord, the somite nuclei of the brainstem, the diencephalic nuclei, and the basal ganglia. The migratory neurons form the cortex in the cerebrum and cerebellum and also form the branchial nuclei and reticular formation that surrounds the periventricular nuclear core of the brainstem, the nuclei of the basis pontis, and the inferior olivary nuclei.

37. The answer is C (2, 4). (*Chapter 2 VI D 3*) The epidural space of the cranium differs from the spinal epidural space because it contains no fat cells or vascular plexus. Although the dura mater forms the inner periosteum of the skull bones, it can potentially separate from the bone and may become distended with blood or pus.

38. The answer is C (2, 4). (*Chapter 2 VI A 1, B, C*) The pia mater is the innermost of the three meningeal coverings of the CNS. With the arachnoid, it constitutes the leptomeninges, but it is separated from the arachnoid membrane by the cerebrospinal fluid (CSF). The pia enters the sulci of the brain, but the arachnoid bridges over the sulci.

39. The answer is B (1, 3). (*Chapter 2 V C 4*) The major cellular components of the blood–brain barrier include the capillary endothelium and the astrocytic end feet, which abut on the external surface of the blood vessels that penetrate the CNS. As the blood vessels penetrate from the pial surface, they receive a connective tissue investment. Even at the capillary level, where the endothelial cells still remain separated from the astrocytic end feet by a basal lamina, a few collagen fibers remain.

40. The answer is C (2, 4). (*Chapter 13 IV F 4*) The anterior commissure interconnects the basal olfactory structures, including the amygdala, olfactory bulbs, and anterior perforated substance. It also connects the neo- or ectocortex of the parahippocampal gyrus and the rest of the temporal lobe. Habenulo–habenular connections run through the anterior commissure where the stria medullaris crosses the midline. The remainder of the neocortical connections, such as those of the parietal lobes, run through the corpus callosum.

41–45. The answers are: 41-B, 42-C, 43-A, 44-D, 45-E. [*Chapter 14 I B 3 d (2); III A 2; V A 4; VI E 2 a*] Many neuroanatomical pathways now can be specified by their neurotransmitters. Thus, selective depletion of the neurotransmitters can be caused by section of the pathways or by destroying the perikarya that produce the neurotransmitter.

Destruction of interneurons of the spinal cord would deplete gamma-aminobutyric acid (GABA) and glycine, inhibitory transmitters produced by the interneurons. Section of the medial forebrain bundle would destroy many of the axons that connect the catecholaminergic and serotonergic nuclei of the brainstem with the cerebral cortex. Destruction of the medullary raphe would destroy the serotonergic neurons of the medulla that project to the spinal cord. Dorsal root section would reduce substance P concentration in the dorsal horns. This neurotransmitter presumably transmits pain impulses from the small fibers in the lateral division of the dorsal roots.

Not only can the neurotransmitters be depleted by actual anatomical destruction of axonal pathways or the destruction of neuronal perikarya, but various drugs or chemicals can also selectively block neurotransmitters either by inhibiting their formation, inhibiting their release, or competing with binding sites on the postsynaptic membrane. By combining anatomical lesions with chemical blockade and direct chemical analysis, various lines of evidence can be developed to establish the transmitters involved in the various layers and regions of the cortex and the different nuclei of the CNS.

46–50. The answers are: 46-E, 47-D, 48-B, 49-A, 50-C. (*Chapter 12 II F*) The thalamus and cerebral cortex reflect each other's functional organization. The thalamic nuclei can be classified according to whether they serve sensory, motor, cognitive, or affective functions.

The calcarine area around the calcarine fissure receives the visual impulses, whereas the transverse temporal gyri and the upper surface of the temporal lobe receive the auditory impulses. The nucleus medialis dorsalis connects with the frontal lobe anterior to the motor cortex. Interruption of this connection results in apathy, indifference, and a reduced reaction to stimuli in general.

The connections from the pulvinar to the parasylvian area and the cortex behind the sensory region of the parietal lobe mediate the language functions of the left hemisphere and the spatial orientation functions of the right hemisphere. Lesions of the cortex, of the thalamocortical or corticothalamic circuits, or of the nuclei that project to the particular region of the cortex tend to give rise to similar neurologic deficits. Thus, lesions of the left pulvinar may cause a thalamic type of aphasia, whereas lesions of the right pulvinar are apt to be associated with loss of awareness of the left half of space. The thalamus also is essential for the general function of consciousness. Bilateral thalamic lesions cause varying degrees of obtundations, including coma.

51–55. The answers are: 51-D, 52-B, 53-A, 54-C, 55-E. (*Chapter 13 VI K 3 a; Figure 13-39*) Some localized lesions of the cerebral cortex cause distinct and clear clinical deficits, whereas lesions of equal size in other regions of the cortex give rise to no obvious neurologic deficit, although they may produce changes in cognitive function, emotion, and general behavior. Lesions, particularly bilateral lesions, of the medial aspect of the temporal lobes, which include the parahippocampal gyrus and hippocampus, cause loss of recent memory.

Lesions that cause aphasia are generally in the parasylvian zone predominantly in the left hemisphere but, in a small percentage of individuals, they are in the same region of the right cerebral hemisphere.

An occipital lobe lesion will cause a contralateral hemianopia due to interruption of the cortex, which receives fibers from the temporal half of the ipsilateral retina and the nasal half of the contralateral retina.

Lesions in the pre- and postcentral gyri cause hemiplegia and sensory deficits, respectively. The sensory deficits from lesions of the postcentral gyrus include hypesthesia and hypalgesia.

Lesions confined to the specific sensory and motor areas of the cortex do not commonly cause overt changes in thought processes, cognitive function, or behavior. Brain lesions that affect only these functions are more difficult to recognize and localize.

56–60. The answers are: 56-E, 57-D, 58-E, 59-B, 60-C. (*Chapter 2 V B 3*) Each of the various glial cell types differs in morphological and functional characteristics. Astrocytes are of two types, fibrous and protoplasmic. The protoplasmic astrocytes are characteristic of gray matter, and the fibrous astrocytes are characteristic of white matter. Astrocytes attach their processes to the pial surface, where they form a continuous inner lining for the pia and act as part of the CNS–cerebrospinal fluid (CSF) barrier. Other processes of the astrocytes abut on blood vessels and form part of the blood–brain barrier. The location and amount of extracellular space in the nervous system is in question. The cytoplasm of the astrocytes is suggested by some authorities as forming the extracellular space for neurons.

Oligodendrocytes occur in the gray matter as perineuronal satellites, with their perikarya near neurons and one or more processes extending to the neuronal surface. In the white matter, the perikarya of the oligodendrocytes line up in rows; in this case, they are called interfascicular glia because they are between the fascicles of nerve fibers. Their processes invest the CNS axons with a myelin sheath.

The microglial cell characteristically is found in gray matter. It was once thought to invade the nervous system from the mesodermal coverings during embryogenesis and to form a perineuronal satellite, which would round up into a macrophage in various pathologic conditions. It is now thought that the cell called a microglial cell actually derives from neural ectoderm like all other intrinsic cells of the nervous system. Macrophages do occur in the brain in response to injury, but they now are thought to migrate in from the blood.

The ependymal cells are a simple columnar epithelium that form a monolayer on the surfaces of the ventricles, aqueduct, and central canal of the spinal cord. These cells also cover the tufts of choroid plexus, which project into the ventricles from the pial surface. In general, they are a rather indolent cell type that does not proliferate readily, but one tumor of the glial series, the ependymoma, does occur. A patient with this tumor has a somewhat better prognosis since the cells are not as proliferative and aggressive as the companion cell the medulloblast, which forms medulloblastomas. Both types of tumors may occur in the posterior fossa, in the midline of the cerebellum, or in the fourth ventricle. The characteristic tumor of the oligodendrocyte is the oligodendroglioma, and the characteristic tumor of the astrocyte is a series of astrocytomas, the most malignant of which are called glioblastomas.

Index

Note: Page numbers in *italic* denote illustrations; page numbers in **boldface** denote tables; page numbers followed by letter A denote the appendix.